Health/Medicine and the
Faith Traditions

Health/Medicine and the Faith Traditions

AN INQUIRY INTO RELIGION AND MEDICINE

edited by
MARTIN E. MARTY
and
KENNETH L. VAUX

FORTRESS PRESS   PHILADELPHIA

Unless otherwise noted, biblical quotations are from the Revised Standard Version of the Bible, copyright 1946, 1952, © 1971, 1973 by the Division of Christian Education of the National Council of the Churches of Christ in the U.S.A. and are used by permission.

Library of Congress Cataloging in Publication Data
Main entry under title:

Health/medicine and the faith traditions.

   Bibliography: p.
   1. Medicine and Christianity—Addresses, essays, lectures.   2. Pastoral medicine— Addresses, essays, lectures.   3. Medical ethics—Addresses, essays, lectures.   I. Marty, Martin E., 1928–   II. Vaux, Kenneth.
   BT732.H43 1982   261.5′6   81-71383
   ISBN 0–8006–1636-7 (pbk.)   AACR2

9401B82   Printed in the United States of America   1-1636

Contents

Contents

Foreword

When Dr. Naurice Nesset, the founder and leader of Lutheran General Hospital, retired in 1979, the medical staff supplied in his honor the initial funding that made this volume possible and thereby expressed their love and respect for the man. Deep appreciation goes to the medical staff of Lutheran General Hospital and its most recently elected presidents: Richard Schulze, M.D. (1979-80), George Nelson, M.D. (1980-81), and Lawrence LeVine (1982-83) for this important support.

Since its inception in 1959, Lutheran General Hospital, Park Ridge, Illinois, has been committed to providing a quality of care that is truly patient-oriented without sacrificing any of the wondrous benefits of modern medicine. "An institution dedicated to the principles of human ecology"* best describes what this hospital is striving to become.

Just as humankind cannot be fully understood by those who exclusively emphasize either bodily or mental attributes, so sick people cannot be made whole again if the essential nature of human beings is not grasped by those who care for them. This volume brings together philosophers, physicians, historians, and theologians who have a broad range of viewpoints about how the faith traditions and medicine have shed light on the question of health and sickness. Yet the contributors share a commitment to promote a greater integration of the marvels of modern medicine with the wisdom of the faith traditions that has evolved throughout the ages. Those who question the need for or advisability of such a synthesis are

---

*Human ecology is the understanding and care of human beings as whole persons in light of their relationship to God, themselves, their families, and the society in which they live.

Foreword

reminded of the increasingly frequent ethical dilemmas with which modern medical technology confronts us. The limitations of the courts in resolving such questions as abortion or continuation of life clearly illustrate this problem. As a psychiatrist for many years, I note with distress the increasing frequency with which the clinical problems of caring for mentally ill people are being redefined as legal dilemmas, for example, the right to receive treatment and the right to refuse it. Yet I wonder whether these dilemmas of today are not related to our inability as a profession in former times to respond more sensitively to the ethical dimensions of psychiatric practice.

On succeeding Dr. Nesset as president, Mr. George Caldwell in 1979 established the Human Values Forum under the direction of Pastor Lawrence E. Holst to promote the implementation of the principles of human ecology in new and creative ways. "Health/Medicine and the Faith Traditions," or "Project Ten" as it is affectionately called, grew out of that forum. Kenneth L. Vaux and Martin E. Marty, as special consultants, have been with the project from the beginning, supplying the necessary inspiration and overall direction, in addition to being co-editors of this volume.

This volume introduces Project Ten. It is an attempt to deal systematically with the contributions of the various faith traditions to ten specific core themes in life confronted daily by the sick and those who care for them. While this volume can stand on its own merits, it is also expected to serve as an introduction to future volumes that will deal with these topics in greater depth.

PATRICK R. STAUNTON, M.D.
Chief of Psychiatry
Lutheran General Hospital
Park Ridge, Illinois

Introduction

This book is for those who find themselves concerned about the interface of medicine and religious faiths. Although it may meet an urgent need for health-care professionals, ministers, and teachers of religion, its aim is to assist the inquiry of all who seek deeper understanding in order to decide about issues of health and disease in the light of beliefs and values. The book is an invitation to an inquiry. The inquiry of medicine into theology and of theology into medicine is one whose time has come. Medical advances force us to declare our deepest metaphysical and ethical values. Religious wisdom must articulate its convictions in this vital realm of experience.

In its attempt to examine the ethics and theology of medicine, the ongoing "Project Ten" (the short name for "Health/Medicine and the Faith Traditions") is looking at ten life "themes" common to both medicine and religion and exploring them in the light of ten world faith traditions. The activities and substance of Project Ten have played a great part in shaping this volume. Chapter 7 explains the aims and themes of Project Ten in more detail.

This book has an advantage over most symposiums. It is not just a miscellany of essays. It was planned in advance; the essays were defined and commissioned as part of a coherent and comprehensive purpose. To engage in the study of medicine and religion we must—

1. Note the social and cultural contexts within which we ask these questions.

Introduction

2. Examine the way the interaction has occurred throughout history.
3. Understand with the aid of philosophy exactly what we are discussing and how it fits other ways of knowing, valuing, and deciding questions.
4. Consider some models of comprehending medical issues within theological frameworks.
5. Bring religious insights to bear on medical concerns.
6. Draw these realms together in a pastoral approach to health care.

The sociological backdrop of the inquiry is sketched in Part One by Martin E. Marty, Fairfax P. Cone Professor of Church History at the University of Chicago and an associate editor of *The Christian Century*.

Two historians on the board of advisers of Project Ten have collaborated with colleagues to produce Part Two, the historical section of the book. Darrel W. Amundsen, known for his splendid summaries of Ancient Near East, Greco-Roman, and medieval medical ethics in the *Encyclopedia of Bioethics*, is Professor of Classics at Western Washington University. For Chapters 3 and 4 he has collaborated with Gary B. Ferngren, Associate Professor of History at Oregon State University.

Ronald L. Numbers and Ronald C. Sawyer survey in Chapter 5 the interaction of medicine and Christianity since the Renaissance. Numbers is Professor of the History of Medicine and the History of Science at the University of Wisconsin in Madison. His study of the religio-medical movements of the nineteenth century has produced a book on Ellen White (*Prophetess of Health* [New York: Harper & Row, 1976]) and numerous essays. His co-edited volume *Sickness and Health in America* (Madison: University of Wisconsin Press, 1978) is a widely used resource book in the history of medicine. Sawyer is a doctoral candidate in the history of science and medicine at the University of Wisconsin in Madison.

A philosophical perspective is given in Part Three by H. Tristram Engelhardt, Jr. When one turns to the literature of philosophy in medicine, indeed in the general field of medical humanities, the name of Engelhardt is well known. Though he is a young scholar, his books, editions, articles, and reviews number well into the hundreds. A Tulane physician and University of Texas philosopher, Engelhardt has taught medical humanities at the Medical College of the University of Texas at Galveston. He is now the Rosemary Kennedy Professor of the Philosophy of Medicine at the Kennedy Institute of Ethics, Georgetown University.

My own essays on theology and medicine (Part Four) reflect a long-standing concern with articulating the religious foundations of medical

Introduction

ethics. At the Institute of Religion in Houston, Texas, I had the privilege of learning with patients, physicians, and nurses at Baylor Medical School and the University of Texas about the depths of belief and values that become evaluative themes in the experiences of health and illness. I presently serve as Professor of Ethics in Medicine at the University of Illinois Medical Center.

In Part Five, two leading American physicians show how the affairs of religion intertwine with those of medicine. Ernst Wynder, M.D., is president of the American Health Foundation and editor of the journal *Preventive Medicine*. All over the world the foundation has under way health studies that are showing the patterns of disease affecting our world as well as causes and potential remedies for those diseases. For this essay Wynder has collaborated with Mary-Carroll Sullivan, R.N., M.T.S., now Research Associate on Project Ten.

Anyone who uses Harrison's reference work in internal medicine will recognize the name of Daniel Foster, distinguished internist and Professor of Medicine. He has also written the popular volume *A Layman's Guide to Modern Medicine* (New York: Simon & Schuster, 1980). Foster's essay (Chapter 10) deals with the need to sensitively consider religious factors within the covenants of medical care.

Part Six presents two essays that draw on the synthetic insights of medicine and religion in order to expound an understanding of pastoral care. F. Dean Lueking, a distinguished Chicago pastor and scholar, writes from the perspective of the shepherd of a congregation, Grace Lutheran Church in River Forest, Illinois. Lawrence E. Holst, Chairman of the Division of Pastoral Care at Lutheran General Hospital, has participated from the beginning in the Clinical Ministry programs in this country. As coordinator of the largest program of hospital ministry in the world, he has a unique vantage point from which to observe the actual day-to-day living expressions of medical ministry.

Dr. Patrick R. Staunton, Chief of Psychiatry at Lutheran General Hospital, has written the Preface, and Dr. David T. Stein, Director of Parish Relations and Lay Training at Lutheran General Hospital and Administrator of Project Ten, has contributed the Epilogue.

The reader is now invited to begin this inquiry with us. Our conviction holds that knowledge is the precondition of virtue. May the reflection on these grand ideas, beliefs, visions, and values translate in your experience and at your place of ministry into deeds of mercy and healing.

Chicago, Illinois   KENNETH L. VAUX

Note: While Fortress Press scrupulously seeks to express itself in language that is free of sexual bias, there are several instances in this book where the generic term "man" has been employed and where the masculine gender has been used to refer to God. These instances should be regarded as the authors' efforts to reflect historical contexts as accurately as possible. Readers should know that not one of these instances escaped our editorial eyes and that we consciously sought not to offend anyone by their inclusion or to violate the policies and standards of the publisher.

MARTIN E. MARTY
KENNETH L. VAUX

PART ONE

The Sociocultural Context

1

Tradition and the Traditions in Health/Medicine and Religion

MARTIN E. MARTY

Connecting health/medicine with religion is not difficult, even if many moderns have forgotten how they intertwine. Connecting health/medicine with religious *tradition* and, worse, specific *traditions* is far more problematic. Most people are religious without thinking about the fact that their way of being so has a long lineage. They may be proud of their identification with Sunni Islam or Polish Catholicism, but they leave to the experts any sense of custodianship for their heritage. And when religious people are striving for health, the last thing in the world most of them wish to do is become self-conscious about lore that, they think, belongs to bearded scribes of centuries gone.

If a tradition seems to be a problem or an irrelevancy to sick people who stand inside an intact tradition, then the situation only worsens when they see themselves in a diffuse and blurry tradition, live at its margins, or even disdain it. An American Methodist, for example, may feel that a Mormon or a Mennonite is very conscious of religious ancestry and the boundaries of his or her faith. But who in Methodism—who even among the professionals—can trace clear lines from Methodist founder John Wesley to First Methodist Church in their town? And among those who can do such tracing, who knows enough about what Wesley and his successors thought and taught about the body, its health and illnesses, to make use of the heritage? Upon first hearing of the possible conjunction between health/medicine and religious traditions, one is tempted to back off. Perhaps some other means of organizing spiritual resources would be more profitable.

The Sociocultural Context

One plausible way to classify information is to follow the alphabet, as encyclopedias do, organizing knowledge "From Abortion to Zygote," as it were.[1] Or scholars may run readers through a sequence of epochs, from primitive and archaic periods through the rise of historic faiths until the modern challenges and the postmodern contemporary world. They may run the risk of losing some readers back in the "begats" of patriarchal times, or somewhere between Moses and Maimonides, before they are able to state issues of today. But historians love them for their efforts, even though they must acknowledge that chronology is not necessarily the only or the best way to present the topics.

People do not live by alphabets or chronology alone. They really *do* live in traditions, *all* of them do, even those who inhabit the tradition of those who rebel against and reject tradition, for tradition derives from the *traditum*, that which is "handed down." Thus every intelligible word all people use is "handed down" from the speech of people who have gone before in a tradition. Religious people share a common story, a divine law or an announcement of good news. They together respond to visions and symbols. Their rites reenact past events and, when celebrated, make these events seem present in living tradition. There are certain things that religious people know are "not done," or others that must be done. They know of inherited taboos or prescriptions, ways of life or behavior patterns. These are all part of tradition and are grasped in the traditions of faith.

Humans are not humans in general. They approach their common humanity through experience in distinct nations, in partly separate races and ethnic groups, and in distinctive religions. Thomas Mann once wrote that the world has many centers. Believers are likely to have their perceptions of health/medicine and religion prismed through life in one of these centers. They may be members of multiple traditions: black Democrat Muslim or white Republican Catholic are possible combinations. Adherents may nuance these complexes further by belonging to differing professional or scientific traditions. A tradition may be oppressively close to them, burdening or suffocating them by the weight of its hold, so that they must shrug it off. A banner in a church speaks to that: "The seven last words of the church: 'We Never Did It That Way Before,'" or the traditions may be fading in the past, corrupted by disuse or fusions. They may seem so inaccessible that the young cannot have identity crises over them because they originally received too little identity from them. But the traditions are there. Hannah Arendt put it well:

4

Tradition and the Traditions

I . . . believe with Faulkner, "The past is never dead, it is not even past," and for this simple reason that the world we live in at any moment *is* the world of the past; it consists of the monuments and the relics of what has been done by men for better or worse; its facts are always what has *become*. . . . In other words, it is quite true that the past *haunts* us; it is the past's function to haunt us who are present and wish to live in the world as it really is, that is, has *become* what it is now.[2]

Religious traditions can come in the form of dietary laws, some of them so intact and vivid to people that *not* to understand the traditions is to induce bloodshed. In 1979 in West Bengal and Kerala, Hindus and Muslims killed one another over sacred cows. In 1980 at Moradabad and throughout Uttar Pradesh, 142 were killed when people in the same two traditions warred over unsacred pigs.[3] Those are issues that apparently have to do only with the well-being of cows and pigs, but to Hindus and Muslims human well-being was at stake. Whites know better than to ask for a drink or to light up a smoke in a Chicago "Black Muslim" restaurant. While orthodox Islam considers this black sect to be heterodox, Black Muslims themselves do not want to be unorthodox in matters of health. Physicians in Cedar Rapids ministering to the Lebanese Muslims who built America's first mosque in 1934 in that relatively small Iowa city must acquaint themselves with the Islamic tradition if they have the well-being of these representatives of the two million estimated American Muslims at heart.

The Hindus may be a smaller minority in North America. Hindu lore, however, though sometimes traduced but always claimed by its followers to be in the tradition, animates many of the "new religions" that prosper among another estimated two million citizens from Berkeley through Boulder to the Benares-on-the-Charles that is Boston. Whoever belongs to or deals with devotees of Eastern religions in America knows that concepts of health and well-being are among the most vivid of any elements that they transport to these shores. Entire catalogs with hundreds of entries offer options for "wholistic/holistic" health, with "holistic," according to one, "representing the more subtle and transcendental aspects."[4] The explorer of such catalogs or the spinner of "self-help" bookracks in airport newsstands would find few evidences that America's was ever a Jewish-Christian culture. Hindu and Buddhist traditions give life to a huge subculture with which other Americans must reckon in the future. Influences from that subculture suffuse the attitudes of many in the surviving majority Jewish-Christian cultures. Mention of Buddhism further

5

points to another intact tradition that derives from the Buddha's "Four Noble Truths" on suffering and healing.[5] Organizing knowledge and inquiry around health/medicine in the Buddhist tradition would not be a difficult task in an American society which often sees itself as tradition-less.

Up close, in nations where they are prevalent, the traditions that live on in the second, third, and fourth largest religions (Islam, with 589 million adherents; Hinduism, with 478 million; Buddhism, with 255 million)[6] might well look complex and diffuse. They would not seem to be nearly as neat as they appear in encyclopedias produced in the United States. But that these *are* traditions of health/medicine with which professionals in health care and religion must reckon or with which believers want to deal, of that there is no question at all. To organize knowledge around Eastern religious traditions, then, does make sense.

Americans in mainstream or majority traditions also have no difficulty with the idea of organizing knowledge of health/medicine around "native religions," a code name for the traditions of Native American or Afro-American survivals and renewals. Those who are not involved in medical or religious work on Indian reservations may seem to have no practical need to learn the American Indian lore. Yet there has been a great revival of curiosity about it on the part of urbanites who were discontented with their own traditions or hoped to learn from others. In terms precisely applicable to the present subject, the "dean of American scholars in this field," Joseph Epes Brown, says that "the new search for the roots of traditions obscured or lost is today symptomatic in varying degrees for both native and nonnative Americans." Brown argues that this is so because of "what may be called a pervasive process on a global scale of detraditionalization or despiritualization" which must be countered.[7]

Near the heart of the Native American tradition is a whole matrix of attitudes toward disease and well-being. Medicine men and shamans received chapter-length treatments in even the most compressed books on the religions of the American Indians. The authors of one such book recognize that from day one, "active missionaries" from Christian Europe in the New World "found serious competition for the Indians' souls from their doctors, or 'medicine men,' as the Jesuits called them."[8] Another apologist, Vine Deloria, Jr., says that "one of the chief past functions of tribal religions was to perform healing ceremonies. . . . Today healing remains one of the major strengths of tribal religions."[9] A recent book, *The Healers: A History of American Medicine*, quite naturally begins with a chapter on the admittedly complex "myth of Indian medicine." Author John Duffy begins the book: "One of the oldest and most enduring of American myths relates to Indian medical skills. . . . We have consistently believed in the efficacy of Indian medicine," and this theme "has been reiterated in recent publications."[10] That tradition has been threatened for five hundred years, but it lives on and still tantalizes and informs.

Far more complicated, compromised, and diffused is another health/medicine tradition rooted in and bearing on religion, that of African "tribalism." The middle-class urban black in the United States has entered the mainstream of medicine and the mainline of religion. African survivals in his or her culture may be almost nonexistent, or mere retrievals of little use to any but dilettantes. A classic debate between Melville Herskovits in *The Myth of the Negro Past* (1958) and black sociologist E. Franklin Frazier in *The Negro Church in America* (1964) posed the issues of survival or the leaving behind of African traditions in the slave, and, later, the free black communities of America. To Herskovits it was important to attack the myth that "the Negro is . . . a man without a past" and to argue that "the civilizations of Africa, like those of Europe, have contributed to American culture as we know it today." Frazier argued back that "the slaves, it seems, had only a vague knowledge of the African background of their parents," though in some "magic and folk beliefs of the rural Negroes in the United States, some African elements have probably been retained."[11]

In any case, African survivals have been most vivid in the Caribbean, where they have been fused with Christian revivalism. There "many revivalist leaders practice healing."[12] Recent Caribbean influxes have helped transport these practices to cities like New York. Advertisements in the back of popular magazines aimed at ghetto blacks are rich in their display of potions, herbal remedies, conjuring items, and other attractions that come from outside the traditions of secular and technological medicine. After the first decade (the 1980s) in two millennia in which the Christian majority will be in the Southern Hemisphere, medical missionaries—the last effective Christian agents in many parts of Africa—will still bring back reports on influences of "tribal" religion in their cross-cultural contacts.

Concerns over disease, famine, population planning and control, and the like are at the center of political debates over Sub-Saharan Africa. All these have to reckon with "traditional religions" in the extremely complex web of tribe, nation, and religion in Africa.[13] Even the most simple and popular explanations of African primal religions find their focus in themes like "one of the most important," that of "the diviner-healer, the person whose priestly role centers on the interpretation of the spiritual situation of the individuals and the cure of psychological and physical ailments." Contrary to Western notions, "rather than being steeped in superstition, the diviner-healers are steeped in the religious traditions of their people. . . . They have acquired the accumulated wisdom of their people. . . . These beliefs, or the primal world view, continue to be widely held." In fact, of all the elements of the African primal religions, "the diviner-healers (and, presumably, the traditions behind them) have been relatively unaffected by the impact of Islam and Christianity. They continue to flourish and to be consulted in times of crisis by many Muslims and Christians as well as by traditionalists."[14] Dr. Michael Gelfand, who worked among the Mashona, southern Bantu, typically praised the *nganga,* who combine divination and herbal medicine and embody the tradition:

> They are keen judges of human behaviour and at the same time botanists of high calibre. Further they believe in their methods just as doctors in England before the sixteenth century believed in Galen's theory of disease. Their general honesty of purpose and desire to help others possibly accounts to some extent for the great attachment of the population to them. Not that dishonest doctors do not exist amongst them, as the African well realizes. But as a general rule the aim of the *nganga* is to help others and restore them to health.[15]

People in the West have gradually come to terms with these African traditions. In 1971, Robin Horton studied "African conversion" noting, in summary, "that Africans took from Islam and Christianity only those aspects of the new religions which met their needs" and that "they continued to emphasize the connection between religious belief and healing and prophecy against the wish of official Christianity which had abandoned these aspects of spiritual activity."[16] Terence Ranger studied twentieth-century logbooks of Christian parishes of the Masasi and Newala and found that "African converts . . . continued to be concerned . . . with health. In default of Christian solutions to [their] problems they continued to apply non-Christian solutions; . . . they turned in case of ill health to the *fundis* and to the Muslim doctors." Ranger says that "the evidence seems to suggest that to many people the sacraments were as desired as rain and health. They wanted both."[17] There are "plural belongers" in Africa just as there are in America, where people may draw upon their Episcopalianism *and* Zen, their Judaism *and* astrology, to fashion syncretisms for well-being. Just as clearly, there are African traditions that from a distance look like *the* African tradition in health/medicine and religion.

Adding Native American and African traditions to the intact lore of Islam, Hinduism, and Buddhism seems to be making the case for traditions easy. After all, these belong for the most part to what the modernized West calls "traditional" cultures. When Westerners in romantic or desperate moves or through acts of cultural generosity reach for them, they do so because they feel that Western traditions are exhausted. *Atanayiita atenda nyina okufumba,* say the Ganda, "He who never visits thinks his mother is the only cook."[18] So the Americans reach to the exotic or esoteric precisely because these *are* embodied and advertised as traditions which, as Ranger said, others can use, "in default of Christian solutions" (here read "Western Christians"). Westerners at large, in the words of Robin Horton, "had abandoned (healing) aspects of spiritual activity."

What about the harder cases, those of traditions that are so complex, so diffuse, so tangled and intertwined, so eroded and recessive because they have survived in pluralistic and secular America, where little operates in their favor? The harder case can be kept simpler for a moment by turning attention to one cluster of American groups we might temporarily label "innovative American religions." In all cases, whatever ancient lineage their adherents claim, to historians and contemporaries these date from the nineteenth century. Nonmembers regard them as novelties. Attitudes relating health/medicine to religion dominate the public perception of their young but robust traditions.

Anyone who lives near to or medically ministers to the 526,961 Jehovah's Witnesses gathered in 7,545 Kingdom Halls will be aware of a clearly defined and bounded tradition. In many respects it is a moderate and compromising one: Witnesses may smoke or drink in moderation, though they meet with increasing discouragement of the practices. They are forbidden sterilization, and there are more frequent expressions against contraception. Hypnosis is ruled out as a sinister and unscriptural procedure. But Witnesses are best known for a both half-literal and over-literal reading of Lev. 17:10 in their New World Translation: "God told Noah that every living creature should be meat unto him; but that he must not eat the blood, because the life is in the blood." This has meant a growing interest not in vegetarianism but in the blood content in meat. Witnesses are told to ask their butcher if blood has been properly drained. They cannot eat blood sausage, wieners, and the like. They are halfway to kosher. The overliteral side that has made their tradition vivid is the reading of "no eating of blood" to mean "no blood transfusions." The prohibition went into effect in 1944, and subsequently there have been many court cases, beginning with *People ex rel. Wallace* v. *Labrenz,* in which the power of the state has been invoked against a basic tenet of an American religious tradition when a life is at stake.[19]

The public has always been aware of a second and by far the most visible and successful of the innovations, the 2,706,000-strong Church of Jesus Christ of Latter-day Saints, or Mormons, who gather at 6,738 places in North America. The public has only recently become aware of the Mormon concern to relate health/medicine to religion, though that concern was present from the first. Founder Joseph Smith and prophet Brigham Young took pains to provide play, recreation, and dancing for converts as ways of making physical health a part of the growth into godhood in which Saints believe. Thus Young: "Complete living requires a sound body. The sound mind in the sound body is the first requisite of any person who desires to live happily and serve well."[20] In a revelation in 1833 at Kirtland, Ohio, Smith passed on a prohibition against smoking and drinking; "Behold," it said of strong drink, "it is not good, neither meet in the sight of your Father. . . ." Then, "Again, hot drinks are not for the body or belly," a prohibition against stimulants in tea, coffee and cocoa. The revelation also praised good eating.[21] All this has added up to the production of a population cohort that reveals markedly lower incidences of cancer and heart disease than most others.

The third visible and curiosity-inspiring bearer of an American innovative tradition is Christian Science, familiar on the American scene for a century, possibly faltering, but holding the loyalty of several hundred thousand citizens. It is not necessary to document the centrality of debate over health/medicine and religion here. Both to the adherents of Christian Science and to its enemies this was a focus, if not *the* focus, of the group founded by Mary Baker Eddy.[22]

Finally, and of ever-increasing importance, is the tradition of Seventh-Day Adventism, one that adds daily to its 3,672 churches and 553,089 domestic members. Like Mormonism and the Jehovah's Witnesses, it is also astonishingly successful overseas. Best known to people at a distance for its Saturday worship, belief in an imminent second advent of Christ, and millennialism, Adventism from the first has shown a preoccupation that went along with these two cardinal beliefs. That preoccupation is health/medicine, based on concepts of well-being propagated by Adventism's re-founder, Ellen Gould White. Her vegetarian movement prohibits use of alcohol, tobacco, and stimulants. Much of it was built on experiments with hydropathy and other cures in sanatariums of the nineteenth century. Were Sabbatarianism and Adventism to wane today, the church could probably propagate itself on the basis of its impressive health care, hospital building and staffing, and demographic statistics of longevity and well-being. While there have recently risen dissenters within, the Adventist tradition is palpable and intact.[23]

In what are often called "world religions" (e.g., Islam, Hinduism, and Buddhism), in misnamed "primitive religions" like the "tribalism" of Native Americans and Africans, and in health-minded American innovative groups there is a great deal of "tangibilification" (to borrow a term from Father Divine) of traditions. Nonmembers stumble over them, bump into them, work around them, plunder them, and in short are aware of the health/medicine aspects if they know only two or three elements of any of these. The hard side of the hard case is what to Asians, Africans, Latin Americans, or Native Americans is the Jewish-Christian nexus, a very tangibilificated tradition.

It is ironic that this tradition, or cluster of traditions, perhaps the most missionary and imperial in the world, does not look like tradition to those who inhabit the world in which Jews and Christians are at home or which they shaped and dominated. It is ironic, we say, but not curious, for the notion is not a subject of curiosity to humanistic or social scientific students of the idea of tradition. They know that "whoever named the water, it was not the fish" that inhabited it. People within a tradition live it and breathe it, taking it as for granted as prose-talkers take prose for granted, without giving the culture a name or recognizing it.

For all the difficulty of naming what is up close, diffuse, and enveloping, there is no reason to despair of efforts to isolate and define most aspects of this dominant Western tradition. Judaism and Catholicism offer the easier examples. When a victorious party in Israel wants to form a coalition with the small but vigorous Orthodox religious parties, it must make compromises on key subjects. These include the practice of authorizing autopsies, various dietary rules that have religious bases, and laws or customs dealing with many intimate aspects of the biological cycle. These political dealings are reminders of the way the Jewish tradition was grounded in a thousands-year-old tradition relating health/medicine to religion. Perhaps nowhere outside the Williamsburg Hasidic colonies in Brooklyn is such a subculture so coherent that medics must take it into consideration. Individual Orthodox members, however, in countless communities, represent the lore and have to be reckoned with.

Judaism after the Enlightenment began making its peace with rationalism and scientific progress. Many Jews moved into the advance guard of modernity and discovery. Much of their transit became a model for other peoples of other faiths. In recent decades, however, after the threat to Jewish survival represented by the Holocaust, the suburban dispersal of the ghetto, intermarriage, small families, and spiritual apathy—and after the impetus to Jewish roots provided by reborn Israel—there has been a measurable retraditioning by self-conscious Jews. Retrievals of tradition must be selective. They are based not on primitive awareness but on what Paul Ricoeur calls a "second naiveté."[24] Now they live not in spite of but through the interpretation of the stories, myths, practices, and lore of their tradition.

Jews—and Catholic or Protestant Christians as well—have learned from a medieval Muslim thinker, Al Ghazali, that "there is no hope of returning to a traditional faith after it has once been abandoned, since the essential condition in the holder of a traditional faith is that he should not know he is a traditionalist."[25] Any project to retrace and recover elements of a tradition connecting health/medicine and religion must be aware of the limits of the endeavor wherever there has been *complete* abandonment and rejection. Where the change has merely meant atrophy or distancing, one might rewrite the first line of Al Ghazali: "There is no hope of *simply* returning. . . ." And as a cautionary word against romantic intellectuals who, to satisfy their need for roots, jerry-build traditions and try to live in them, there is the scorching word of sociologist Max Weber:

> Never as yet has a new prophecy emerged . . . through the need of some modern intellectuals to furnish their souls with . . . guaranteed genuine antiques. . . . They play at decorating a kind of domestic chapel with . . . sacred images from all over the world, or they produce surrogates . . . which they peddle in the book market. This is plain humbug or self-deception.[26]

Hopes of avoiding self-deception, then, will have to be directed at efforts to discern survivals or tradition and in making visible what has been neglected in them. At least there can be what Charles Peguy called *ressourcement,* a resourcing by going deeper into traditions with whose surface people too casually live. Some measure of the "trying on" of tradition, in the spirit of the second naiveté, a suspension of some critical wariness in the hope of drawing on the inherited wisdom of a people, can be informing and therapeutic.

That this *ressourcement* has gone on and proceeds apace in the Jewish community is visible in literature from Harry Friedenwald's two-volume *The Jews and Medicine* in 1944[27] through more recent books such as *Jewish Medical Ethics* and *Modern Medicine and Jewish Law.*[28] Jewish themes in medical ethics are surfacing at medical schools. No self-respecting symposium on health/medicine and religion would neglect this intricate, at times Sinai-solid, at times gossamer-frail, tradition. Jews tend to be concentrated in northeastern cities; it is said that two-thirds to three-fourths of them live in a thirteen-county area around and including New York City. The interplay of tradition and abandonment in that region is often an urgent topic in medicine and health care, but the Jewish dispersal is sufficiently concentrated in clusters elsewhere to make the tradition a practical matter, not only an intellectual one, for outsiders as well.

Now for "the Christian tradition." While 6,250,340 Jews in North America are reminiscent of or potential bearers of a tradition open to 14,336,520 people around the world (statistics of world religion are maddeningly imprecise, yet published with delicate precision), the first Christian cluster presents an anomaly. There are 76,444,600 at least nominal embodiments of the tradition of Eastern Orthodoxy; 4,750,000 are in North America. Eastern Orthodoxy is five times as large as Judaism in North American population, yet it is safe to guess that it has generated not one-hundredth of the literature that American Jewry has produced or inspired and is all but invisible to Americans who do not live in urban enclaves of Russians, Serbians, Greeks, and the like.

Yet Orthodoxy, where it is gathered, does count for much; it makes demands on medical personnel and imposes claims on those who study health/medicine and religion or who would profit from traditions not their own. Eastern Orthodoxy, more than any other Christian group, is custodian of the very term "tradition." This churchly cluster expounds clear bodies of ethical injunctions based on holy tradition. Many of these have to do with issues of health and medicine. In the *Encyclopedia of Bioethics,* Stanley Harakas shows the bearing of this tradition on health care, the rights of patients, human experimentation, abortion ("a long

13

history of opposition"), organ transplants, drug addiction, mental health, aging, death, dying, euthanasia, human sexuality, fertility control, population, genetic counseling, and genetic screening.[29] In all these cases a cursory reading suggests that Orthodoxy has some distinctive understandings of our subject. Score another for a tradition intact.

Roman Catholicism? Must one defend the weight and visibility of that tradition? Even the most half-aware citizen knows that the Catholic tradition has things to say and do about abortion, birth control, and euthanasia. Catholics have been known for their pioneering in the creation of hospitals and other institutions of care. With 49,812,178 members in 24,161 places, and with a North American "population" including nominal Catholics of millions more, the Catholic tradition is accessible to all. It impinges on the lives of American non-Catholics everywhere. While pluralism and other forces of modernity take their toll on Catholic loyalties and clarities, a worldwide tradition that lays claim to the Bible, the early Christian fathers, Augustine and Aquinas, down through impressive modern moral theologians, needs no defense for its place among the traditions. Comic Lenny Bruce once said that in America, Catholicism is the only "*the* church." It is not the only "*the* tradition," but few find it difficult to associate the word "tradition" with Catholicism.

Almost all the problems that have to do with the very notion of organizing "health/medicine and religion" around traditions as people in North America experience them and as thinkers expound them are climaxed in the issue of what to do with Protestantism. You cannot pretend away its nominal North American population of 98,857,500, its long history, and an endlessly divided body of believers and hangers-on. Yet if because they are geographically remote, Islamic sects like the Shiite and Sunni and scores more can be amalgamated into the "Muslim tradition," no such luxury is available to North Americans who struggle with the two hundred and more varieties of Protestant denominations. Each of these is virtually split down the middle over controversy. Yet whoever wants to do justice to power relations, to serve people in health/medicine and religious professions, to honor a history and open a lore, or even to be a fair-minded phenomenologist accounting for the appearances of things as they are, must stumble into, over, or around the phenomenon of Protestantism.

Historically focused reference books like the *Encyclopedia of Bioethics*, where condensation and codification are necessary luxuries, go back to the sixteenth-century roots and draw a line between two Protestantisms, those that derive from Luther and those that derive from Calvin. The index is revealing as to topics demanding separate inquiry:[30]

Calvin, John	Luther, Martin
on abortion	on abortion
on after-life	on after-life
on contraception	on calling
on ensoulment	on contraception
on marriage	on ensoulment
on miracles	on marriage
on sickness	on sickness
virtue, theory of	virtue, theory of
Calvinism	Lutheranism

The score is even, with Calvin meriting separate notice on "miracles" and Luther on "vocation."

A current exploration, "Health/Medicine and the Faith Traditions" (nicknamed Project Ten), sponsored by Lutheran General Hospital, Park Ridge, Illinois, in the 1980s is giving separate space to Lutheranism within Protestantism. There are several reasons for this, however hazardous it may appear to be, chiefly because it inspires the possibility of calls for "equal time." What about communions like the Anglican, which is open to Catholic and Protestant traditions, or the Baptist, which reveals distinctive views of the disciplines of faith and the statistical muscle and regional power to be especially visible in the United States?

Isolating Lutheranism is an experiment. The project on traditions, by separating out the largest Protestant communion, with seventy to eighty million members worldwide, is dealing with one that claims precisely to define confession and a putatively intact theological tradition. Lutheranism has given much attention to these. A study of this faith may reveal the extent to which such a communion ever had, keeps clear, has available, or makes use of its theological, liturgical, and practical traditions on the urgent topics of health/medicine. If Lutheranism does, what can be learned by a scrutiny of its distinctiveness and its shared features can be extrapolated upon for research and employment by Anglicans, Baptists, and others.

There is also a historical reason, implied in the reference to the index of the *Encyclopedia of Bioethics:* Both in the public eye and in cultural history, Luther and Lutheranism made up an original half of the Reformation, the Germanic-Scandinavian version that spread later to North America and, selectively, around the world. To these add a theological rationale. Typical of hundreds of possible citations is one by Bernard Ramm, who teaches at the American Baptist Seminary of the West. He speaks of "the sacramental gulf" separating the Lutheran from the Reformed half of the original Reformation. *"Ihr habt einen anderen Geist"* (You have a different spirit), Luther insisted across the table from the Swiss Reformer Huldreich Zwingli in 1529.

The differences of spirit, Luther and Lutherans insisted, went beyond the debated point of sacraments to Christology and other themes. Says Ramm: "No other theologian of the Reformation as much as Luther stressed the incarnation and the enhumanization of God." His was a more "physical" sort of Protestantism, a more "substantial" and thus less "spiritual" version. "That 'different spirit' divided the Reformation then, and the division remains within the church today."[31] If so, the tradition *should* have distinctives relating to "enhumanization" and "physicality," since peoples' bodies are involved in health/medicine. Do Lutherans possess distinctive things to think about or enact when they start hospitals, authorize deaconesses, send out their medical missionaries, engage in bedside care, nurture their children, and write denominational statements on abortion, stewardship of the earth, population control? At this stage the Lutheran General project planners, whose advisers on the first day were called together by a Presbyterian and soon included people of Jewish, Catholic, agnostic, Muslim, Adventist, and nondescript or, as American colonials would say, "nothingarian" traditions, leave the issue in question form and will report later on answers.

That leaves majority Protestantism, the Swiss-Lowlands-French-part-Germany, Transylvanian, British Isles, Puritan-North American and the rest of the world version, in the general camp of non-Lutheran Reformation influence. The code word for all this is "Reformed," and behind its traditions, ranging from Baptist through Puritan to Anglican and centering in Reformed and Presbyterian bodies, there was the inaugurating spirit not of Luther but of John Calvin. Americans have come to be at home with calling this tradition merely "Protestant."

They have also, by squinting their eyes half shut and looking as if from the distance of Mars, succeeded in simplifying their vision of its many subtraditions into two traditions. One we could call "neo-Reformation," or "re-Reformed," but shall call "Evangelical." In its conservative, sometimes traditionalist, fundamentalist, pentecostal, and self-named neo-evangelical or later evangelical thicket, there has always been the claim that it is most literally steadfast about reproducing sixteenth-century

Calvinist Protestantism. Besieged by evolution, higher criticism, and progressive views of history late in the nineteenth century and early in the twentieth, and written off in secular and liberal religious cultures as a throwback that was to be passed over by Enlightenment and modernity, evangelicalism has survived and is, alongside Islam, the most expansive religious complex in the world.

To refer in this cluster to "pentecostal" may mean drawing upon what old Calvinists would have said was an "Arminian heresy." It is also rich in disturbing ecstasies and open to supernatural miraculous healings. Or one may point to more scholastic Calvinists. They remember that Calvin thought that startlingly miraculous interventions in matters of health/medicine ended with the apostolic age. Admittedly, then, as these two illustrations show, the tradition is tangled like all others. But in the scholasticism, the literalism, the resistance to modernism, the most ready resort to biblical infallibility, the reliance on Reformation-era documents and—most relevant in the present topic—the willingness or eagerness to see a sovereign God supernaturally intervening in providential care of humans, there is a tradition. Those inside it recognize one another under code names like "born again" or "evangelical." Those outside it are likely to be witnesses to, called to conversion, or forced to reckon with specific moral and ethical standards which may often counter the mainline of the culture.

That leaves, then, the mainstream of Reformed or Calvinist modernity in North American culture, the most blended and thinned out but also most "up close" tradition of them all. This one raises almost all the problems for the others. In it swim not the fish who could not have named the water but the oceanographers and depth-explorers who described the science of all the other swimmers and gave names to the processes. We can call this "Mainline Protestant." While this includes the few survivors of turn-of-the-century "modernist" Protestantism, they are only a minority. These wanted a simple and complete accommodation to science, reason, enlightenment, and modernity even at the expense of ancient Scripture, Reformation confessions, or ageless theological traditions.

By "mainline" we mean most open to modernity's changes, most experienced with pluralism, least defensive about secular experiment. Modernity can be seen as a process of the "chopping up" of life—scholars call it differentiation, diffusion, and refinement—and "choice" or voluntaryism.[32] The mainline of Euro-American Protestantism was, as they say, "present at the creation" of modern humanisms and scientific discovery. Its pioneers took and they gave, resisted and overaccommodated. They kept some continuities to the Bible, Augustine, Calvin, and the Puritans, and they kept being transformed. They eventually yielded space to the neo-Reformation revivalists, who kept displacing them, and they grudgingly shared space with Roman Catholics, Eastern Orthodox, other continental Protestants, Jews, and nonbelievers in what was once their empire and near-monopoly.[33] Today they probably make up half of churchgoing Protestant America, but their nominal adherents and their "alumni association" make them the dominant group.

The role of this mainline or modern Protestant tradition in health/ medicine and religion topics is protean. Inquirers can grasp it everywhere and yet somehow nowhere. It is interstitial, filling the gaps of a secular culture, and tentacular, barnacled to other vessels of modernity. One aspect of this Protestantism is extremely reliant on biblical witness interpreted through critical understanding. It has spawned "neo-Orthodox" movements of selective retrieval from the Reformation era. The mainline has been one of the most theologically fertile lineages in Christian history and has established most of the major university centers for religious inquiry in North America.

How does one comprehend such an elusive sprawl of a tradition, and where does one confront it? Perhaps the observer must take a look from the greatest distance. One could say that modern Protestantism more than any other religious tradition invented the modern hospital, which is reliant upon science and pluralism. When belligerent reactors in the Third World, of whom Ivan Illich is one of the more eloquent and notable, engage in reaction against modern medicine, health care, and hospitals, they may use code words like "imperial" or "colonial," "capitalist" or "technological," "Western" or "modern." But insofar as there is a religious ethos behind this whole thrust, the mainline and sometimes secularized Protestantism is at its heart. And if people in this Third World sometimes express appreciation for the mixed blessings of technology and modern medicine because they cut into infant mortality, diminish pain and suffering, extend life and help make it more enjoyable, they also recognize that this medicine came in a two-package deal. Colonialist *and* Christian, capitalist *and* Protestant, welfare planner *and* social Christian were usually teamed.

The vision up close, however, is one of diffusion and confusion. It is possible, for example, to picture the president of, say, a Lutheran-based hospital, who has moved blithely and without pain to that hospital while remaining a member of Methodist and/or Presbyterian denominations and while dealing with ecumenical staffs, never being offended or cheered, inconvenienced or convenienced by the mainline and semi-secular Protestant tradition. It is entirely plausible, because this tradition does not appear in the form of what John Courtney Murray called a "Thing"; it is plausible to think that traditions do not come to most people of the world, or that *his* tradition is not very clearly perceived by the world's people at a distance as far from him as Islam is from his hospital.

One could explain the form this tradition took at great length, but it is valid to cite only one accounting, the best-known recent one. Sociologist Talcott Parsons, the theorist of modernity who concentrated on the meanings of differentiation and diffusion, the "chopping up" and spreading out of tradition, addressed the issue. With Max Weber, Parsons distinguished ways of looking at the world into "otherworldly and innerworldly," the latter leading to "mastery over the world in the name of religious values." Where modern Protestantism took shape, it was such mastery that it aspired to. While "otherworldly" types who excluded the "innerworldly" looked only for pure, spontaneous, selfless acts of love, Parsons saw also the "institutionalization of Christian ethics to become part of the structure of society itself." Thus institutionalized, it is hard to be seen any longer as a separate tradition, but it *is* a tradition!

Second, Parsons comes to his field of expertise—differentiation. This differentiation, or chopping up, for example of church from state, or the worship day from the work day, or sacred explanations from secular explanations (these are my illustrations, not his), while it *changes* the forms of religious influence, does *not lead to their disappearance*, only their diffusion. Modern Protestants are interested both in the survival of their churchly base for certain functions of life and in a religious influence on society, even if that is expensive to the churchly base, goes unrecognized, and may take even new forms. Thus Parsons sees a "Christianizing" —here we should call it a "Protestantizing"—of secular society, effected by this aspect of the church's "influence on a life which remained by the church's own definition secular . . . but still potentially at least quite definitely Christian."

For Max Weber and Parsons, what mattered less was the way Reformers like Luther took away the legitimation of the monks' and nuns' calling; what mattered more was the way their heirs now endowed the "secular life with a new order of religious legitimation as a field of "Christian opportunity.' " Therefore, "far from weakening the elements in secular society which pointed in a direction of 'modernism,' the Reformation . . . strengthened and extended them."

Broad publics are aware of this process as Weber saw it issuing in "the Protestant Ethic and the Spirit of Capitalism." Americans have known that this version of Protestantism helped produce what Ernest Tuveson called a "redeemer nation," or that it blended with the Enlightenment to call forth a public or civil religion. Only in recent decades has it become clear that Protestantism also had much to do with encouraging scientific, technological, and industrial ventures of the sort that have a bearing on health/medicine. Some of this awareness has come about because of attacks by environmentalists, ecologists, and "wholistic/holistic" apologists on the "secularized Protestant" use and misuse of the Bible to create a world of dominance at the expense of nature and the distinctively human.

As for humanitarian causes, to Parsons the Protestantism that issued from the Reformation was "not primarily one of 'giving in' to the temptations of worldly interest, but rather one of extending the range of applicability and indeed in certain respects the rigor of the ethical standards applied to life in the world." To Parsons and others at home with modernity, "we are deeply committed to our own great traditions. These have tended to emphasize the exclusive possession of the truth. Yet we have also institutionalized the values of tolerance and equality of rights for all." Parsons was not complacent about what others saw to be collapse in modernity. He simply did not think the tradition was at fault. It was confronted with new and almost insuperable problems.[34]

Weber, Parsons, and their kin among celebrators of the Protestant ethic diffused in the culture have a host of critics among neo-traditionalists today. Thus John Murray Cuddihy has written of "the ordeal of civility" occasioned when modernity asked people to minimize their offensive traditions:

> Parsons, as an intellectual descendant of Calvin, has displayed, according to the conventional wisdom, an all but sovereign indifference to the high cost of this "passing of traditional society," . . . this "passage from home." . . . Members of the Protestant core-culture, like Parsons, theorize from within the eye of the hurricane, where all is calm and intelligible. But for the underclass below, as for the ethnic outside, modernization is a trauma. Parsons views modernization—correctly, I contend—as a secularization of Protestant Christianity. . . . Differentiation slices through ancient primordial ties and identities, leaving crisis and "wholeness-hunger" in its wake.[35]

Tradition and the Traditions

Those who would speak for "the underclass below" or "the ethnic outside," those who have "wholeness-hunger," appear also within the Protestant core-culture. They advocate a return to the distinctive sources of the tradition. The modern Protestant tradition lives between these open-to-the-secular and return-to-the-source appeals. In both cases it is urgent that its bearing on health/medicine and vice versa be explored, for the sake of those in the tradition and those affected by it.

If this appeal for organizing knowledge and inquiry of health/medicine along the lines of the traditions people actually inhabit and bear has any weight, it remains finally to reflect on the meaning not of the traditions but of tradition itself. The inquiry mentality gives subtle encouragement to traditions. Tradition, it is clear, does not mean denomination or church body. If it did, the results would be less promising or threatening, certainly to all who do not share a particular tradition. But something more potent and dangerous is here: the "hooking in" of religion to all the other dimensions of life, about each of which people feel very deeply.

Traditions do not only give life or address health/medicine. They also kill. If Hindus and Muslims kill one another over sacred cows and desecrating pigs, if Muslims and Jews threaten one another over biblical claims on a Holy Land, if tribal Africans are at war with one another, if Protestants and Catholics kill one another in Northern Ireland and Muslims, Christians, Druses, and Jews all kill others in Lebanon, they are acting out of traditions. Says Harold Isaacs of these traditions as they turn tribal:

> We are experiencing on a massively universal scale a convulsive ingathering of people in their numberless grouping of kinds—tribal, racial, linguistic, religious, national. It is a great clustering into separatenesses that will, it is thought, improve, assure, or extend each group's power or place, or keep it safe or safer from the power, threat, or hostility of others.[36]

No one should want to activate *such* tribal traditionalism in relatively civil North American communities. Self-assertion of traditions could create havoc in hospital boards and community health centers. It is already disrupting debates over sex education in high schools. The potential for incivility is evident already in the conflicts over abortion and euthanasia in American public life. But it can be argued that the destructive side of traditions will also find its expression without encouragement. An inquiry into health/medicine and the religious traditions stands some chance of compensating by bringing out the constructive side.

The Sociocultural Context

Why the accent on constructive tradition today? In health/medicine, people are in trouble. We know little, and each year we know more about how little we know about bodies and their well-being. Medicine, once sure of its scientific future, is becoming more open to wholistic inquiry, thanks to pressure from patients, outside criticism, and second thoughts by medical and health professionals. Meanwhile religious professionals, once sure that they could best serve by blocking scientific research or retarding it, are becoming more open to modest hearings from medical experts and the people who are clients of both, adherents to plural communities in health/medicine and religion.

Stated positively, in medicine and religion, where experts have been good, they have dealt only with specialists. The patient needs to know that the languages of rabbi and surgeon are at least intelligible to the other, since both are born of specialized concerns for a general patient. Those who would promote preventive care and general well-being are developing both scientific and religious resources, but these have been related only selectively.

Tradition has come back into its own, at least selectively, as part of a search for identity and, more, for social location. Differentiation chopped up not only the world, but also the psychic life of people in it, leaving them with wholeness-hunger. They seek their roots, their groups, a common life, a community of memory and hope, which will always be grounded somehow in traditions. To know who one is, to recognize meaning in one's social environment, is therapeutic, a mark of well-being or, in religious terms, of salvation. To pursue distinctive traditions provides security; to have traditions encounter one another stimulates necessary risk. There is always the chance that in an inquiry into health/medicine and the religious traditions people will learn the merits of borrowing, grafting on, and profiting from others as they impart of their own. In every aspect of such transactions, bearers of tradition will see them change.

Tradition is often honored for its own sake, not for its content. Inquiry therefore must move beyond the *politesse* of recognizing that there *are* traditions to the question of what they contain and would propagate. British visitor D. W. Brogan tells of a "frightened citizen who, rescued from a lynching bee, protested: 'I didn't say I was against the Monroe Doctrine; I love the Monroe Doctrine, I would die for the Monroe Doctrine. I merely said I didn't know what it was.' "[37] People are often caught in the grind of Islamic or Catholic or Mormon traditions without knowing what they are. Often the people in them do not know. Hence, inquiry is urgent.

Traditions are always in flux. A convert to Presbyterianism acquires a tradition and may soon become more expert at its boldnesses and subtleties than will many an uncurious lifelong Presbyterian. Traditions experience syncretism, a mixing because of migrations, intermarriage, mass media of communication, internal reform. They may be inert, waiting for a charismatic leader who transforms them by saying, "It is written, but I say unto you . . . ," as Max Weber pointed to such leaders.[38] They may be full of potential and waiting for a virtuoso leader who renews by saying, "It is written, and I insist. . . ." Surviving traditions are not stagnant ponds but living streams.

Today intellectuals are reexploring the *idea* of tradition. Yet specific studies like this one on health/medicine and religious traditions can make a contribution by pointing to the *realities* of traditions. Edward Shils calls his *Tradition* the first "comprehensive book about tradition and traditions," the first which "tries to see the common ground and elements of tradition and which analyzes what difference tradition makes in human life."[39] Be that as it may, the interest that inspired such a book is an indicator of the appropriateness of an inquiry into traditions. Not many years ago a "now" generation, afflicted with self-chosen amnesia as much as its successor is with nostalgia, was iconoclastic about tradition. It rejected the *traditum* as being part of a despised parental world, of "power structures," establishments, corrupt institutions. What was needed was the vision of utopia, a trashing of the old to clear the ground for the new.

In the midst of those years Eugene Goodheart wrote cautionary words that have a bearing on explorers of religious traditions:

> The *tabula rasa* [mental clean slate] is a presumption of innocence. It is not the result of genuine discovery, for instance, that the Christian and classical traditions are no longer part of us. The enactments of our personality and character are involuntary, often compulsive. We are not free to choose what we are or even what we will do. We cannot simply wish away traditions that we have grown to dislike. The very dislike may be conditioned by the fact that they still possess us, if we do not possess them. . . .
>
> To keep the traditional culture alive in us is not necessarily to affirm or celebrate it. Nor is it necessarily an act of pious pedantry. If the tradition contains within itself permanent human possibilities, then it is necessary to keep alive as a kind of repository of options. Indeed, it may be especially necessary to do so at a moment when men feel secure in nothing, for they

may be able to keep the life possibility going simply by worrying about the
reality of lives lived in the past.[40]

Goodheart has written a kind of charter for inquiries that have become
vital. Individuals need no instruments except libraries to begin their own
search for traditions as "repositories of options." Churches and synagogues would explore "what's in it for them" that they stand in certain
theological or liturgical heritages. Is there health and well-being as a
potential in such lineages? Are they contributing to the strength of their
communities or "sitting on" the traditions? Have they learned from
others? Medical schools and theological seminaries alike have reason to
enlarge their newly enjoyed explorations of health/medicine ethics to see
how these relate to specific traditions. Intellectual leadership is called for
and will be found. The test will be the contribution of the people who
live in traditions, or in the impact that inquiry has on their health/
medicine and their religion. More and more of them are likely to find
that though they did not possess traditions, the traditions still possess
them and still carry promise.

NOTES

1. "Abortion" and "zygote" are the first and last entries of Warren T. Reich,
ed., *Encyclopedia of Bioethics*, 4 vols. (New York: Free Press, 1978).

2. Hannah Arendt, "Home to Roost," in *The American Experiment: Perspectives on 200 Years*, ed. Sam Bass Warner, Jr. (Boston: Houghton Mifflin, 1976),
p. 75.

3. Martin E. Marty, "Religion," in successive *The World Book Year Book*
volumes (Chicago: World Book–Childcraft, 1980, 1981), 1980 volume: p. 463;
1981 volume: p. 465.

4. For samples, see Leslie J. Kaslof, *Wholistic Dimensions in Healing* (Garden
City, N.Y.: Doubleday & Co., Dolphin Books, 1978), foreword, and passim;
Shirley L. Radl and Carol A. Chetkovich, . . . *And the Pursuit of Happiness* (New
York: A & W Pubs., 1978).

5. Hajime Nakamura, "Buddhism," in Reich, ed., *Encyclopedia*, 1:137.

6. International statistics are compiled by Franklin H. Littell for *1981 Britannica Book of the Year* (Chicago: Encyclopaedia Britannica, 1981), p. 785. American statistics supplement these throughout the essay. They are taken from
Constant H. Jacquet, Jr., *Yearbook of American and Canadian Churches 1981*
(Nashville: Abingdon Press, 1981); see alphabetized notations on church groups.

7. Joseph Epes Brown, "The Roots of Renewal," in *Seeing with a Native Eye:
Essays on Native American Religion*, ed. Walter Holden Capps (New York:

Harper & Row, Forum Books, 1976), pp. 26–27; Capps introduces Brown as "dean" on p. 5.

8. Åke Hultkrantz, *The Religions of the American Indians* (Berkeley: University of California Press, 1967), p. 84.

9. Vine Deloria, Jr., *God Is Red* (New York: Grosset & Dunlap, 1973), p. 263.

10. John Duffy, *The Healers: A History of American Medicine* (Urbana: University of Illinois Press, 1979), p. 1.

11. Albert Raboteau, *Slave Religion: The "Invisible Institution" in the Antebellum South* (New York: Oxford University Press, 1978), pp. 48–54, discusses the debate. See Melville Herskovits, *The Myth of the Negro Past* (Boston: Beacon Press, 1958), pp. 298–99; and E. Franklin Frazier, *The Negro Family in the United States* (Chicago: University of Chicago Press, 1966), p. 7; and E. Franklin Frazier, *The Negro Church in America* (New York: Schocken Books, 1964), p. 21.

12. George Eaton Simpson, *Black Religions in the New World* (New York: Columbia University Press, 1978), p. 113.

13. Frederick T. Sai, "Medical Ethics, History of: Sub-Saharan Africa," in Reich, ed., *Encyclopedia*, 2:897–900.

14. Robert Cameron Mitchell, *African Primal Religions* (Niles, Ill.: Argus Communications, 1977), pp. 38–43.

15. Michael Gelfand, *Medicine and Magic of the Mashona* (Johannesburg, 1956), p. 97. See also John Taylor, *The Primal Vision: Christian Presence Amid African Religion* (Philadelphia: Fortress Press, 1963), pp. 147–48.

16. Robin Horton, "African Conversion," *Africa* 41 (April 1971), cited by T. O. Ranger and I. N. Kimambo, *The Historical Study of African Religion* (Berkeley: University of California Press, 1976), pp. 15–16.

17. Terence Ranger, "Missionary Adaptation of African Religious Institutions: The Masasi Case," in Ranger and Kimambo, *Historical Study of African Religion*, p. 230.

18. Taylor, *The Primal Vision*, p. 26.

19. Barbara Grizzuti Harrison, *Visions of Glory: A History and a Memory of Jehovah's Witnesses* (New York: Simon & Schuster, 1978), p. 98. See also William J. Whalen, *Armageddon Around the Corner: A Report on Jehovah's Witnesses* (New York: John Day, 1962), pp. 196–98, with several citations on health from *The Watchtower*.

20. John Widstoe, ed., *Discourses of Brigham Young* (Salt Lake City, 1925), p. 56, cited by Thomas O'Dea, *The Mormons* (Chicago: University of Chicago Press, 1957), p. 144.

21. The Joseph Smith quotations are from section 89 of the Doctrine and Covenants in O'Dea, *The Mormons*, pp. 145–46.

22. On the relation of Christian Science to the mainstream culture, see Stephen Gottschalk, *The Emergence of Christian Science in American Religious Life* (Berkeley: University of California Press, 1973).

23. On the origins of this tradition, see Ronald L. Numbers, *Prophetess of Health: A Study of Ellen G. White* (New York: Harper & Row, 1976).

24. Paul Ricoeur, *The Symbolism of Evil* (Boston: Beacon Press, 1967), p. 351.

25. The Al Ghazali quotation appears in a context which elaborates his position in Ernest Gellner, *Legitimation of Belief* (Cambridge: Cambridge University Press, 1974), p. 147.

26. Ibid.

27. Harry Friedenwald, *The Jews and Medicine*, 2 vols. (Baltimore: Johns Hopkins Press, 1944).

28. Immanuel Jakobovits, *Jewish Medical Ethics: A Comparative and Historical Study of the Jewish Religious Attitude to Medicine and Its Practice*, 2d ed. (New York: Bloch Publishing Co., 1975); and Fred Rosner, *Modern Medicine and Jewish Law* (New York: Yeshiva University Press, 1972).

29. Stanley S. Harakas, "Eastern Orthodox Christianity," in Reich, ed., *Encyclopedia*, 1:347–53.

30. Reich, ed., *Encyclopedia*, 4:1855, 1891.

31. Bernard Ramm, "The Sacramental Gulf," *Eternity* 32 (July–August 1981): 36–37.

32. John Murray Cuddihy, *The Ordeal of Civility: Freud, Marx, Lévi-Strauss, and the Jewish Struggle with Modernity* (New York: Basic Books, 1974), pp. 9–14, on "differentiation"; on choice, see Peter Berger, *The Heretical Imperative* (Garden City, N.Y.: Doubleday & Co., 1979).

33. For this story, see Martin E. Marty, *Righteous Empire: The Protestant Experience in America* (New York: Dial Press, 1970), and Robert C. Handy, *A Christian America: Protestant Hopes and Historical Realities* (New York: Oxford University Press, 1971).

34. See the introduction by James F. Childress and David B. Harned, eds., to "Christianity and Modern Industrial Society" by Talcott Parsons in their *Secularization and the Protestant Prospect* (Philadelphia: Westminster Press, 1970), pp. 43–44, and the Parsons essay, pp. 44, 46, 49, 55, 69.

35. Cuddihy, *Ordeal of Civility*, pp. 9–10.

36. Harold R. Isaacs, *Idols of the Tribe: Group Identity and Political Change* (New York: Harper & Row, 1975), p. 1.

37. D. W. Brogan, *The American Character* (New York: Vintage Press, 1956), p. 156.

38. Weber discussion is in Michael Hill, *The Religious Order* (London: Heinemann Educational Books, 1973), p. 2.

39. Edward Shils, *Tradition* (Chicago: University of Chicago Press, 1981), p. vii.

40. Eugene Goodheart, *Culture and the Radical Conscience* (Cambridge, Mass.: Harvard University Press, 1973), pp. 9, 15.

2

The Intertwining of Religion and Health/Medicine in Culture: A View Through the Disciplines

MARTIN E. MARTY

Modernity. produces divisions. It separates the spheres of life. The processes of modernity tend to chop up aspects of existence that most people wish they could keep together, to see whole. They call forth experts and specialists who learn to treat one part of human need without touching another. Through the whole experience, most people have a strong drive that calls them to look for wholeness.[1]

One dimension of modern life where the "chopping up" or differentiation is apparently most vivid is the point where religion and concerns over health/medicine now usually diverge. If you are physically sick you go to the hospital, but if you have a spiritual need you may turn a different corner down a separate lane and go to the church. The collegian who chooses to minister to diseased people majors in science and may go to medical school or specialize in nutrition. On the other hand, the young person who chooses to serve the demands of the soul ordinarily majors in the humanities and then goes on to seminary or acquires special theological outlooks for use as a lay person. The professionals in both these circles go to their own meetings, read papers that have little to do with anything outside their fields, and stop understanding or caring about concerns expressed elsewhere. They often narrow their range of interest not out of malice or arrogance but simply because that is what the pressures of modern life call them to do.

Scholars tell us that it was not always so. Histories that cover the first thousands of years of human experience do not need separate chapters for religion over against health/medicine. They do not, that is, until the last chapter, which covers events in the most recent century or two. Before this time, in most of the world, the witch doctor was the doctor, the priest was the medicine man, the food on the table was the food of the spirits or the gods. Not many moderns would wish to go back completely to the existence they call primitive, though some romantics make the effort and many wise ones learn from people in simpler settings. But citizens who live in cultures that are marked by science and technology often sense that with all the gains in medicine and the narrowing of religious explanations they have also lost something.

The concept of chopping up or separating which characterized the spheres of religion and medicine created difficulties for the editorial panels who planned this book. Taking the reader behind the scenes to an editorial council is the best way to illustrate this. Some would say, "If we make the essays really useful to doctors, can ministers and priests read them? After all, the language of physicians is very technical." Then, from the other end of the table: "But we want people on *both* sides to read the book. Suppose we direct all the concerns at ministers; how will we hold the attention of doctors?" If the issues had to reach no further than that first division, life could still have remained comparatively simple for the planners. But in the second round they had to become more realistic. Is the world of the "doctors" so unified and simple? Will a nurse care about the same things as a hospital administrator, and will a psychiatrist read essays aimed at surgeons? If the medical world seems specialized, then what about the world of religion? How can the same book address Muslims and Methodists? And "Ministers" are diverse experts who live in separate worlds; the world of the Christian Science practitioner differs vastly from that of the Pentecostal faith healer. Both are distanced from the concerns of the Harvard Divinity School student who uses theological resources for a thesis in bioethics.

At the point of near chaos, someone at an editorial planning session then dared to verge on *true* chaos. At this point the minutes of the meeting might well record the following questions: "Do you want an inquiry into religion and health/medicine that would try to reach only the professionals, the technical people? What about lay people in both medicine and religion? They have most at stake, since it is their health and spirit about which the writers profess to care. They are seeking wholeness. Who will address *them?* Do they always have to content themselves with separate and simplistic books and conferences?"

At the stage where all such questions were on the table, when essayists and editors were ready to pack up in despair, to go home and write only for the people on their side of the various divides, a matter of conscience kept pressing: "Stay with it!" Someone has to begin with that lay person, for we are all laity in respect to medicine *or* religion *or*. . . . The planners knew from their own experience that there is profit when experts who had previously gone separate ways begin to respond to each other.

Begin the design, then, with a hypothetical person in a hospital. She is surrounded by various specialists who are really helping her but each of whom speak distinctive languages that do not translate well. One expert looks at her as a subject of medical care for whom surgery and the right prescriptions are urgent demands. The same patient as a private and desperate entrepreneur must do her own connecting with a second set of people who have a bearing on her possible recovery, even if they are not professionals. These are the people who, we might say, make up the specialty of providing her with a context. Among them are family, friends, representatives of clubs and religious groups, senders of bed jackets and greeting cards. They help her come to terms with the threatening environment of beepers and tubes and hospital routines.

On the mail pile next to the bed are the first of what will seem an endless sequence of letters representing other specialties like economics or law. Here are the hospital bills, forms to fill out, insurance statements. If something goes wrong, there may be malpractice suits; if there has been an automobile accident, lawyers will be called in. Theirs is not the language of medicine, but they will "call in medical experts to witness" about possible whiplash or the effects of internal injuries.

As if these were not worlds enough, the patient often has still another world with which to contend or on which to draw: the world of religion. She lives in a universe of moral discourse, whose experts may not know much in a technical way about medicine, economics, or law. She asks, for example, "Will I live? . . . Should I have an organ transplant? . . . Why is God, a good God, doing all this to me? . . . Am I guilty of something? Should I—cough! cough!—have heeded the warnings about cigarette smoking? . . . Shall I listen to my cousin who wants to take me out of the hospital to a faith healer? . . . Teach me to pray!"

Suddenly a relatively unequipped person has urgent reasons to connect disparate worlds, in the present case the worlds of religion and health/medicine. She must integrate kinds of expertise as they affect her and translate languages of specialists who cannot make sense to one another.

The Sociocultural Context

At this point in their imaginings and hypotheses the temptation is strong for editors and essayists to betray their own vocations. It is not too difficult to step out of their distinct roles and in doing so leave behind their learning and conscience. They could, theoretically at least, become celebrities by inventing and patenting a new therapy or a new religion, one that is cut off from centuries of scientific research or religious traditions. If they succeeded, they might have their moment in the sun or the television studio lights, their week on the best-seller lists. After that would come the exposure of their fraud or their failure. They would then be seen as the dabblers and chatterers they really were. Serious people know better than to expect "wholeness" on such cheap terms. They do not trust the minister who takes up surgical tools, or the anesthetist who engages in "mystico-transcendental therapy." The specialists, we must presume, live in separate worlds not because they are malicious or selfish but because they are dedicated to helping by becoming very good at a part of what concerns that patient.

This picture of "chopped up" life may be too bleak and sterile, too finely etched. Fortunately there is a good deal of blurring in real life. No doubt, for beginnings, the majority of people in specialties of health/medicine are themselves personally religious, as the vast majority of the human race is, by whatever strict definitions of religion one would use. Certainly the majority of people in religious life and work are concerned about health/medicine, be it their own or that of others in their communions or cultures. Where the two sets of people, concerns, expertise, and language do separate out of hostility, peacemakers can come on the scene to reduce hostilities. Where they are divided because they have customarily ignored each other, it is possible that they can have their curiosities about one another's worlds quickened. Where they possess latent insights or knowledge about what it takes to deal in more inclusive ways with a patient or a parishioner, they will best live out their vocations if they develop these latencies until they become patent and visible.

Having criticized dabblers and chatterers, it is proper for me to be asked how anyone can address the issues of reducing hostility or ignorance between these separate worlds and how to promote knowledge and understanding across them. In this inquiry we have chosen to do so by inviting in not dabblers and chatterers but people who are all specialists. They have their roles. The minister is partly differentiated from the clinical counselor, though both are in the world of religion. The physician who preaches prevention and the physician who teaches medicine are asked to address the subjects from the viewpoint of their very precise kinds of expertise. And in this book another range of specialists has been called in: historians, philosophers, theologians, and ethicists. I want to talk about them and their world, their approaches and methods, their disciplines and what these have to offer.

It may seem jarring, ironic, or paradoxical to visit such specialists to see how *they* handle the general, to visit people in different disciplines to assess the connections they make, or to visit victims of modern "separation" to gain insight into the quest for wholeness. But broadly defined disciplines in the social sciences and the humanities, three each of which we shall visit briefly, do include people who have reached beyond confinement to find methods for addressing the intertwinings that make up culture. It is not our purpose to see what each discipline has had to say about health/medicine in isolation or about religion in its segregation. Instead, the questions are, "What have these disciplines done to bring together the concerns that a patient, a lay person, has? If they have done little in recent times, why is this so? If they wish to do more, how do they go about doing so?"

The hypothetical—or actual—lay person might through it all profitably keep asking, "What's in it for me, if I come to better understandings of how religion and health/medicine can or should intersect in culture? Are there better ways for one to get handles on these connections than are apparent? Such seemingly self-centered questions can keep the inquiry from remaining merely academic. They can help professionals stay alert to their need to aid in the task of being responsive beyond their fields of expertise. This introduction to six "bridge" disciplines, then, is not an inquiry for inquiry's sake but an observation that might help participants in those disciplines in "the helping professions" to be reminded of that larger vision which the patient or lay person brings. From some point of view or other, at some time or other, we are *all* such patients and lay persons and should have the most profound motivations for pursuing the inquiry.

THREE OF THE SOCIAL SCIENCES

A social science that has illumined the connections between religion and health/medicine for a century is anthropology. This is a largely modern discipline, though it has roots as far back as Plato and Aristotle—which seems to be true of all disciplines. A person lying in a hospital in an industrial society or reading a health magazine or going to synagogue probably senses little or no link to anthropologists, whose field of study seems quite remote. Popularizer Robin Fox put it well when he dealt with the stereotype:

> If you meet an anthropologist and decide to ask him a question, you will probably pick one of three topics: primitive people, early man, or race. If you know there is to be an article by an anthropologist in a Sunday magazine, you assume it will be about one of these three things.[2]

The hospital patient is not "primitive" or "early" or preoccupied with race—at least not at the moment. He or she is sophisticated, "contemporary," and preoccupied with medicine. Yet it is the world that once was called "primitive," now often described as "native," which has a bearing on many aspects of the search for health. Physicians and researchers readily admit that in some respects we are "not much further along than the medicine men," that understandings of modern medicine are often quite primitive, and that some drugs in expensive pharmacies encapsulate what herbal witch doctors "knew" long ago or know now, far away. Many people in medical professions have respect for the way native peoples learn to live with the rhythms of nature or to heal with the fruits of the field. Meanwhile very modern religionists are relearning the power of symbol and myth or of rite and ceremony in healing or keeping people whole.

Whoever thinks that modern industrial societies have no room for the kind of medicine anthropologists care about would do well to look in the back of any number of popular magazines. Potions, aphrodisiacs, and herbal cures are offered to millions. For that matter, staying for a moment with the concept of the primitive, it is present on cultural levels other than those of the popular magazines. From time to time therapy from that world even becomes faddish. Thus during the years of the "counterculture" in the late 1960s, collegiate dropout sons and daughters of professors and physicians tried to adopt Native American or African medicine in their rural communes. Their impulse may have been romantic, but it was not wholly misplaced. The large industry that offers "wholistic" or "holistic" approaches to health also trades to a considerable extent on the kinds of medicine that attracted the old-time anthropologist.

What anthropology has to offer, both in the stereotype that Robin Fox portrays and in more complex recent versions, is a realization that on the most profound human levels, people have perceived how intertwined

Religion and Health/Medicine in Culture

religion and health/medicine are in the basics of culture. Today, however, anthropologists do not confine themselves to the world of primitives. Under the impetus of Claude Lévi-Strauss and other "structural anthropologists," some scholars have even collapsed meaningful distinctions between primitives and sophisticates, between native and technical medicine. To them the universe is so structured, and the human mind to match it, that certain forms and responses pervade all cultures. The patient in a modern hospital may be filled with tubes while the Trobriand Islander is not. But there is little difference based on "cultural evolution" between the ways the two comprehend and address their sufferings and hopes.[3]

Not all anthropology is structuralist, which means in part that not every anthropologist denies differences between "primitive" and "modern" or between "prelogical" and "logical" mentalities. Some anthropologists have more of a sense of history than Lévi-Strauss. Cultural evolutionists and structuralists are not the only other parties to schisms in the discipline. Students of religious sects have not really run into denominational conflict until they have seen how biological anthropologists war against cultural anthropologists, or how distant are those who study ethnography from those who trade in symbols. For our connections, however, it is chiefly cultural anthropology that offers most promise.

Anthropology from the first was concerned with both religion and health/medicine. It knew no schism between them because the people it studied seemed to do little differentiating or separating between the spheres of life.[4] To the cultural evolutionist, the great move to modernity was the differentiation, the specialization, the chopping up of life already mentioned, the breaking of connections between sacred and secular and thus the segregating of religious from medical spheres of life.[5]

As "primitive" cultures change, thanks to the invasion of missionaries, commercial interests, technology, or even anthropologists with tape recorders, anthropologists have conducted research into the industrial cultures as well. Thus people like Mary Douglas, Victor and Edith Turner, and Clifford Geertz have studied the menu and diet, the pilgrimages, or the patterns of cleanliness in Europe and America, as if standing outside their own culture the way they stand outside those of the Javanese or Balinese whom Geertz has also studied.[6] What their researches confirm is that there are certain basic ways of relating to symbols that cut across layers and levels of culture.

The Sociocultural Context

The great service that cultural anthropologists today are performing in our field of inquiry is this: They have brought tools from the "primitive" world and used them on complex "modern" cultures, only to find that there are unities that specialists overlook, that "wholistic" approaches are deeply rooted in the human response. They have found it necessary greatly to enlarge the understanding or definition of religion itself.

Some people in the medical profession might casually ignore or disdain the present study of intertwinings on first hearing simply because they equate "religion" with "organized religion." They know that in the bowels of the hospital there is a sometimes frequented chapel, used by a segment of the hospital population and presided over by a special caste of professionals who remain remote if not bizarre. They know that some patients will want to consult a religious professional or chaplain, that dietary laws or medical practices of, say, Jehovah's Witnesses or Seventh-Day Adventists present obstacles to their medical approaches.

To such professionals it often comes as a surprise that, thanks to anthropology and sometimes sociology, religion is seen as having seeped far beyond institutions or as never having been confined in them. To the anthropologically informed person, the physician in the white coat looks like and may be a sort of priest in one of the "denominations" within the religion of science. Checking in to the physician and making the rounds of the wards are highly ritualized acts, informed by meanings that patients see in them. The hierarchy of medical professionals is as formal as the hierarchy of a church. Belief in the processes of medicine may often be as important in curing as belief in God or the dogmas of a church is important for spiritual health.

The anthropologist, then, promotes our present inquiry by expanding the notion of religion, sometimes as far as Clifford Geertz does. To him, in a modern classic definition,

> religion is (1) a system of symbols which acts to (2) establish powerful, pervasive, and long-lasting moods and motivations in men by (3) formulating conceptions of a general order of existence and (4) clothing these conceptions with such an aura of factuality that (5) the moods and motivations seem uniquely realistic.[7]

Some experts in health and medicine may feel that this kind of definition goes too far; for that matter, some people in religious studies feel that way too. Such scholars may wish to include an element that numbers of their colleagues add: that religion needs some sense that an outside Power or powers, a Person or forces, somehow would transact with the world of nature and humans and demand some sort of response. This has been a convenient addition in most Western definitions of religion, but many Buddhist sects are thoroughly religious without this sense. Even some Western faiths, including Ethical Culture and Secular Humanism, which have been pointed to by the Supreme Court as "religions," do not have the theistic or deistic elements.

Anthropologists do not say to the peruser of potion advertisements, "Go back" to the primitives and use these potions or herbs. They may say that there is less difference between the sacred potion and the secular medicine than you once believed. And they are likely to add that the hospital ritual and the temple ritual can converge for the sake of healing. But anthropologists need not themselves be goads or counselors. They perform their service by showing how on all levels of culture, religion (broadly defined) is present as an aid or an obstacle in healing. Just as creatively, or devastatingly to the religious reactionary, anthropologists may complicate their existence by showing how a comparison of cultures deprives them of uniqueness. Some professors of religion protest that social sciences like anthropology are reductionist, which means that to them religion is "nothing but. . . ." It is nothing but magic or super-stition or witch-doctoring or voodoo or a composite of ritual instincts. "Nothing-buttery" is one of the risks in the social-scientific studies. Reductionism will not go away because religious people build walls around themselves. But it is clear by now that there is no single response of religion to anthropology, and vice versa. It is equally clear that connec-tions between religion and health/medicine will become especially vivid to those who acquire something of the anthropologists' eyes.

A second social science, older than anthropology, presents similar options and challenges. Sociology, born earlier in the nineteenth century in the work of Auguste Comte and Karl Marx and refined later by Max Weber and Emile Durkheim, promoted new understandings of what it is to be social human beings. Even to name Karl Marx is to suggest how "connections" between religion and the rest of culture—in his case the social or economic more than the medical—are intertwined. Religion to his kind of sociologist and many others was "nothing but" a projection of divine beings to meet human needs. The name of Max Weber, on the other hand, points to a different but related kind of awareness. Weberian sociologists have proposed that just as "consequences have ideas" so also "ideas have consequences." That is, if to Karl Marx the fact that if one is a middle-class aspiring European one is also likely to find it advisable to be Calvinist, or that if one is an enchained industrial worker one will find release and relief by "otherworldly" religious hopes, so Weber deals with a different set of theories and findings. Weber projects that if one believes deeply in one's calling in life and in the stewardship of time and the industrious use of resources and has come to this outlook by a profound but ever-changing belief in the Calvinist system, one is likely to find a way of life called capitalist. Religious belief in both cases is taken seriously but appraised less for its theological truth than for its societal utility.

The sociologist is not always the grand theorist. Sociologists are adept at many kinds of inquiry that have bearings on religion, on medicine, and on connections between religion and health/medicine. They can engage in survey research or interviews, in polling and statistical analysis, to help religious leaders understand patterns of institutional growth and loyalty. Or they can help point to needs for new hospitals or reasons for conflict between physicians and nurses. "Medical sociology" is a reasonably well populated corner of the profession not of medicine but of sociology.[8]

Neither "medical sociology" nor "sociology of religion" in their full sense is the present point. The methods each has developed and the basic theories they propound illumine the inquiry. The present point is that both specialties in this social science are poised to show connections the public often fails to see. It is disappointing to see how spare and sparse religious references have been to date in the medical sociological literature. Religious sociology has spent energies on topics that are less urgent than medical understandings in the religious sphere. What professionals from both camps discover is a web of relations in individual lives for which there is little institutional carry-over.

Thus in a culture like that of North America well over 90 percent of the people say they believe in God, and more than 60 percent are members of religious institutions and over 40 percent regularly participate in and attend them. The symbols that attract adherents and the behavior patterns that issue from them, both so accessible to the sociologist, include arrays of concepts that deal with health/medicine. For medical or health professions to overlook these is to miss the location of the patient. Meanwhile, religious people who fear sociology because they might find that belief in these symbols or that to which symbols refer are "nothing but" a sign of social class attachments, and are thus driven off, will fail to understand how much people's faith is embedded in contexts. They will overlook the ways in which the human environment does help determine, if it never wholly determines, human response. One would be ill-advised to begin the practice of medicine in a Muslim part of Africa without learning something sociological concerning what Islam teaches about health and medicine and what Muslims practice. To say that is to pay tribute to that which sociology studies: If religion were nothing but "truth exempted from history," we would not expect such cultural dispositions. One need only deal with the epidemiology or symptomology of a set of people or the symptoms of a person or patient—and that would be that. Knowing that the understanding of connections is different among the Muslims from that among Orthodox Jews in New York, Lutherans in Minnesota, or Seventh-Day Adventists in southern California is to begin to recognize the potential in blending the wisdom of medical and religious sociology. For the individual to become aware of these cultural and social contexts and environments can also be a step toward better health, toward cure. One need not be wholly imprisoned by traditions or circumstance if one is aware that all humans are somehow in traditions and circumstances. More on the positive side, sociology, by pointing to context and environment, can also point to resources forgotten within a tradition or accessible beyond it.

A third social science that has seen connections between religion and health in culture and that has also been tempted to see religion as "nothing but" is psychology. Psychology as a discipline bridging social sciences and the humanities is not quite the same thing as psychology used in therapy. Here we are speaking only of the cluster of academic subdisciplines that in formal ways seek to understand and connect religion and health/medicine through psychological inquiries.

The case of psychology in the context of intertwining religion with health/medicine is more like anthropology than sociology. That is, although sociology was born with ties to "sociology of religion"—all the founding giants took up the subject—their focus was less on medical aspects of personal and social life as these related to religion. Anthropology did devote itself to these connections. So, in different ways, did psychology. One need only mention the names of Sigmund Freud, C. G. Jung, and William James to see the intertwining made vivid. In *Varieties of Religious Experience* (1902), William James went to great pains to show the legitimacy of the religious category in the context of science. Jung liked to say that among his patients in the second half of life, psychological problems were in virtually all cases somehow religious. And Freud, the genius of greatest influence, saw religious connections at most important psychological junctures.

Freud saw the id, the superego, and the ego involved in constructing religion. He tried to account for the beginnings of religion in the psychological history of the human race, as his books *Moses and Monotheism* and *Totem and Taboo* demonstrate. If that was true of the social dimension, so too personally, religion was constructed in each individual, a point Freud tried to establish in *The Future of an Illusion*. God was a projection, a creation of the "as if," a necessity for people who had to fashion a benign universe out of what was in fact a hostile one.

Today only a few Freudian fundamentalists agree with Freud's root observations; most scholars believe they were ill-founded and even simply wrong. But these giants did succeed in setting enough terms that scholars in psychological studies still grapple with religious archetypes (Jung), myths (Freud), or experiences (James).[9]

A half century or more after the founding theories, various forms of religious connections are potent in the literature of analysis and therapy. Thus Joel Kovel devotes a full chapter to "the mysticotranscendent approach" to therapy in a catalog of theories.

> For many, the transcendent approach—whether offered by any of the Eastern meditative practices, including Yoga, Zen, Sufism and Tibetan Buddhism, or by variants of the Judeo-Christian mystical tradition—has offered the solace of belief and a coherent approach to the world, while promising relief from neurotic tension. . . . Obviously a religious elaboration will go a long way toward structuring the transcendent state of mind, and it will introduce powerful social effects related to the institutionalization of the religion. These factors cannot fail to have important emotional consequences whether or not the objective superstructure of the religion has any validity on its own terms. It was William James who observed that more alcoholics have been cured by religious conversion than by all the medicine in the world. For all the immense apparatus of modern psychiatry, I suspect the same observation would hold true today.[10]

Not all religious proclamation or observance, not even all therapy, is friendly to modern psychological theories. And psychology is also, for the most part, a specialized and highly secularized discipline. The behaviorist in psychology, like the sociobiologist in sociology, has little room for reckoning with the "mysticotranscendent" realm or can reduce it through "nothing-buttery" until the believer or adherent loses interest.

Still, given its roots as a discipline and the kind of effects Kovel referred to, there is plenty of connecting going on where psychology plays its part in health/medicine and religion. Michael Argyle and Benjamin Beit-Hallahmi, who stand far apart from the assumptions of religious people, have no difficulty filling a book with survey data on the intertwining of our subjects. Their data includes measurements of religious activity, factors in environment and situation ("parental factors," "marital status," age and religion, sex differences, personality types, "adjustment"), and the like. And they conclude with a catalog of theories. For origins, Freud's "father-projection" appears alongside "cognitive need" theories, in which people must make sense of a chaotic universe. As for maintenance, "relief of guilt," "fear of death," and "deprivation and compensation" are typical. Finally, the co-authors cite "theories of consequence," having to do with how individuals find personal integration or at-homeness in society. Even though theirs is a mere two-hundred-page summary work, the literature is so rich that their bibliography takes up thirty-five pages—a sign of the scope of literature about the connections.[11]

THE HUMANITIES

Alongside the social-scientific approaches to inquiry are those disciplines called "humanistic." Here we need only point to their roles. Everyone who seeks to understand how health/medicine and religion intertwine in culture will inevitably make use of these to some extent. First, history. Both medicine and religion have pasts, and telling the story of how they developed somehow throws light on what they are and do today. The professional student of these pasts, the scholar who tells stories for a living, is called a historian. But the professional does not have a monopoly on using the past. What people call "old wives' tales" about cures are really representations of the past, and the person who brings them up is, while doing so, acting as a historian. On the other hand, the people who criticize "old wives' tales" by showing how later developments in medicine and religion proved them untrue and unhelpful in curing are also acting as historians because they use evidence of the past to inform the present.

Similarly, it is virtually impossible to deal in any continuous way with the connection between health/medicine and religion in cultures without making use of texts. Here the study of literature comes into play. People can make inquiries about their own time and place while relying only on what is oral. As soon as there is any interest in looking at what people have thought and done somewhere else, texts are necessary. These texts need not always be in formal, printed books. They can be ancient prescriptions preserved on papyrus or pottery shards or even on tombstones that give testimony about longevity rates or cholera epidemics. In whatever form, they tell us more than nonliterate evidences like burial positions, deformed skeletons, or crude mortars and pestles found by archaeologists.

Especially in the field of religion, texts, usually called scriptures, are of special importance. So it is that inquirers into these connections are in some way or other literary critics, students of language and literature. Some are professionals who make sophisticated studies of the structure or theory of language. But nonprofessionals are also students of literature when they ask such questions as "What does the word of God in that book have to say about the body?" or "Why does a Buddhist scripture differ from a Hindu one?" or, most complex of all, "Why do Adventists and Catholics read such different meanings into or out of the Bible?"

Alongside historical and literary studies is a third prime humanistic discipline, philosophy. Philosophy, which means literally "love of wisdom," is the intellectual pursuit of meaning through ideas and expression in language. As in the other two cases, not all philosophy is done by professional scholars in colleges, universities, or research centers. The simple victims of disease who ask why they suffer something malignant in a universe that they regarded as benign are philosophers. Patients who cry out at a "good God" for allowing evil to happen eventually fall into silence and then, if faith endures, find some way to continue affirming. In religious terms, that turn is an act of faith, but it is also somehow a use of philosophy, for it expresses a kind of wisdom that comes by experience and reflection.

While philosophy, like history and literature, is too rich, varied, and important to be left only to academics and researchers, it is also a formal and professional discipline that scholars can and must refine through the centuries. Not all their refinements will strike people seeking health as having much to do with their struggles. There are philosophers who go out of their way to see that their inquiries do not touch questions that are vital to nonphilosophers. For them philosophy is a language game as rewarding as chess, and rewarding in the same way, following only its own rules. Anglo-American universities may even be dominated by such ways of seeing philosophy in our time. Like Islam or Buddhism or

Christianity, fields of learning have many denominations and sects. But over the long pull of history a significant number of disciplined thinkers regularly return to questions of what is true, beautiful, and good and are of help in connecting religion with health/medicine. Much of the discipline of medical ethics is, in this sense, philosophy.

We also should not in our imaginings leave the philosophers off alone somewhere in the realm of ideas. Even the most remote and abstract of them in their personal lives stand on a common footing or lie in beds of perplexity alongside other victims of pain and disease.

> For there was never yet philosopher
> That could endure the toothache patiently.[12]

SINCE THIS PROJECT IS HUMANISTIC . . .

The humanities include more than history, literature, and philosophy. In the United States a National Endowment for the Humanities in its original charter included "language, linguistics, literature, history, jurisprudence, philosophy, archaeology, comparative religion, ethics, the history, criticism, theory, and practice of the arts" along with "those aspects of the social sciences which have humanistic content and employ humanistic method along with the study and application of the humanities to the human environment. . . ."[13] Because the present inquiry is largely humanistic, it is valuable to reflect on what such a vision has to do with religion and meanings. Distancing between religion and other spheres of life is a problem that current inquiries have set out to overcome. Study of the humanities was long thought to distract people from religion, and in all fairness it must be said that it no doubt often did. We must examine this problem to throw light on the need for new inquiry about religious connections with culture.

In one recent discussion, a philosopher interested in history, Frederick A. Olafson of the University of California, San Diego, writes:

> The relationship between humanism and religious belief is one that has given difficulties for centuries and has caused a good deal of personal anguish to those humanists like St. Jerome and Petrarch who have aspired to be sincere Christians. That there is some deep source of conflict here seems undeniable; but it would just as certainly be mistaken to define humanism as atheistic or even antireligious.[14]

There have been, it is true, "forms of religious belief that are radically incompatible with humanism because they proclaim the nothingness of man and transfer to their gods every possible form of agency or achievement with which man might otherwise be tempted to credit himself." Thus, in the instance of medicine, there are forms of religious faith in the modern world—extreme forms of Christian pentecostal healing movements, for example—that repudiate the humanistic study of medicine because they repudiate medicine. Mundane human achievements count for nothing in the world of pure transcendence and total miracle.

Olafson knows, however, that even if such outlooks were once standard, today most faiths have changed their views and accept the human part in divine-human relations with a warmer embrace.

> There are also religions that teach that there is something, however limited, that human beings as individuals and as societies can do and that thus concede a measure of significance and value to the achievements of human culture and even allow a modicum of human pride, as well as of shame, stemming from the contemplation of what has been done.

Olafson notes that "some measure of human self-assertion has maintained itself, however covertly, even within the most inhospitable and man-denying systems of belief."

Olafson's statement is too modest. Humanism of the humanities sort has a high place among "the religions of the book" (Judaism, Christianity, and Islam) in many periods of their development. These faiths kept the lights of learning on when there were Dark Ages around them, when "barbarians" were at the gate. Still, his is a good reminder of the mistrust of humanities and humanism among fundamentalists of many stripes in many cultures and faiths. Such mistrust in the past often inhibited the development of medicine in the interest of dogma or religious control. In the more recent past it has kept people from being curious about the *meanings* of developing medicine and care for the body. In the West, religious history has often been the history of synagogues, mosques, and churches, the history of theology and liturgy. It has too seldom paid attention to the lives of ordinary worshipers, most of whom have believed that their faith has something to do with their bodies and their health. Too seldom do the texts that speak of such concerns receive the analysis that more formally "religious" ones do. And philosophically grounded studies of "bioethics" from a religious point of view have often, until recently, been at the curricular margins of seminaries, at the sparse ends of ministerial bookshelves. Change is at hand, however, and in the literate religious camps there is an eagerness to see connections, to overcome barriers, not known at many earlier periods in history.

Religionists, however, know that there are problems from the other side as well. Perhaps neglect of religion by humanistic scholars of health and medicine, be they historians, critics, or philosophers, is more difficult to trace. In the case of religious antihumanism, it was rather simple: Give all to God and there is nothing left for humans. Why study them? Be caught up in the One and the All, as are mystics who try to "get out of the body." And why should you care about being "in the body" or curious about it? But the humanities, as studied in the secular academy where most physicians and health-care experts are trained, should have fewer profound reasons for ruling out religion. Yet, historically, health-care professionals were aloof; only recently has there been a making of connections, an overcoming of old suspicion and hostility. Much more must occur before members of literate cultures can get the full benefits of these connections.

The suspicion and hostility developed in humanities chiefly on two grounds, and there have been parallels in social sciences as well. When, four or five centuries ago, humanists began to break free of formal religious control, religious leaders struck back. Like the scientific community, the humanistic community has vivid if stereotyped recall of the Galileo case and its counterparts, wherein religious enforcers would not allow humanistic or scientific inquiry to proceed unhampered. To this day, thanks in part to fundamentalist encroachments presumably on the soil of all faiths, humanists have reason to remain wary of certain kinds of religious expression. The visitor need not walk far down the corridors of a medical school to find a person who was once bruised by church or community leaders, parents or pastors. Perhaps they had slapped the fingers of future medical researchers who in their adolescence had reached for the "forbidden books" section of their small-town library or denominational college. Such victims do not always forget the slights or the repressions, and they carry over their own experiences into cases against all religion, mistrusting its every expression.

If on the negative side this freeing from repression led to suspicion, hostility often developed from a more positive sense of liberation on the part of many humanistic scholars who are interested in health and medicine. Looking back into history or into their own lives, they recall a sense of people being cooped, cramped, and crisped in tight shells, huddled under carapaces of religious symbols that allowed for no light or breath. They saw humans receiving speculative answers dogmatically given to questions not being asked and being denied questions that would illumine the human story. To walk out from under the canopies of the sacred into fields of free inquiry was such a movement of freedom that they looked back only with distaste. The religion some of them once serenely ignored they later disdained.

In America, at least, one could give several accountings of these moves among humanistic scholars. What happened to rule out religious understandings of health/medicine at crucial stages? We might date the great turn within the past century, when the modern university was born. The colonial college and the higher academies of the pre–Civil War period were almost all run by the churches. At the turn of the century they came more and more to be tax-supported state schools. It seemed out of place to many in such schools to do religious inquiry in a nation which believed, it was said, in "the separation of church and state."

So at state universities there were no theological schools or religion departments. In a time of increasing specialization of learning, it was difficult for anyone to bridge gaps because one partner, the religious, was missing from campus humanistic contexts. And it was on campuses that most inquiry occurred. Now it is possible to report that in an ever more pluralistic and, some say, more secular America, there is encouragement to overcome artificial barriers put up by unimaginative believers in "separation." The U.S. Supreme Court, in the very decisions that ruled out Bible-reading, prayer, and devotion from the schools, "ruled in" the study of religious connections in culture.

In *Abington Township School District* v. *Schempp*,[15] the second of two famed "school prayer" decisions, the Supreme Court argued:

> One's education is not complete without a study of comparative religion or the history of religion and its relationship to the advancement of civilization. . . . Nothing we have said here indicates that such study of the Bible or of religion, when presented objectively as part of a secular program of education, may not be effected consistent with the First Amendment.[16]

Since that period the lonely religion departments at schools like the pioneering University of Iowa have found company in several hundred tax-supported departments. Meanwhile, private universities and denominationally related schools saw some expansion of religious inquiry during the 1960s, when humane use of the humanities was in favor on campuses.

Religion and Health/Medicine in Culture

Since then there have been cutbacks in the humanities and some shifts of student interest toward immediately practical preprofessional courses, which sometimes leave little time or curiosity for humanistic understandings. But the exclusionist principle, at least, has changed. The principle by itself does not solve everything. It takes time for religious scholars to attune themselves to every cultural need, and there is still much to do as humanists learn to look for connections between religion and health/medicine in the texts and traces they study.

A second reason for the broken connection in the academy, where most inquiry has gone on, had little to do with the separation of church and state. Instead it simply resulted as a practical effect of the specialization that went on when universities became modern and differentiated. While many scientists rightly think of history, literature, philosophy, and other disciplines as being ancient, they did not cohere around the name "humanities" until the twentieth century in America. The first use we can find was by Texas professor Thomas Fitz-Hugh in 1898, and it was only around World War II that there was self-conscious interest in the humanities.[17]

During these decades the ideal of integrated liberal arts suffered. More than many would like to admit, students were compelled to choose early between "science" or "the humanities." They had to become familiar with separate castes of faculties, separate sections of libraries, and to make a choice. The student who intended to be a physician or a dietitian went on one track, while the student who would be a philosopher or historian went on another, sometimes parallel but more often diverging or contrary track. Never again did they meet. They spoke different languages and lived in different worlds.

Within the humanities the same kind of specialization went on. Historians found demands so great that they would master their discipline while neglecting not only science but also literature and philosophy. Within their discipline they would become "cliometricians" who used statistics, or "psychohistorians" who employed psychological methods to study the past, or "positivists," "ordinary storytellers," or whatever. They stopped talking to one another. One might be a historian of culture and completely overlook the role of disease in culture. Or one would be an expert on one country or county, one century or moment, and lose curiosity about all others. I once met an expert on "the middle years of Michael the Drunkard" (b. 838, d. 867 in Constantinople) who professed no expertise and little competence in the ruler's "early" or "late" years. Presumably he could study the policies of Michael without getting into the question of whether being "the Drunkard"—in the zone of health/medicine—had an effect on his statecraft.

To this day it is a subject of curiosity for a historian to show interest in the history of disease, unless he or she is a specialist in the study of the medical past. Most reviewers remarked how noteworthy it was for "general" historian William McNeill to have written *Plagues and People*, on civilized disease pools of Eurasia or the ecological impact of medical science and organization since 1700. Yet even far-ranging McNeill gave only a couple of pages to the religious connections. He noted how cholera spread through Muslim pilgrimages to Mecca, or commented on Jewish and Muslim prohibitions against eating pork as a religious instance of inhibiting infections. Books like his, however, give rich clues to areas of research on "connections" still ahead.[18]

Not all the past failure to exploit these clues is the result of anti-religious bias among humanists or antihumanistic bias among scientists. Within the secular academy there are tensions and strains among and within the disciplines. In our present inquiry into the religious connections, it is important to remember that good and valid reasons of structure or outlook play their parts as well. Take, for example, the contrast in impulses between scientist and humanist as they relate to time. George Steiner, a notable critic, commented on this in a popular magazine article:

> Even at the sharpest edge of autistic engagement, the scientist is oriented toward the future, with what it contains of morning light and positive chance. . . . Today's high-school student solves equations inaccessible to Newton or to Gauss; an undergraduate biologist could instruct Darwin. Almost the exact contrary holds true for the humanities.

The humanist, especially in the field of religion, is likely to be looking backward. The wisdom in Plato or Aristotle, in Maimonides or Asoka or Calvin, is more telling than some forward-looking efforts by would-be relevant people of mere talent, not genius, in our own time. How dampening to the scientist is this vision:

> The proposition that there is to come in the West no writer to match, let alone excel, William Shakespeare or that music will not produce again the phenomena of prodigal quality manifest in Mozart and Schubert is logically undemonstrable. But it carries a formidable weight of intuitive credibility.

Religion and Health/Medicine in Culture

> The humanist is a rememberer. He walks, as does one troupe of the accursed in Dante's "Inferno," with his head twisted backward. He lurches indifferent into tomorrow.[19]

No good purpose is served by pretending away these forward versus backward-looking turns of the head. Understanding them will help inform the question of why it is often so difficult to bring together the medic and the parson, the biochemist and the pastoral counselor, the laboratory technician and the priest. Yet the person in search of continuing health or relief from disease cannot profit from the luxury of seeing the two cohorts march in opposite directions in the corridors or confine themselves in laboratories on the one hand or chapels and temples on the other.

Humanistic inquiries that dominate this book on religion in its intertwining with health/medicine will seem to touch only one segment of the lives of people engrossed in diet, politically involved with getting votes for or against abortion amendments, or dying patients. The humanities have their place, a limited place. But those limits can be large. Something of the boundaries and promise of the humanities comes through on the first page of a report in 1980 by the Commission on the Humanities:

> Through the humanities we reflect on the fundamental question: what does it mean to be human? The humanities offer clues but never a complete answer. They reveal how people have tried to make moral, spiritual, and intellectual sense of a world in which irrationality, despair, loneliness and death are as conspicuous as birth, friendship, hope, and reason. We learn how individuals or societies define the moral life and try to attain it, attempt to reconcile freedom and the responsibilities of citizenship, and express themselves artistically. The humanities do not necessarily mean humaneness, nor do they always inspire the individual with what Cicero called "incentives to noble action." But by awakening a sense of what it might be like to be someone else or to live in another time or culture, they tell us about ourselves, stretch our imagination, and enrich our experience. They increase our distinctively human potential.[20]

On the terrain of the humanities, thus defined, more and more scholars of religion have begun to feel at home. It is not necessary to spell out in detail here just what is involved when humanistic scholars of religion take up their disciplines. Instead, there are examples. Kenneth Vaux shows how the humanistic discipline of theology informs the history of medicine. Darrell Amundsen and Ronald Numbers are historians in action, providing a perspective through time on religion and medicine. Tristram Engelhardt uses a philosophical approach to the intertwinings. Every contributor, including physicians, is somehow serving as a literary critic of texts. They complement the efforts by practitioners, each of whom has come to the present point through study of the humanities, and the medical scientists, who demonstrate how humanistic one can be within their professions.

What they here present are only beginnings, illustrations, clues, and goals for their own future work, for a specific project that will pursue their leads, and for independent scholars and practitioners. They serve their purpose well if they lead people in the medical and health services camps to see how complex the ties have been. And they double their effect if they help guide people in the religious professions and fields of study, the rabbis and theologians and their kin and kind, to see how concern for the body in the dimensions of health/medicine are interwoven into the web of spiritual interests with which they feel more immediately at home.

While the professionals set out on their inquiries, research scholars and librarians are busy assembling awesomely lengthy bibliographies. These reveal what has been done. They are also turning up canyon-sized gaps, each suggesting what we must still inquire about. These are not merely gaps in learning, voids in scientific pursuit, or charters of humanistic research. They are also the situations of life wherein most people spend much of their time. The testimony of such lay people and the physicians or religious leaders who serve them are prime data for the understandings that are on the horizon, the excitements that are ahead. What will be confirmed is that many a philosopher has the toothache and shows a comprehension of pain and the lure of health. At the same time, many an ordinary citizen with a toothache also reveals some grasp of philosophy that philosophers should admire, of spiritual groping that religious professionals will find valuable, for in the end the intertwinings in culture come to their focus in the people who make up the culture. They will not tolerate inquiries that never touch their lives. If professionals and specialists fail to take their testimony or to minister to their curiosities and needs, the field will remain open for charlatans and quacks. The present inquiry is evidence that such exploiters will not have the field to themselves, that men and women of dedication and skill are ready to take up an inquiry that can be not only "humanistic" but also "humane."

Religion and Health/Medicine in Culture

NOTES

1. This view of modernization is reinforced in John Murray Cuddihy, *The Ordeal of Civility: Freud, Marx, Lévi-Strauss, and the Jewish Struggle with Modernity* (New York: Basic Books, 1974), p. 10; "Differentiation is the cutting edge of the modernization process, sundering cruelly what tradition had joined. . . . Differentiation slices through ancient primordial ties and identities, leaving crisis and 'wholeness-hunger' in its wake."

2. Robin Fox, *Encounter with Anthropology* (New York: Dell Publishing Co., 1975), p. 10.

3. The literature of Lévi-Strauss and structuralism is enormous and need not concern us here. Those who seek a lucid introduction to an arcane field would find Edmund Leach, *Claude Lévi-Strauss* (New York: Viking Press, 1970) useful. Its short bibliography is also helpful, though there has been an explosion of literature in the ensuing decade.

4. Access to 1,135 studies of what used to be called "primitive," and now is often referred to as "native" medicine can be found in Ira E. Harrison and Sheila Cominsky, *Traditional Medicine: Implications for Ethnomedicine, Ethnopharmacology, Maternal and Child Health, Mental Health, and Public Health— An Annotated Bibliography of Africa, Latin America, and the Caribbean* (New York: Garland Publishing, 1976).

5. For a succinct summary of cultural evolution as it bears on religion, see "Religious Evolution" in Robert Bellah, *Beyond Belief* (New York: Harper & Row, 1970), pp. 20–50.

6. Relevant examples are Mary Douglas, *Purity and Danger: An Analysis of Pollution and Taboo* (London: Routledge & Kegan Paul, 1966), and sections in *Natural Symbols: Explorations in Cosmology* (New York: Random House, 1972). See also sections on miracles in Victor Turner and Edith Turner, *Image and Pilgrimage in Christian Culture* (New York: Columbia University Press, 1978).

7. Clifford Geertz, *The Interpretation of Cultures* (New York: Basic Books, 1973), p. 90.

8. See Linda H. Aiken and Howard E. Freeman, "Medical Sociology and Science and Technology in Medicine," in *A Guide to the Culture of Science, Technology, and Medicine,* ed. Paul T. Durbin (New York: Free Press, 1980), pp. 527–37 and passim.

9. A fair-minded but critical summary of Freud's views of religion and culture intertwined is in John Bowker, *The Sense of God: Sociological, Anthropological and Psychological Approaches to the Origin of the Sense of God* (Oxford: Clarendon Press, 1973), chap. 6, pp. 116–34. The entire Bowker work is relevant to the social-scientific half of this chapter, and it includes a useful bibliography.

10. Joel Kovel, *A Complete Guide to Therapy: From Psychoanalysis to Behavior Modification* (New York: Pantheon Books, 1976), pp. 148–49.

11. See Michael Argyle and Benjamin Beit-Hallahmi, *The Social Psychology of Religion* (London: Routledge & Kegan Paul, 1975), chap. 11, pp. 178–207, deals with "theories of religious behaviour."

12. William Shakespeare in *Much Ado About Nothing*, act V, scene 1, line 35.

13. *Division of Education Program Guidelines* (Washington, D.C.: National Endowment for the Humanities, n.d.), p. 3.

14. Frederick A. Olafson, *The Dialectic of Action: A Philosophical Interpretation of History and the Humanities* (Chicago: University of Chicago Press, 1979), pp. 255–56.

15. 374 U.S. 203 (1963).

16. The case is reprinted in Arthur B. Frommer, *The Bible and the Public Schools* (New York: Liberal Press, 1963), p. 78.

17. Laurence Veysey, "The Plural Organized Worlds of the Humanities," in *The Organization of Knowledge in Modern America 1860–1920*, ed. Alexandra Oleson and John Voss (Baltimore: Johns Hopkins University Press, 1979), pp. 51–106.

18. William H. McNeill, *Plagues and Peoples* (Garden City, N.Y.: Doubleday & Co., 1976); there are also some comments on religion in Frederick F. Cartwright, *Disease and History* (Ithaca: Cornell University Press, 1972).

19. George Steiner, "The Cleric of Treason," *The New Yorker*, December 8, 1980, p. 185.

20. Report of the Commission on the Humanities, *The Humanities in American Life* (Berkeley: University of California Press, 1980), p. 1.

PART TWO

The Historical Setting

3

Medicine and Religion: Pre-Christian Antiquity

DARREL W. AMUNDSEN
and
GARY B. FERNGREN

Four basic relationships between religion and medicine have existed throughout history: (1) medicine has been a manifestation or function of religion; (2) medicine and religion have been functionally separate but allied and complementary; (3) they have simply coexisted; and (4) they have enjoyed both a hostile and a competitive relationship. In some cultures only one of these relationships existed; in others more than one appeared at different levels of society, with one being dominant. When it is not hostile to secular medicine, religion influences, or attempts to influence, secular medical practice, while individual secular physicians or groups of physicians may be committed to religious beliefs that in varying degrees influence their understanding of disease, method of treatment, and ethics. At the same time, religion fulfills a strictly spiritual or pastoral role that complements the efforts of medical personnel. Further, it is sometimes appropriate to speak of a religious medicine (distinct from secular medicine and religion proper) which exists when the religion, or a cultic variation of it, offers an alternative medical or healing opportunity.

Perhaps in every society another factor has related in various ways to both religion and medicine: magic. Magic may be defined as any attempt to manipulate and control nature and destiny by practices and substances thought to possess inherent supernatural power. By contrast, religion may be defined at its most primitive level as any attempt to win the favor or avert the disfavor of superior powers or beings, thus enabling man to coexist with these superior entities. In some cultures magic is so intertwined with religion that we speak of magico-religious practices—including magico-religious medicine. While it is possible for religion and medicine to coexist, magic by its very nature impinges upon human concerns which properly belong to medicine, thus conflicting with any medical system not magico-religious. It is significant that magic has retained its basic characteristics over the centuries while both religious and medical systems have changed a great deal.

As we study the intertwining of religion, magic, and medicine from primitive times through the end of classical antiquity, basic questions emerge. What causes illness? Why did I become ill? If religion (or magic) provides an answer to these questions, what effect will the answer have on the sufferer's actions? Where will the sufferer go for help? What do the different people whose help the sufferer may seek think of illness and of the ill? When such people or professions are secular, how do they view their role in relation to religion? Likewise, how does the religious system view disease, the ill person, and any secular involvement in attempts to restore the sick to health? How does the religion view illness? Is sickness seen only as an evil? Or is suffering seen as something that can educate or ennoble?

PRELITERATE PEOPLES

The ethnological and anthropological investigation of contemporary primitive peoples has yielded rich understandings of ancient preliterate cultures. While ancient and contemporary characteristics may not be identical, certain features are shared by such a diverse variety of contemporary primitive peoples that they may be attributed without undue caution to ancient preliterate peoples as well. One of these features is the essentially magico-religious understandings and treatment of most diseases. As a general rule, primitive peoples do not distinguish among religion, magic, medicine. The first two often are one and the same, and medicine is subsumed under them.

In a primitive culture, when a person became ill, the nature or cause of the illness had to be determined. A wide variety of diagnostic techniques, usually involving divination, the interpretation of dreams or omens, and oracles, were practiced. The diagnosis disclosed both the cause *and* the disease, since in primitive societies the cause was the disease. The diagnosis thus revealed what or who caused the affliction. The explanation was that either a demon (or other spiritual force, such as a deity or ghost) had entered the sufferer (often because the latter has broken a taboo) or an individual had maliciously employed magic (perhaps sorcery) against the sufferer. We typically call the person conducting the diagnosis a medicine man or a witch doctor or a shaman.

While the shaman was not always the chief, he was almost invariably the most learned man in the tribe or village. His learning involved both an intimate knowledge of the supernatural and an ability to use such knowledge beneficially. In many ways he was the precursor of modern medical practitioners. But Henry Sigerist sagely observes that "it is an insult to the medicine man to call him the ancestor of the modern physician. He is that, to be sure, but he is much more, namely the ancestor of most of our professions."[1] In his person a variety of functions involving the welfare of the community were combined. And he performed most, if not all, of these functions through magico-religious means. The means brought to bear in the healing of the sick may have included incantations, prayers and sacrifices, dances with music and drums, transfer of disease to animals or plants, and so forth. Such treatment was psychotherapeutic; its high degree of success seems to have depended upon a strong belief by healer, patient, and community in the efficacy of the magical process.

Primitive people did not attribute all disease to possession or magic; rather, they were well aware that there were some common ailments, such as coughs, an upset stomach, or a bee sting, which they or a family member could easily alleviate. Other conditions beyond his or his family's capacity to treat may well have been seen to result from an identifiable cause. For these he may have had recourse to a herbalist (who was sometimes also the medicine man). The usually empirical treatments for such complaints, along with minor surgical procedures (primarily treatment of wounds), and the setting of fractures, may strike us as "natural" and "rational," devoid of any magico-religious elements. But even here magical performance was indispensable, for it alone rendered the surgical procedures effective and activated the powers in the drugs. Among preliterate peoples, then, medicine simply cannot be extricated from the magico-religious fabric of their society.[2]

THE ANCIENT NEAR EAST

Preliterate peoples were essentially prehistorical. The invention of writing made possible the creation of written sources that distinguish some cultures as historical (beginning roughly 3000 B.C.). While preliterate societies and Ancient Near Eastern cultures shared some characteristics respecting the roles of religion, magic, and medicine, they also diverged. Further, cultures of the Ancient Near East (Egypt, Mesopotamia, and Persia) varied among themselves. Egypt and other civilizations that inhabited Mesopotamia have much more in common with one another than with Persia.

Both Egypt and Mesopotamia lived under an absolute, despotic, but sometimes benevolent monarchy. The king, the center of life, irresistibly drew everything to himself, tying together all of life's facets. The monarchy was founded on and justified by a religious system that permeated society. In Egypt and Mesopotamia every aspect of life was molded by religion. All activities, even commercial and economic activities, depended upon the gods. The two spheres, human and divine, were brought together by the monarch, who in Egypt was a god descended among humans but in Mesopotamia was a human being who mediated between the two spheres. Herein lies a major difference between the Egyptian and the Mesopotamian attitudes toward life. Mesopotamian culture was characterized by anxiety, uncertainty, and fear that the divine will might not be comprehended. Thus the harmony of the two spheres was marred by a fear that the cosmic order, and thus the social order, might at any time fall prey to chaos. Egypt, by contrast, was marked by constant serenity and happy resignation to the predestined order, because, with the Pharaoh a god, the divine will was always knowable.

Both Egyptian and Mesopotamian religions were naturalistic and polytheistic, founded on the worship of cosmic forces. The supreme good in life was harmony with the divine, a constant harmony between man and deified nature. People felt secure only when they saw themselves at peace with the transcendent world. As the maintenance of this relationship was their responsibility, they expended much energy in attempting to preserve and, when necessary, restore that harmony between themselves and the divine. The religious world view of such societies was steeped in magic.

Injury and especially illness created disharmony, a dissonance between man and his total environment. Although in the case of injury one might turn to the supernatural in seeking to know why the accident or assault occurred, the immediate cause would be readily evident. Not as certain was the cause of illness. As with primitive peoples generally, so also with the Egyptians and Mesopotamians was disease usually viewed etiologically rather than symptomatically. Spirit intrusion was both the cause and the disease; the intruding spirit was the morbid element residing in the patient. The intruding spirit must be removed, but first it must be identified, and the reason for its intrusion discerned.

In Egypt the supernatural authors of disease were the gods, the dead, or spirits. Spirits were thought to be sent through the malevolent magic of one's enemies; the dead might seek vengeance for various reasons, and the gods might exact punishment for offenses. Spirit intrusion caused by magic or by the dead would be countered by magical means. Punitive illnesses sent by the gods usually could be removed only by the gods who had inflicted them. A god might punish a person for a variety of offenses, many of which were simply cultic or ritual violations having no discernible moral overtones. There is little evidence to suggest that in Egypt the idea of sin as a moral failing was viewed as a cause of disease. Quite different was the case in Mesopotamia, where there appears to have been a much stronger sense of sin as a moral failing that precipitated divine retribution.

As in Egypt, so also in Mesopotamia, spirit intrusion was viewed both as the cause of disease and as the disease itself. Given the distinctives of Mesopotamian religion, we should call these spirits demons. In Sumer before the Akkadian conquest (ca. 2500 B.C.), it was held that demons might attack through sorcery or as agents bringing about the fate of the afflicted or simply at random. A sufferer would seek (indirectly) the assistance of the great gods. He would petition his own personal god, a minor deity seen as particularly interested in the man or his family. The personal gods, of whom there were a multitude, were seen as weaker than the demons. Accordingly they could only intercede with the great gods on behalf of their special devotees.

Some centuries after the Akkadian conquest, two significant changes began to take place. One was that the personal gods came to be viewed as more powerful than the demons and thus able to thwart their designs. The second was that a conviction began to grow that illness was divine retribution for mistakes, failings, and ultimately sins in a sense not seen distinctly in the Egyptian sources. If a demon succeeded in entering a man, it was because his personal god had turned away and permitted it to happen. The anger of one's personal god was thought to have been precipitated by an offense, either ritual/cultic or moral. There was, in Mesopotamia over the centuries, an increasing sensitivity to moral probity, as evidenced, for example, in the "mirror of confession,"[3] which listed a wide variety of sins ranging from disrespect of parents to abuse of the weak. The linking of sickness and sins was exploited in the Code of Hammurabi, where the god Ninkarrak is mentioned as inflicting sickness on those who do not obey the law.

When a man's sin is made responsible for his suffering, it is inevitable that the problem of the apparently unjust suffering of the righteous will arise. Between 2000 and 1700 B.C., a poem entitled "Man and His God" (usually called "the Babylonian Job")[4] was composed in Mesopotamia. It was the first known attempt to deal with the problem of human suffering—similar but greatly inferior to the Book of Job. In this poem a man presents his case to his personal god. He is plagued by sickness and other forms of suffering. He is aware of no wrong on his part. Instead of blaspheming his god, he comes humbly to him with tears, glorifies him, and laments and wails before him, until his personal god is moved to pity and the sufferer's tears are turned to joy. Two lessons are learned: (1) the gods' values cannot be measured by human standards and (2) man's only recourse is to trust and hope. In this piece we have an instance of a man seeking healing directly from God. This method, namely personal prayer, seems to have been the most common religious—and perhaps the only strictly religious—recourse for the ill in Mesopotamia. Reliance upon such petition exclusively may well have been only a last resort for those who already had availed themselves of the skills of those engaged in what we can loosely label medical services. These services were extended by two distinct but complementary professions: the *āšipu* and the *asû*. The *āšipu* was a magician and exorcist as well as a priest. The *asû* was not a priest but was closer to what we would call a physician and surgeon. These two did not in any way stand in opposition to each other, nor do they appear to have been competitive rivals. The *āšipu* was concerned with diagnosis and prognosis; he would attempt to identify the demon, determine the intentions of the god, indicate whether the illness was fatal, and estimate its length. If the prognosis was unfavorable, he would withdraw from the case. He used few if any drugs, but quite reasonably attempted to cure through prayers, libations, and so forth. The incantations usually involved Gula, a goddess of healing, or Damu, a god of healing.

Distinct from the *āšipu* was the *asû*, who was not a priest. Where the *āšipu* was concerned with etiology, the *asû* concentrated on therapy directed toward the relief of acute and pressing symptoms. The *asû* was both a pharmacist and a prescriber of drugs, employing also a wide variety of empirical methods, for example, lotions, suppositories, cataplasms, and enemas. He was basically a craftsman, although his treatment was not entirely devoid of magic in that he would sometimes use incantations as an aid to his treatment. In this there seems to be a borrowing from the *āšipu*, although the inverse appears not to have been true. Whether the Mesopotamian who became ill sought the assistance of the *āšipu* or the *asû* probably depended upon whether the ailment was one for which (what we would call) a natural cause was readily apparent, in which case a person might well consult the *asû* directly. Undoubtedly some went first to the *āšipu* and then to the *asû*, either at the recommendation of the former or as a result of refusal to treat the case. Some texts refer to both the *āšipu* and the *asû* working together on the same patient. The craft of the *asû*, the therapeutic technique, was an independent tradition, although it probably had its roots in the empirical medical practices of earlier primitive stages. In a primitive society, however, these were often performed by the medicine man, whereas in Mesopotamia such procedures were functionally—if not always ideologically—separate from magico-religious procedures.

In Egypt people who became ill had a variety of healers to whom they could go. Their recourse to religion took a different form from that in Mesopotamia, where appeal to one's personal god was probably always appropriate. Afflicted Egyptians who chose to avail themselves of the services of priests could go to those of Thoth, the divine physician of the gods, or Isis, or a wide range of other gods, including the deified Imhotep, who were at least peripherally concerned with healing. If suffering from disease of the eyes, they could receive assistance from the priests of Dovaou, who apparently used palliative or healing medicines, probably combined with magico-religious practice.

These, however, were not the main sources of healing. There was a triumvirate of medical practitioners to whom recourse was most frequently had. These were the *wabw*, the *swnw*, and the *sa.u*. The *wabw* was the priest of Sekhmet, a goddess of healing. The role of the priests of Sekhmet is a matter of dispute. Some scholars maintain that they were surgeons, others that they were originally only mediators between the patients and Sekhmet, who gradually had acquired empirical techniques, particularly the use of drugs, which they combined with their magico-religious practices. The *sa.u* was the sorcerer or exorcist who used primarily charms, incantations, and so forth, addressing the disease directly, which was held to be the agent as well. Sometimes, however, the *sa.u* would employ drugs as part of the treatment.

The Historical Setting

The third, the *swnw*, was the physician in roughly the same sense as the *asû* in Mesopotamia. The *swnws* were united by their common worship of their patron deity Thoth, although they were not priests. As with the *asû*, the practices of the *swnw* included the use of incantations or prayers employed to intensify the healing power of the remedy applied. The roots of their empirical therapy are probably the same as those of the *asû*.

We know much more about the medico-surgical techniques practiced in Egypt than those of Mesopotamia because of the preservation of several medical papyri, most notably *The Edwin Smith Surgical Papyrus*.[5] In this papyrus, there is an interesting case in which the surgeon is advised not to be diverted by the mystery of the symptoms. Without reference to the supernatural cause, he is to attempt to deal with the symptoms themselves and conquer the ailment. This, however, should not be considered a rejection of the validity of magico-religious practices. At times two or even all three of these professions (that is, of the *wabw*, the *swnw*, and the *sa.u*) would be combined in one person. There was no rivalry among the three roles. In Egypt and Mesopotamia, magical, religious, and what we would call rational medicine existed side by side, overlapped, sometimes blended, yet were different although complementary systems, all compatible with one another and with a cultural ethos into whose very fabric a magico-religious consciousness was woven.[6]

A new empire arose with the Persian conquest of nearly the entire Near East in the second half of the sixth century B.C. During the reign of Darius (521–486 B.C.), Zoroastrianism was adopted as the Persian national religion and some significant changes occurred in the perception of the relationship of health, disease, and healing with religion. Although there is dispute over some aspects of its development, Zoroastrianism was fundamentally a dualistic system. Ahuramazda was the spirit of light, the creator of good; Ahriman was the spirit of darkness, the creator of evil. Aligned under them were a variety of benevolent spirits or malevolent demons. In such a system many previously (or potentially) confusing or ambiguous relationships became easily defined. Suffering and disease are evils; they are caused by Ahriman. Joy, health, and healing are good; they come from Ahuramazda. The various means and professions addressed to the restoration of health accordingly are auxiliaries of Ahuramazda, fighting against the forces of Ahriman. The ill, who are victims of Ahriman, are polluted and in need of purification; and the act of healing is itself a form of purification. Indeed, it is safe to say that healing occupied an important and central position in Zoroastrianism, because in the battle between the forces of good and evil all healing arts were essentially purificatory. Thus all healers were priests. There were three classes of healers, in the following order of status: (1) priests who healed by the holy word, practicing magico-religious medicine by incantations and the like; (2) priests who healed by pharmacological means; and (3) priests who engaged in surgery.

Given the distinctive character of Zoroastrian dualism, medicine had a religious mission in Persia[7] which was qualitatively different from the role of medicine in Egypt and Mesopotamia. All three were distinct from the unique ethos of Israel.

PRE-CHRISTIAN JUDAISM

Ancient Near Eastern cultures, other than that of Zoroastrian Persia, saw the earth, the sky, indeed the entire cosmos, as divinities. Israel was a notable exception, holding a very different view: There is only one God, the Creator of all things. He is not part of nature, but is above and outside it and is a distinct and totally independent being. All creation, including man, draws its existence and destiny from God. Pre-Christian Judaism has more in common with Zoroastrianism than with the other religious systems of the Ancient Near East, but the differences are far greater than the similarities. While Zoroastrianism is basically dualistic, with man playing a significant role in the battle between good and evil, in Judaism, as reflected in the Old Testament, the cosmos is under a single direction. Although there is a force of evil, it is so far subordinate to God as to pose no significant challenge to God's authority. In addition, both justice and compassion are essential to God's character and are manifested especially in his relationship with his covenant people.

A close relationship between sin and illness was believed to exist at two levels: (1) because of Adam's sin all physical evils (including illness) entered the world; and (2) illness is visited upon people because of their sins. According to the Old Testament, the world was without flaw before the Fall, but with Adam's disobedience sin was introduced into the world, ushering in physical suffering, pain, and finally death (Gen. 3:16–19). That after the Fall physical, though not moral, evil proceeds from God as the omnipotent ruler of the universe is repeatedly expressed in the Old Testament. Thus disease and injury are a consequence of sin, but they are also clearly within the realm of God's control. In Deut. 32:39, God says: "I kill and I make alive; I wound and I heal." Disease, as a manifestation of his wrath against sin, could be seen on both an individual level and a national level. In the former category many examples can be cited. Miriam was smitten with leprosy for questioning Moses' special relationship with God (Num. 12:1–16). Judah's firstborn was evil, so God took his life (Gen. 38:7). The child Bathsheba bore to David was sick and died on his seventh day because of David's sins of murder and adultery (2 Sam. 12:15–18). When Elisha's servant Gehazi accepted a reward from Naaman, Gehazi and his descendants were smitten with leprosy (2 Kings 5:25–27). Jehoram, king of Judah, was struck with an incurable disease of the bowels for leading his people into idolatry (2 Chron. 21:11–18). God inflicted leprosy on Uzziah, king of Judah, for entering the temple to burn incense (2 Chron. 26:16–21). On a wider scale, when David sinned by holding a census contrary to God's will, he was given the choice between seven years of famine, fleeing for three months before his enemies, or three days' pestilence upon his land. He chose the latter, and the "angel of the Lord" stretched out his hand and slew with plague seventy thousand Israelites (2 Sam. 24:10–25). When the Philistines captured the ark of the covenant, God smote them with what appears to have been hemorrhoids until the ark was returned (1 Sam. 5:6–12). This punishment of the Philistines is an example of the promise of God to lay diseases on those who hate the children of Israel (Deut. 7:15).

Much more important than isolated examples of God's inflicting disease is the promise of health and prosperity for the covenant people if they are faithful to him, and of disease and other suffering if they spurn his love. This promise runs through the Old Testament. "If you will diligently hearken to the voice of the Lord your God, and do that which is right in his eyes, and give heed to his commandments and keep all his statutes, I will put none of the diseases upon you which I put upon the Egyptians; for I am the Lord, your healer" (Exod. 15:26). This positive assurance is amplified by its negative correlate elsewhere when God promises to inflict upon them, if they are unfaithful, "sudden terror, consumption, and fever that waste the eyes and cause life to pine away" (Lev. 26:16), pestilence, inflammation, the boils of Egypt, ulcers, scurvy, an incurable itch, "extraordinary afflictions, afflictions severe and lasting, and sicknesses grievous and lasting . . . all the diseases of Egypt . . . every sickness also, and every affliction which is not recorded in the book of this law" (Deut. 28:21, 22, 27, 28, 59–61). To Jeremiah, God says that "sword, famine, and pestilence" he will send upon the unfaithful remnant (24:10) and, to Ezekiel, that Jerusalem will bear "four sore acts of judgment, sword, famine, evil beasts, and pestilence" (14:21). Habakkuk says of God that "before him went pestilence, and plague followed close behind" (3:5). Hosea cries out to his people, "Come, let us return to the Lord; for he has torn, that he may heal us; he has stricken, and he will bind us up" (6:1). The Psalmist brings the promise down to an individual level. "He who dwells in the shelter of the Most High, who abides in the shadow of the Almighty, will say to the Lord, 'My refuge and my fortress. . . .' For he will deliver you . . . from the deadly pestilence. . . . You will not fear the terror of the night . . . nor the pestilence that stalks in darkness. . . . No evil shall befall you, no scourge come near your tent" (Ps. 91:1–10). Passages often considered as messianic offer the hope of healing, physical as well as spiritual (e.g., Isa. 53:4–5; 61:1–2; Mal. 4:2). When the Messiah has come, no one in Jerusalem will say, " 'I am sick'; the people who dwell there will be forgiven their iniquity" (Isa. 33:24).

The mental and physical anguish that sometimes accompanies contrition for sin is spoken of repeatedly in the Psalms, for example, Psalm 38: "There is no soundness in my flesh because of thy indignation; there is no health in my bones because of my sin. . . . My wounds grow foul and fester because of my foolishness. . . . I am utterly spent and crushed; I groan because of the tumult of my heart. . . . Do not forsake me, O Lord! O my God, be not far from me! Make haste to help me, O Lord, my salvation!" (vv. 3, 5, 8, 21–22). The acknowledgment of and repentance of sin is essential for such healing, as in Psalm 32: "When I declared not my sin, my body wasted away through my groaning all day long. For day and night thy hand was heavy upon me; my strength was dried up. . . . I acknowledged my sin to thee, and I did not hide my iniquity; I said, 'I will confess my transgressions to the Lord'; then thou didst forgive the guilt of my sin" (vv. 3–5). This forgiveness and consequent healing is not the result of appeasing a hostile deity through ritual and offerings, as is graphically demonstrated in Psalm 51, especially in verses 16 and 17: "For thou hast no delight in sacrifice; were I to give a burnt offering, thou wouldst not be pleased. The sacrifice acceptable to God is a broken spirit; a broken and contrite heart, O God, thou wilt not despise."

Suffering in general and sickness in particular were seen not simply as punishment but rather as chastisement that was not vindictive but corrective. This view, however, did not make them easier to endure for people who searched their hearts and could find no specific sin to be confessed. The sons of Korah in Psalm 88 presented a litany of their sufferings, for which they saw no explanation: "O Lord, why dost thou cast me off? Why dost thou hide thy face from me? Afflicted and close to death from my youth up, I suffer thy terrors; I am helpless. Thy wrath has swept over me; thy dread assaults destroy me" (vv. 14–16). But the classic case is that of Job. Small comfort was provided by his friends, one of whom said, "Behold, happy is the man whom God reproves; therefore despise not the chastening of the Almighty. For he wounds, but he binds up; he smites, but his hands heal" (Job 5:17–18). Such an appraisal, although completely in accord with Old Testament thought, becomes for Job merely a heartless cliché that rubbed salt into the wounds of a man who was sorely tried but in the end was vindicated by God, who asks Job who he is to question God's ways. Thus the righteous sufferer must resort to mystery and acknowledge God's inscrutable ways and ultimate goodness. It is God's goodness and mercy, especially in the afflicting of the chosen people, that is clearly displayed throughout the Old Testament: "Blessed is the man whom thou dost chasten, O Lord," says the Psalmist (94:12). This sentiment is echoed in the Book of Proverbs: "My son, do not despise the Lord's discipline or be weary of his reproof, for the Lord reproves him whom he loves, as a father the son in whom he delights" (3:11–12). The condition of contrition, submission, and dependence upon God into which the responsive sufferer is brought by personal affliction is seen as a greater good than the indifference wrought by sustained prosperity and uninterrupted health. Consider the case of the irascible trickster Jacob, whose miraculously inflicted injury was not healed but rather was used to make him depend upon God and achieve a spiritual maturity commensurate with his new name, Israel (Gen. 32:24–32).

Although space does not permit a detailed analysis of the relationship of illness and sin, suffering and spiritual growth, what has thus far been said should be sufficient to demonstrate that illness in the Old Testament is viewed in its moral and spiritual dimensions rather than in its physical nature. Since the most important issue was a person's relationship with God, and prayer was the chief means of healing, the spiritual climate was not only inimical to the use of magic but utterly repudiated its authority and employment. Diverse forms of magic were prohibited in the Mosaic code. Those practicing divination (soothsayers, augurs, sorcerers, charmers, mediums, wizards, and necromancers), if discovered, were to be put to death (Exod. 22:18; Deut. 18:10). The use of magic was not completely eradicated, however, and it appears to have increased during times of apostasy. King Manasseh practiced soothsaying and augury and dealt with mediums and wizards (2 Kings 21:6), but the prophets called down God's judgment on those who were engaged in various types of magic, including sorcery, enchantments, witchcraft, divination, and soothsaying (e.g., Isa. 3:2–3; 47:9, 12; Jer. 27:9; Ezek. 13:17–23; Mic. 5:12). Isa. 28:15 implied that some apostates were involved in a magical pact that was thought to render them immune to death. However, some apparently superstitious folk-practices are mentioned, such as the use of mandrake to remove sexual barrenness (Gen. 30:14–16) and the belief that an aged man could prolong his life by drawing heat from a maiden's body (1 Kings 1:1–4).

Given the essentially religious character of the understanding of disease and suffering evident in the Old Testament, one would not be surprised to find a sacerdotal medical practice among the Jews like that which prevailed elsewhere in the Ancient Near East, although devoid of pagan magical elements. But this is simply not the case. There appears to be no evidence for priests functioning as physicians or surgeons, much less as diviners or exorcists. The only involvement of priests in matters pertaining to health was in an area in which Israel was unique in the Ancient Near East, and that is in the enforcement of a relatively sophisticated code of personal and social hygiene. In this capacity, priests were involved in various procedures for purifying those contaminated by childbirth, leprosy, seminal discharge, menstruation, and contact with a cadaver (Leviticus 12, 13, 15, and 21). Quite exceptional was the "jealousy ordeal" detailed in Num. 5:11–31, which has an affinity with a variety of magico-religious practices of some preliterate pagans. The closest that the priests of the Old Testament came to occupying the role of physician occurred when faced with the disease called leprosy.

More involved than priests in medical concerns were prophets whose role sometimes included prognostication or healing, and sometimes restoring the dead to life. In all but one recorded instance of healing by a prophet, some "natural," if not necessarily empirical, supplementary means were employed. That such procedures were not expected, at least by foreigners, was demonstrated by the story of Naaman. When the leprous Naaman, commander of the Syrian army, came to Elisha to be healed and was told by a messenger simply to dip himself in the Jordan River seven times, he indignantly replied, "I thought that he would surely come out to me, and stand, and call on the name of the Lord his God, and wave his hand over the place, and cure the leper." When Naaman did what Elisha had commanded, however, he was healed (2 Kings 5:1–14). Both Elisha and his predecessor Elijah were credited with raising a child from the dead; in both instances the prophet, after beseeching God to restore the boy to life, stretched himself out upon the body (1 Kings 17:17–24; 2 Kings 4:18–37). In the second instance it is specified that Elisha warmed the child's body by putting his mouth, eyes, and hands upon the other's respective members. When Hezekiah, king of Judah, became dangerously ill, the prophet Isaiah came to him and informed him, "Thus says the Lord: Set your house in order; for you shall die, you shall not recover." When Hezekiah wept bitterly and prayed to God for recovery, Isaiah returned and told Hezekiah that God would add fifteen years to his life. Isaiah then instructed some unspecified attendants to take a cake (i.e., a poultice) of figs and apply it to the boil (probably a carbuncle) "that he may recover" (Isaiah 38 and 2 Kings 20). The only instance of prophetic healing without some "natural" means is recorded in 1 Kings 13:1–6. When Jeroboam, an idolatrous king of Israel, ordered an unidentified "man of God" (i.e., a prophet) to be seized, his extended arm was paralyzed. Upon a requested entreaty to God by the prophet, Jeroboam's arm was restored.

It should be noted that when Isaiah came to the ill Hezekiah his purpose was not to heal but to give an unfavorable prognostication. Other instances of prophets' prognosticating are found in the Old Testament. Ahijah, a blind prophet, was consulted about the fate of the ill son of King Jeroboam (1 Kings 14:1–17), and Elisha, upon arriving in Damascus, was questioned by an envoy of the Syrian king about the outcome of the latter's illness (2 Kings 8:7–15). That prophets were frequently consulted for prognosis, at least by kings of Israel and Judah, is also suggested by an incident recorded in 2 Kings 1. Ahaziah, king of Israel, had fallen and seriously injured himself. He sent messengers to inquire of Baal-zebub, the god of Ekron, whether he would recover. "But the angel of the Lord said to Elijah . . . 'Arise, go up to meet the messengers of the king, . . . and say to them, "Is it because there is no God in Israel that you are going to inquire of Baal-zebub, the god of Ekron?" Now therefore thus says the Lord, "You shall not come down from the bed to which you have gone, but you shall surely die." ' " (2 Kings 1:2–4).

The condemnation of King Ahaziah for consulting Baal-zebub, god of Ekron, concerning his illness is predicated upon the same principles as those governing the judgment upon Asa, king of Judah. Asa was seriously ill with a disease of the feet (probably gangrene), "yet even in his disease he did not seek the Lord, but sought help from physicians. And Asa slept with his fathers . . ." (2 Chron. 16:12–13). Many biblical scholars take this as a condemnation of resorting to secular medicine as such, but a more likely explanation is that the physicians whom Asa consulted were foreign physicians whose procedures, even if empirical, would have been magico-religious in nature. Would there have been physicians in Judah whom he could have consulted, whose practices would have been consonant with Jewish religious principles? This question cannot be answered with certainty since there is no evidence for the existence of a distinct medical profession among the Jews during the Old Testament period. The Hebrew word for physician is the participle of the verb *rapha*, the original meaning of which appears to be "one who sews together" or "one who repairs." Its first participial occurrence is in Gen. 50:2, where Egyptian physicians are said to have embalmed Jacob. The use of the participle is sometimes metaphorical, as in Job 13:4, where Job refers to his friends as "worthless physicians." The verb itself is often used literally in the sense of healing from disease or injury, as in several of the passages cited above (e.g., Gen. 20:17; Num. 12:13; 2 Kings 20:5–8), but also in a much broader sense, as in Deut. 32:39, Job 5:18, and 2 Chron. 30:20. When Jeremiah writes, "Is there no balm in Gilead? Is there no physician there?" (8:22), although he is speaking metaphorically, he assumes the existence of both balm, as a therapeutic substance, and those who would apply it, namely physicians, literally, ones who repair or heal. When Joram, king of Israel, was wounded in battle, he returned home "to be healed" (2 Kings 8:29; 9:15; 2 Chron. 22:6). It is reasonable to assume that healing in this instance involves not merely convalescence but some kind of active treatment as well. Indeed, it is inconceivable that at any time the Israelites had no knowledge at all of the rudimentary treatment of wounds and uses of herbs for various ailments in which natural causality is evident. In the Book of Exodus we find the stipulation that if a person injures another in a quarrel, if the injured party survives, the one who inflicted the injury is held financially liable "for the loss of his time, and shall have him thoroughly healed" (21:18–19). The last clause indicates that the expense of medicines, and perhaps of the one dispensing or applying them, was to be borne by the guilty party. Several incidental references imply the existence of binders of wounds (Isa. 3:7), knowledge of the setting of fractures (Ezek. 30:21), and the use of various therapeutic substances (Isa. 1:6 and Jer. 51:8).

Even though in the Old Testament, God is represented as the only healer and God's people are to refrain from resorting to magical or pagan healing practices, the use of natural or medicinal means is not only not precluded but even employed in ostensibly miraculous healings. Medical knowledge was probably limited to folk remedies, however, and there were very likely no systematized therapeutics, much less a distinct medical profession similar to that of the magico-religious-empirical practitioners that existed elsewhere in the Ancient Near East. Not until the intertestamental period do we have evidence for a Jewish medical profession.

By the second century B.C. the Jews, both in Palestine and abroad, had been exposed to Greek "scientific" or "rational" medicine that had nothing in its theory or practice inherently antithetical to Jewish religious scruples, and Jewish medical practitioners were apparently not uncommon. While space does not permit us to trace these developments, we shall look at one significant piece of literature from this period. A particularly valuable source of information for many aspects of Judaism of the second century B.C. is the apocryphal book known as the Wisdom of Jesus ben Sira, also called Ecclesiasticus, written in Hebrew in Jerusalem early in the second century B.C. and translated into Greek by the author's grandson several decades later in Alexandria. This work is concerned in great part with human conduct and ethics as they should be regulated by religious principles.

Although the vast majority of people at all times and in all places have highly valued good health, the Old Testament has little if anything to say directly on the subject. But in ben Sira there are such statements as the following, strikingly Hellenic in tone: "Better off is a poor man who is well and strong in constitution than a rich man who is severely afflicted in body. Health and soundness are better than all gold, and a robust body than countless riches. There is no wealth better than health of body . . ." (30:14–16). Since he recognizes health as so highly desirable, it is not surprising that ben Sira urges, "Before you fall ill, take care of your health" (18:19). How he recommends that people take care of their health falls into two categories. Since it is God who "grants healing, life, and blessing" (34:17), ben Sira advises, "Before falling ill, humble yourself, and when you are on the point of sinning, turn back" (18:21). Such an outlook is consonant with the perspective of the Old Testament. But ben Sira adds a second group of injunctions: "Jealousy and anger shorten life, and anxiety brings on old age too soon" (30:24); and "In all your work be industrious, and no sickness will overtake you" (31:22). In addition to these and other sound maxims, he goes on to warn that "over-eating brings sickness, and gluttony leads to nausea. Many have died of gluttony, but he who is careful to avoid it prolongs his life" (37:30–31). There follows in chapter 38 a discussion of the role of physicians, beginning with the command to "honor the physician with the honor due him, according to your need of him, for the Lord created him" (38:1). For the next fourteen verses, ben Sira's argument runs along these lines: Healing comes from God, and the physician's lot is admirable and dignified. Since God created medicines from the earth, "a sensible man will not despise them." God gave people the skill to compound medicines, and through this God is glorified (38:2–8). There is now a change in ben Sira's emphasis: "My son, when you are sick do not be negligent, but pray to the Lord, and he will heal you. Give up your faults and direct your hands aright, and cleanse your heart from all sin. Offer a sweet-smelling sacrifice. . . ." However, "give the physician his place, for the Lord created him. . . . There is a time when success lies in the hands of physicians, for they too will pray to the Lord that he should grant them success in diagnosis and in healing, for the sake of preserving life" (38:9–14).

There is nothing suggested by ben Sira that is in any way discordant with the attitudes enunciated in the Old Testament. But ben Sira enlarges upon earlier principles and attempts to resolve the tension that might be thought to exist between a reliance upon God and the use of natural means that were primarily acquired from pagan sources. His advice on prophylaxis is also noteworthy. In preliterate societies and in the Ancient Near East (including Israel), health was thought to be preserved by punctilious attention to divine commands, as nearly all disease was seen in terms of divine causality. While a limited cause-and-effect relationship along "natural" lines in certain conditions was undoubtedly recognized, it remained for the development of a "rational" medical theory to introduce into lay consciousness a broader recognition of "natural" causality, leading to "rational" prophylaxis and treatment. In ben Sira there may be seen some evidence of the possible influence of a "rational" medical system that had emerged in Greece during the fifth century B.C.[8]

GREECE

The kaleidoscopic nature of Greek religion precludes a summary description. It possessed no creed or dogma and hence had no concept of heresy; it had no sacred scriptures and no religious figures that obtained universal authority. Much religious activity was of a local nature, rooted in the Greek polis or city-state and enjoying little influence beyond a city's boundaries. There were deities that gained widespread worship, and religious institutions (such as the Delphic oracle) that enjoyed influence over a wide geographical area. But without theologians to systematize belief, there was much disparity, not merely of time and place but even within the same community. Greek religion can perhaps best be described, in Gilbert Murray's phrase, as an "inherited conglomerate," a centuries-long accumulation of religious beliefs, myths, rituals, and practices that contained many layers and inconsistencies. As polytheists, the Greeks were not exclusive in their attitudes to foreign gods. They not only respected the deities of other peoples with whom they came into contact (and often identified with their own gods), but even adopted them into the Greek pantheon.

The Greeks of Homer's time, like the peoples of the Ancient Near East, believed that the gods played an active role in all aspects of life, including sickness and health. Like the cultures of the Near East, they too looked for supernatural causation in disease. Death or disease might result from arrows sent by Apollo (*Iliad* 1.9–52) or be caused by a *daimon* or other divine power (*Odyssey* 5.394–97). Whatever disease results from supernatural intervention in human affairs, it is viewed as divine displeasure for having violated a taboo or offended or provoked a god by insulting his honor in a way that is sometimes discoverable and sometimes not. Diseases sent by the gods can be neither avoided nor healed unless the anger of the gods can be appeased by sacrifice or purification. Disease was regarded as a shameful condition that required the affected person to be isolated.

Beginning with Hesiod, who like Homer probably lived in the eighth century B.C., we find another attitude to disease that is quite different from Homer's. In Homer, disease, thought to be sent by a god, comes from outside the individual, but it is not the result of possession either by a god or by a demon. After Homer, however, we see the development of ideas of possession and the need for ritual purification. These ideas are found in the worship of Apollo and the Olympian gods and in the cult of Dionysus. In the former, the Delphic oracle taught the necessity of purification for pollution; in the latter, the idea was introduced that a worshiper could be possessed who manifested hysterical behavior such as outbursts of ecstatic dancing, sexual license, and engaging in a sacrificial rite called the *omophagia*, which consisted of tearing an animal to pieces and devouring it raw. Divine possession could manifest itself in less sensational ways, such as prophetic or poetic inspiration. It was natural that the concept of possession be extended to disease.

According to Hesiod in *Work and Days*, in early times evil or toil or diseases did not exist (90–92). Evil and disease came into the world as *daimones* who escaped from Pandora's box as punishment of the human race for Prometheus's seizure of fire. "But the rest, countless plagues, wander amongst men; for earth is full of evils and the sea is full. Of themselves diseases come upon men continually by day and by night, bringing mischief to mortals silently; for wise Zeus took away speech from them" (*Works and Days* 100–104).[9] *Daimones* is a term that is difficult to define. The word can refer to any divine agency, but it is often vague and imprecise in its meaning. Some *daimones* were kindly, others were harmful, like those to whom disease was attributed.

> The ancient Greek saw divine causation everywhere. Some events he ascribed to specific named deities, Olympian or other; but in the case of many events the answer to the question "why has this happened to me?" was "A *daimon* has sent this." Popular belief might assign particular functions to some *daimones*—each human being might have his own—but an infinity of these unseen powers remained for causing good or harm in general. . . . The word well illustrates the tangle of supernatural causation within which the ancient Greek passed his life.[10]

Disease was also thought to be caused by *keres* and *alastores*. *Keres*, like *daimones*, were malignant invisible powers that caused illness, misery, and death. They were neither personifications nor abstractions, but concrete though vaguely defined supernatural powers. The *alastores* were also evil spirits that were believed to bring vengeance for homicide.

Since possession by a god or other divine power was believed to cause illness, the early Greeks turned for healing to a group particularly suited to the healing of heaven-sent illness—the *iatromanteis*, or "medicine men," of early Greece. The *iatromantis*, a physician-seer, was a common feature of archaic Greek society (ca. 800–500 B.C.). He wandered from city to city employing magic and religious means to avert disease and pollution. The *iatromantis* used herbs, spells, charms, exorcism, and various methods of purification. The Cretan poet Epimenides was an *iatromantis*, summoned to Athens in the sixth century B.C., when the Athenians were suffering from a plague, to purify the city from pollution that had been incurred by a sacrilege committed when a magistrate killed several men who had sought sanctuary at a temple. The Greeks believed that certain acts could pollute a whole people or city. This view was very much a part of the widespread ancient belief that the gods might bring some kind of punishment upon a whole society for an offense committed by one person. Society was viewed as an aggregate of citizens who were kinsmen in the widest sense and who might therefore share in the misfortune one of its members by experiencing his or her guilt or fate. Hence an entire city or army might be afflicted by plague or other natural disaster as a punishment for the offense of an individual. Pollution could be introduced by a variety of actions, even those that were unintentional and therefore lacked moral guilt; for instance, accidental homicide or exposure to cadavers. A polluted person must be exiled or shunned to avoid contamination, and the pollution incurred could be removed only by purification. Doubtless the ancients' belief in pollution provided an explanation for disaster, an explanation that was based on the observation that even unintentional actions can upset the "moral order" and thus bring about consequences for society as a whole.

Of course a disease might be divinely caused for reasons other than pollution. The Greeks believed that the gods sent disease for a variety of reasons. In Homer it was sent for an insult or offense against a particular god; in post-Homeric belief, as the Greeks sought to relate justice to theology, they expected Zeus to punish injustice. It was a natural inference, one frequently made, that prosperity was a sign of divine favor and that suffering and disaster were indications of the gods' displeasure. Evidence of the gods' displeasure was often seen by writers like Herodotus in divine nemesis that struck people down if they enjoyed too much success, and in a view of the gods as jealous of prosperity that produces hybris, an overweening pride. Yet, as it was apparent that the righteous do not always prosper but often suffer injustice, while the wicked avoided deserved punishment and even flourished, the idea arose that a person could be punished for the deeds of ancestors (for punishment had to be meted out in this life, there being little expectation of reward or punishment in an afterlife).

Side by side with a religious explanation of disease and attempts to avert it by means of an *iatromantis*, there existed from Homeric times a secular approach to medicine that is found in the practice of physicians. Physicians exist in the *Odyssey*, called *demiourgoi*, "men who work for the people." They were itinerant members of a craft like seers, carpenters, and heralds. They were not medicine men, but they treated wounds, relying on skill, observation, and experience. From the sixth century B.C. we hear of physicians in Greece, concentrated particularly in Asia Minor and the Greek colonies in Sicily and south Italy. However, we know next to nothing about physicians between the time of Homer and that of Hippocrates. Presumably knowledge of medicine was transmitted by apprenticeship like any other craft. Near the end of the sixth century B.C., medical schools developed in various places in the Greek world, including Croton, Rhodes, Cyrene, Cnidus, and Cos. These were not schools in the modern sense but groups of physicians and students who served as apprentices under them. It was in the medical center on the island of Cos off the coast of Asia Minor that the famed Hippocrates lived in the fifth century B.C. Although he became known as the "father of medicine" and is the subject of much legend, we know almost nothing about him. There are extant only two contemporary references to him, both in the dialogues of Plato. He probably first became a subject of widespread interest during Hellenistic times, when a number of anonymous medical works came to be attributed to him, works known as the Hippocratic corpus, numbering some sixty or so treatises. None can be attributed to Hippocrates with any certainty. They represent a disparate group of medical writings, most of which were probably composed in the fifth and fourth centuries B.C. They reflect a variety of points of view: Some preserve the teachings of the Coan school, others the views of the Cnidians. Some were written by physicians and are of a clinical nature, while others were composed by lay writers to appeal to a widespread interest in medicine and medical theory among the general public; still others were composed by professional teachers of philosophy or rhetoric and are more theoretical.

It was in the fifth century B.C. that Greek medicine began to take on the form of a science as well as a craft. A science requires the existence of a body of theoretical knowledge. Until the late fifth century B.C. this can hardly be said to have existed in medicine. There were, of course, many empirical techniques that had been collected and transmitted, but these could not be called a body of knowledge. The medical practitioner could undoubtedly identify symptoms and supply details about illnesses; he might be skilled at treatment, which consisted of applying traditional remedies. But there was no attempt to understand disease in general terms, to frame general theories that could be applied to particular cases. It was the addition of the theoretical aspects of medicine and disease that led to the creation of "scientific" medicine in antiquity. Such medicine tried to explain disease in terms of natural causation. This approach went beyond the skill and competence of the ordinary practitioner. Those physicians who attempted a more general understanding of disease and its etiology turned to philosophy, for it was believed that a correct understanding of human nature could be gained from philosophy, which alone could furnish universal formulations.

In the Hippocratic corpus we see the earliest attempts to provide a theoretical basis for the practice of medicine. Most Hippocratic treatises reveal an approach to medicine that is both rational and empirical: rational in its freedom from magic and superstition and in its belief in the natural causes of disease, and empirical in the collection of case histories with careful descriptions of symptoms. Many of the medical theories found in the Hippocratic corpus were taken over from the pre-Socratic philosophers, who attempted to formulate cosmologies that explained the world in terms of natural processes rather than in mythological categories. The theory of the four humors, for example, was borrowed from Empedocles. Traces of the older mentality can still be found in some of the Hippocratic treatises that are not wholly free from "primitive" concepts of disease, but they reveal a wedding of speculative philosophy to medicine which provided the theoretical underpinning that made medicine "scientific" in classical Greece.

The rational approach to medicine is seen in an interesting Hippocratic treatise, *On the Sacred Disease*.[11] Madness was often regarded by the ancients as a punishment of the gods. Thus Herodotus wrote that the madness that afflicted the Persian king Cambyses was explained as the result of his offending the Egyptian god Apis (*Persian Wars* 3.29–30). Epilepsy was similarly thought to be caused by divine possession, a view that is rejected by the writer of *On the Sacred Disease*. He begins the work by stating, "I am about to discuss the disease called 'sacred.' It is not, in my opinion, any more divine or more sacred than other diseases, but it has a natural cause, and its supposed divine origin is due to human inexperience and to their wonder at its peculiar character." His rational outlook is sharply distinguished from the traditional view:

> My own view is that those who first attributed a sacred character to this malady were like the magicians, purifiers, charlatans, and quacks of our own day, people who claim great piety and superior knowledge. Being at a loss, and having no treatment that would help, they concealed and sheltered themselves behind superstition and called this illness sacred, in order that their utter ignorance might not be manifest (chap. 2).

Near the end of the work he says, "There is no need to put the disease in a special class and to consider it more divine than the others; they are all divine and all human. Each has a nature and power of its own; none is hopeless or incapable of treatment" (chap. 21).

The theology underlying the statement that all diseases are both sacred and human does not reflect popular opinion, according to which certain diseases like epilepsy are caused by particular gods or divine forces. It is rather derived from the pre-Socratic philosophers. This view precludes the direct interference of the gods in the natural order but regards every natural event as divine. The physician is freed by this view to seek natural causes of disease. Hence, the writer of *On the Sacred Disease* can explain epilepsy as being due to "the things that come and go from the body, from cold, sun, and from the changing restlessness of winds" (chap. 21). This naturalistic explanation of disease became one of the hallmarks of the Hippocratic physician, but it did not indicate a purely mechanistic understanding of nature.

How did Greek laymen of the classical period react to this "scientific" approach to disease? Did they retain the supernatural etiology of disease? With the growth of rationalism in the latter half of the fifth century B.C. and the widespread influence of the sophistic movement, naturalistic explanations must have displaced the older views for many. A significant lay interest in medical questions developed, and a number of Hippocratic treatises were addressed to a general audience. They must have done much to spread the new naturalistic views of medicine. And of course those who sought help from Hippocratic physicians would have expected them to help by rational treatment.

Was there a "conflict" between religion and the new emphasis of Hippocratic medicine? Since the time of Homer, physicians were a feature of Greek life. Even in the archaic period, when plague and disease were widely thought to be the result of divine punishment or

The Historical Setting

daimones, medical treatment was recognized as a legitimate approach to illness, the treatment of wounds, and the setting of fractures and dislocations. There is no reason to assume that in the fifth century B.C., when rational medicine came to predominate, secular medicine was viewed with suspicion. Since Hippocratic writers did not deny the divinity of nature, they did not offend popular belief. When they described disease as the result of natural processes, they were not excluding recognition of divinity, for nature itself was regarded as divine. Their theology was rational but not atheistic. Medicine was recognized as a divine art that had been given to humanity by a god. It was trusted and looked to for aid. "I have discovered regimen, with the god's help, as far as it is possible for mere man to discover it," concludes the author of *Regimen* (chap. 93). The Hippocratic attitude toward religion is not hostile. "In fact, it is especially knowledge of the gods that by medicine is woven into the stuff of the mind," according to the author of *Decorum*. "Physicians have given place to the gods, for in medicine that which is powerful is not in excess. In fact, though physicians take many things in hand, many diseases are also overcome for them spontaneously. . . . The gods are the real physicians, though people do not think so" (chap. 6). Prayer is not rejected. In *Regimen* we read, "Prayer indeed is good, but while calling on the gods a man should himself lend a hand" (chap. 87). However, there is little advice in the Hippocratic corpus for the physician or patient to resort to prayer alone for the healing of disease. The reason is not hostility to religion, but rather the belief that prayer should be used to thank the gods rather than to ask them for favors.

Side by side with the development of rational Hippocratic medicine in Greece in the fifth century B.C., there existed a tradition of religious medicine in which patients sought healing directly from a god rather than from a physician. Those who sought divine help for healing could appeal to a wide variety of gods, demigods, and heroes. Originally there were no special gods of healing; any deity could be invoked by the sick. Many local cults of healing grew up around holy places that were regarded as the burial place of heroes, mighty dead people, real or imaginary, who were thought to give aid in time of need and who might be appealed to for healing. One such hero, Asclepius, came to be the chief healing god of Greco-Roman antiquity. Asclepius is mentioned in the *Iliad* as a mortal, the "blameless physician," who was taught medicine by Chiron. Hesiod and Pindar speak of him as the son of Apollo and Coronis, who became famous as a physician and even restored the dead to life, for which he was slain by a thunderbolt of Zeus. Later legend made him a god. His cult seems to have originated at Tricca in Thessaly, but it spread to Epidaurus, perhaps in the sixth century B.C., and it was here that it first attained real prominence. From Epidaurus the cult spread throughout the Greek world, to Athens in 420 B.C., to Pergamum in Asia Minor, and to Cos in the fourth century B.C., to Crete, to Cyrene in North Africa, and in 291 B.C. to Rome, where the god was worshiped under the Latin name Aesculapius. Asclepius gradually came to attract to himself the healing functions of many of the other Greek gods and heroes. Perhaps he owed his success as the healing god par excellence to his association with Apollo and the support of the Delphic oracle, or to the zeal of his priests at Epidaurus in promoting his cult. It is noteworthy that the rapid spread of the cult of Asclepius began in the fourth century B.C., when there was a marked decline in the traditional civic religions and a growth of cults that offered the personal spiritual comfort which had been lacking in the state cults. The worship of Asclepius appealed to the rising individualism in Greece and evoked a personal devotion to the god that was not often found in the formal civic religions.

There existed in Greece from early times a group of physicians called Asclepiads, who claimed descent from Asclepius; they were found at Cos and Cnidus, among other places. Since one of the chief sanctuaries of Asclepius was on the island of Cos, the birthplace of Hippocrates, it used to be believed that Hippocratic medicine grew out of the healing associated with the temple of Asclepius on Cos and that the Asclepiads were priest-physicians. There was a tradition in antiquity that Hippocrates came to realize the importance of gathering clinical cases and employing dietetics from accounts of cures that were posted in the temple at Cos.[12] The origin of rational medicine in Greece was thought to be found in religious medicine that was practiced by the priests of Asclepius. This theory has been shown to be untenable by the archaeological excavations at Cos, which revealed that the sanctuary of Asclepius was not founded until the fourth century B.C., that is, after the age of the development of Hippocratic medicine, and therefore cannot have been the cradle of Greek rational medicine. Emma and Ludwig Edelstein, in their definitive study of Asclepius,[13] have suggested that Asclepius began as a culture-hero, and became the patron of physicians who practiced their art as wandering craftsmen. The term Asclepiads, "sons of Asclepius," came to be adopted by those who practiced medicine and considered themselves descendants of the hero, who gave them the protection that they needed as itinerant physicians and was a god to worship who was not tied to a particular place. The Asclepiads were never priest-physicians. Eventually Asclepius's reputation was spread by physicians until he became the chief healing god and came to eclipse others. He was deified perhaps at the end of the sixth century B.C. In the fifth century his cult began to spread from Epidaurus to the rest of Greece, and in the fourth century it was brought to Cos, where the Coan physicians adopted him as their patron. Once sanctuaries of Asclepius were established in Cos and elsewhere, Hippocratic medicine and temple-healing flourished side by side. The cult spread all over the Mediterranean world until there were over four hundred temples and shrines dedicated to Asclepius, either alone or with other gods.

As the chief healing god of Greece, Asclepius was sought out by the sick who came to his temples seeking miraculous healing, often for diseases that physicians could not cure. When sick people arrived they first had to undergo a rite of purification, for spiritual purity was required of those who wished to approach the god. Over the entrance to the temple at Epidaurus were these words: "Pure must be he who enters the fragrant temple; purity means to think nothing but holy thoughts." Sacrifices were offered (usually cakes and fruits) and the worshiper could read case histories written on marble tablets in the sanctuary telling of instances of miraculous healing. Excavation has brought to light three of these tablets at Epidaurus that date from the fourth century B.C. They relate some seventy case histories of supposedly miraculous cures. The tablets were doubtless intended to encourage the faithful to trust the god for healing. The actual process of healing involved incubation—the practice of having patients spend the night in the *abaton*, the holiest part of the temple, where they were to lie on a couch and wait for a dream or vision of the god, in which Asclepius would appear to heal or advise them. The god often appeared holding a staff with a snake coiled around it, which became associated with him. Sometimes he merely touched patients, sometimes he operated on them or administered medicine, and sometimes a sacred serpent or dog would lick the wounds. When patients awoke the next morning they might find themselves cured. Many cures took place; of this there can be no doubt. Those who were healed left votive offerings, which have been found in considerable numbers at the sanctuaries of Asclepius and testify to actual cures. The most interesting of these are models of terra cotta of eyes, ears, limbs, and other organs that had been healed.

Pre-Christian Antiquity

What kinds of disease were cured by Asclepius? Henry Sigerist suggests that most will probably have been either those suffering from chronic diseases or displaying the symptoms of hysteria.[14] The latter are known to respond well to faith healing, but the cure is usually not permanent. In this regard the "miraculous" healings furnish evidence of ancient psychotherapy. Women who were childless sometimes sought help. Several cases recorded on the marble tablets are clearly fictional, like that of the woman who gave birth to a child she had carried for five years or the woman who received a new eye in her vacant eye-socket. The incubants sometimes dreamed of operations or the administration of medicine by Asclepius, who seemed to heal as a physician might be expected to, that is, by surgical or other medical means.

Eventually around the temple of Asclepius at Epidaurus and elsewhere there grew up a complex of buildings constructed to adorn the sanctuary and entertain visitors, for example, theaters, stadiums, gymnasiums, sanatoriums, baths. There were guest houses for patients who required a long stay. The athletic facilities were used for the celebration of the festival of Asclepius. By Roman times the nature of the cures performed in the sanctuaries of Asclepius changed. They ceased to be immediate and miraculous; instead the incubants were told in dreams what kind of regimen or prescription was recommended by the god for the recovery of their health. The god recommended exercise, fasting, riding, swimming, gymnastics, ointments, and the use of purgatives, as well as more exceptional treatments. Hence temple cures became much more a matter of rational therapeutics and less a matter of miraculous healing.

One might expect to find an antagonism between secular and religious medicine as represented on the one hand by physicians and on the other by the numerous sanctuaries of Asclepius. Yet such antagonism seems to have been lacking. Asclepius was the patron of both physicians and patients. He presided over the practice of secular medicine. Those who took the so-called Hippocratic oath swore by Asclepius and other healing gods. In Athens, physicians sacrificed to Asclepius and Hygieia (the personification of Health, who was a child of Asclepius) twice each year for themselves and their patients. Galen calls himself a servant of Asclepius, "since he saved me when I had the deadly condition of an abscess," and elsewhere speaks of Asclepius's healing a man who was so badly swollen "that it was impossible for him to move himself."[15] Physicians generally accepted the validity of divine dreams and had no

79

philosophical objections to miraculous healing. Rather, religious medicine was viewed by the physicians as complementing their own work.[16] When Greek physicians believed they could no longer help a patient, they refused to give further treatment. The patient was regarded as beyond the point at which rational medicine could help; it was expected that the patient might now seek the direct help of the god Asclepius. Physicians were not jealous of the ability of the god to heal in cases where they could not, particularly in chronic cases, which physicians were reluctant to treat. Hence one cannot speak of a "conflict" between religious and secular medicine, for both were aspects of healing that came from the same god. The two traditions existed side by side, probably with little contact.

During the Hellenistic period, after the death of Alexander the Great in 323 B.C., a number of foreign deities poured into Greece from the Oriental world, for instance, Isis and Serapis from Egypt and Mithra from Persia. These cults spread rapidly throughout the Mediterranean world, challenging the primacy of Asclepius as a healing god. But the cult of Asclepius continued to retain its position. The popularity of the god owed much to his claim to be the god of both the rich *and* the poor. In a world in which society felt no obligation for the welfare of the poor, those who could not afford the fees of physicians could seek the aid of Asclepius. It was the god's claim that he took care of the poor; moreover, he was satisfied with small thank-offerings, which the poor could afford. In a society conspicuously lacking in charitable concern for those in need, the sanctuaries of Asclepius seem to have offered, in Roman times, inexpensive medicine for those who could not afford the services of a physician. This may be the reason for the growth of rational therapeutics in his sanctuaries in the second century after Christ. The hostels that began to be attached to the temples may have represented forerunners of the hospitals and poorhouses established later by the Christians. Here the sick could spend long periods of convalescence. It is no wonder that Asclepius was called the "most philanthropic of the gods" and was regarded by early Christians as the chief competitor of Christ because of his remarkable similarity in role and teachings to the Great Physician. Some of his sanctuaries were still in existence in the sixth century after Christ.

What role did magic play in Greek medicine? There is little evidence of magical practices (incantations and the like) in secular medicine from Homer to Galen (second century A.D.). Sophocles says that a good physician does not sing incantations over pains that should be cured by cutting (*Ajax* 11.581–82). The writer of *On the Sacred Disease* speaks disapprovingly of "magicians, purifiers, charlatans, and quacks" who resort to purifications and incantations in treating epilepsy. Yet the Greeks, like everyone else in antiquity, believed in magic, and magical practices were undoubtedly sometimes employed for healing, particularly when rational methods were unsuccessful. According to Diodorus, everyone resorts to incantations and prayers when the art of the physician fails to cure (frags. 30, 43). Not all physicians were free from magical practices, and some employed incantations and recommended the use of amulets. These physicians were probably a minority. The Roman author Pliny the Elder states that no one doubts that magic had its origin in medicine (*Natural History* 30.1), but there is no evidence that there was ever a connection between the two in Greece. In this regard Greek medicine differs essentially from medicine in Egypt and Mesopotamia, where there was no definite boundary line between magic and medicine.

ROME

The practice of religion in Rome as in Greece was largely an official activity for the whole community. The Romans believed that they were surrounded by supernatural beings, initially conceived of as spiritual powers of a vague and undefined nature called *numina*. Later these beings were personified, and Roman religion, originally animistic, developed into a polytheism. Even then they evoked no personal devotion, for they were gods of the state. The Romans saw themselves as under the care of certain gods, whose worship was maintained by the state. The official cults of Rome were administered by elected priests who maintained traditional rituals and took care of the temples. The official religion was supported by funds provided by the state; it was the duty of each citizen to take part in the public worship of the gods. The purpose of this worship was to maintain the *pax deorum*, "the peace of the gods," that is, to ensure the continued favor and blessings of the gods on Rome. To this end a scrupulous observance of every traditional rite was required. The official worship of the gods was based on the idea of a contract between the community and the gods for the mutual advantage of both. This concept was summarized by the Latin words *do ut des*, "I give in order that you might give." A failure to honor the gods by worship and sacrifice might result in losing the blessings that had been given in the past or being punished by some heaven-sent calamity. Hence the Romans approached the gods with reverent fear rather than affection; they were so concerned with proper form that their worship tended to be excessively mechanical and formal. In addition to the great divinities that protected Rome, Romans worshiped the spirits and *numina* that protected their particular households or presided over some aspect of their lives. The Romans assigned a spirit to every object or activity, and out of this swarm of *numina* each Roman would appease or seek the protection of those most relevant to his or her situation.

Since the Romans believed that if religious duties were neglected or carried out in a faulty manner the gods might withdraw their favor from the community or express their displeasure by sending disasters or prodigious events, the Romans took great care to provide regular festivals and to maintain the accustomed prayers and sacrifices to the gods. If a calamity or natural disaster occurred, it was generally regarded by the Romans as a sign of divine anger that required some sort of expiation in order to restore the *pax deorum*. The Romans lived in constant fear of displeasing some divinity. Divination was an important aspect of Roman religion, and for this purpose a college of augurs had the duty of discovering, by observing certain signs, whether the gods approved of a proposed action. In the case of existing or pending disaster, such as famine, pestilence, or war, the Roman senate might order additional sacrifices, supplications, vows, festivals, or other measures to appease the wrath of the gods. These were usually undertaken after consulting the augurs or sacred books.

In spite of the Roman tendency to assign a separate deity to each function, the early Romans appear to have had no specific gods of either disease or healing. Rather they relied on a variety of gods to protect them from disease. Thus Mars, the god of war, is appealed to in an early Latin hymn, the "Carmen Arvale," to permit no plague to come upon the Romans. And in an ancient prayer preserved by Cato the Elder (234–149 B.C.), Mars is called upon to protect from visible and invisible diseases and to bring health and strength to one's home and family (*De Agri Cult.* 141). Certain deities were frequently appealed to specifically in matters of health, for example, Carna, an Italian goddess of the underworld who had special care of the vital organs. She was asked to preserve the liver, heart, and other vital organs, and she practiced magic that could be sought to avert disease.

Pre-Christian Antiquity

It was not always possible for the Romans to determine which gods had sent a plague; in prayers, to avert the disease, the formula "whether you be a god or goddess" was sometimes employed. The Romans also personified disease, hoping to appease it with worship and sacrifice and so avoid its further spread. Thus Febris (Fever) became a goddess who was thought to be favorable to humankind and to provide magical remedies for disease. Three temples were built in her honor in Rome. Other personifications of disease included Cloacina and Mefitis, who were invoked for protection and healing from vapors and poisonous gases.

For much of their early history, the Romans explained disease and disaster as being the result of supernatural causation: The gods had been offended and it was necessary that they be propitiated. As early as the reign of the Roman king Servius Tullius (traditional dates, 578–535 B.C.) prodigies occurred, accompanied by a pestilence, that were regarded as the result of the neglect of certain religious rites. In 462 B.C., when Rome was attacked by plague, the senate ordered the people to beseech the gods to remit the disease. Widespread pestilence was responsible for the introduction of a number of foreign deities from Greece and elsewhere when Rome's own gods failed to avert disease. In 431 B.C. a temple was dedicated to Apollo in recognition of his aid in ending a plague that had raged for two years. He was worshiped as Apollo Medicus (Apollo the Physician) and came in time to replace many of the traditional Roman gods as averters of sickness. Apollo came to be credited with having discovered the art of healing. His cult was later spread throughout the Latin West.

In 293 B.C., when pestilence broke out in Rome, the Sibylline books were consulted; they recommended that an embassy be sent to Epidaurus to bring Asclepius to Rome to stop it. It was not until 291 B.C., however, that the Romans sent the delegation. Although the priests at Epidaurus hesitated to honor the request, the god himself appeared in the form of a serpent in the temple before making his way to the ship, which carried him to Rome. The serpent left the ship at the Tiber Island, and it was there that the Romans dedicated a temple to him as Aesculapius in 291 B.C. The cult of Aesculapius apparently was not prominent in Rome during the Republican period (i.e., until the end of the first century B.C.). But the introduction of his cult was nevertheless significant, for he was viewed not merely as an averter of disease, like Apollo, but as a healer of individuals. During the late Republic, several other foreign gods of healing were introduced into Rome, offering healing by the use of magic, divination, or incubation, but we know little about them. The healing practices of Aesculapius in Rome were apparently quite similar to those of Greece. Sacred serpents and dogs were kept at his sanctuary, and although the practice of incubation is not mentioned before the end of the first century A.D., it is likely that it was employed. Inscriptions recording cases of healing have been found, but they date from the second century. They involve dream oracles, and the suggested remedies are of a theurgic nature. The cult came to enjoy great popularity in the first century A.D. and eventually spread throughout the West. Large numbers of votive offerings have been found at his sanctuary in Rome. The use of magic seems to have been a characteristic of healings by Aesculapius, probably representing an adaptation of the cult to Roman practices.

Until the migration of Greek physicians into Rome, the Romans apparently had neither physicians nor rational medicine. Pliny the Elder says that for six hundred years they were "without physicians . . . but not without medicine" (*Natural History* 29.5).[17] He explains this curious lack by stating that "it was not medicine itself that the forefathers condemned, but the medical profession, chiefly because they refused to pay fees to profiteers in order to save their lives" (29.8). Plague was averted by propitiating the gods; in individual cases of illness the Romans combined magic and divination, much of it inherited from the Etruscans and Sabines, with folk remedies. The *paterfamilias*, who was the oldest living male in the family and the head of the household, usually acted as de facto physician for the members of the household. Typical of these practitioners of Roman popular medicine was Cato the Elder, who made himself familiar with medical matters in order to be able to treat his family. Plutarch says that Cato

> had compiled a book of recipes and used them for the diet or treatment of any members of his household who fell ill. He never made his patients fast, but allowed them to eat herbs and morsels of duck, pigeon, or hare. He maintained that this diet was light and thoroughly suitable for sick people, apart from the fact that it often produced nightmares, and he claimed that by following it he kept both himself and his family in perfect health. (Plutarch *Life of Cato* 23.)[18]

Cato gives a good deal of medical advice in his handbook on agriculture. Included are many folk remedies probably derived from the Italian peasantry; these are mixed with supplications, prayers, sacrifices, and ritual processions for the protection of his family, crops, and herds. He makes much use of treatments that employ cabbage; magical incantations are also regularly employed.

For the Romans every aspect of life—conception, gestation, birth, growth, marriage, childbearing—was under the protection of a god or *numen*, whose protection must be sought. There were many native goddesses to whom a Roman matron could appeal for protection in childbirth, but most of these were eventually replaced by either Juno Lucina or Diana. A variety of magical formulas or incantations were recited to ensure a safe childbirth, and sometimes the laying-on of hands was employed. This was a means of transferring the power of a god or goddess for healing (or, in the case of childbirth, for safe delivery). The right hand was applied, signifying a good influence. A variety of other gods and goddesses could be appealed to. A curious prophylactic ceremony, probably going back to very early times, took place on the Roman festival of the Lupercalia, held in honor of the god Faunus. The priests of Faunus, clad only in goatskins, ran around the Palatine hill striking women with strips of goatskin to promote fertility.

The first person to practice medicine in Rome as a distinct profession was the Greek Archagathus, who settled in Rome in 219 B.C. He was treated with great respect, but his excessive use of surgery and cautery eventually made him unpopular (he came to be called *"carnifex,"* "the executioner") and produced a disgust with the entire profession. There must have been some demand for Greek physicians, however, for they continued to come to Rome. Cato feared that the Greeks "are a quite worthless people, and an intractable one, and you must consider my words prophetic."

> When that race gives us its literature it will corrupt all things, and even all the more if it sends hither its physicians. They have conspired together to murder all foreigners with their physic, but this very thing they do for a fee, to gain credit and destroy . . . I have forbidden you to have dealings with physicians. (Quoted by Pliny *Natural History* 29.7.)

Yet in spite of conservative opposition, Greek physicians came to enjoy increasing popularity. For example, the physician Asdepiades, in the first century B.C., gained a wide reputation, which he largely passed on to his successors. Another Greek import, the cult of Asclepius (Latin, Aesculapius), which on its introduction into Rome first attracted the lower classes, by the time of the Empire came to appeal to the upper classes and even emperors. But Roman traditional practices, consisting of magic and folk medicine, continued to exist even after the introduction of religious and rational medicine from Greece. This is illustrated by the compilation of folk and magical remedies made by Pliny the Elder in his *Natural History.* Romans also continued to consult soothsayers when ill.[19]

The religious beliefs and general culture of the Romans underwent a significant change in the last two centuries before Christ, mainly as a result of Rome's conquest of Greece and the eastern Mediterranean. There was a tendency of the upper classes to abandon the traditional religion for either skepticism or philosophy, usually of Stoicism or Epicureanism. But many ordinary people found the worship of the traditional Roman gods no longer satisfying. It was too formal and mechanical to satisfy the private needs of the large number of Romans who had left farming for the cities. As Rome conquered the Mediterranean world to create an empire, vast numbers of slaves poured into Italy, especially from the East, and many of these brought with them their native religions. Astrology, which had spread from Babylon to Greece, became very influential in Italy by the first century A.D. The belief was common that one's destiny was fixed at birth by one's stars. Magic too enjoyed great vogue in Rome. Magicians abounded and sold charms to curse enemies, exorcise demons, or heal diseases. But perhaps the most striking phenomenon of Roman religious life was the penetration of Italy and the western Mediterranean by a group of cults known as the mystery religions. These were religions that came from Egypt and Asia but had been modified by their contact with Greek civilization after Alexander's conquest of the Persian Empire. Once the mystery religions invaded Rome they quickly submerged Roman traditional religion, for they gave a personal satisfaction that the old religion was unable to offer. They often featured elaborate ceremonies that appealed to the emotional needs of their adherents, and they offered a promise of personal immortality through communion with a god. They had a universal appeal to all classes, rich or poor, slave or free, citizen or foreigner. The most influential cults were those of the Great Mother (*Magna Mater*), Cybele, the Egyptian gods Isis and Serapis, and the Persian god Mithra.

Hence the Roman Empire, which by the end of the first century B.C. spanned the entire Mediterranean, became an amalgam of religious traditions, the variety of which was reflected in approaches to healing.

Pre-Christian Antiquity

Healing played an important part in many of the Oriental cults, whose priests employed a variety of means to cure the sick, including astrology, magic, divination, and the use of herbs. The most prominent of the oriental healing gods was Serapis, whose methods of healing were much like those of his rival Aesculapius. The priests of the Oriental cults came to exercise a strong influence over the adherents of their faith. They were versed in sacred knowledge and came to be looked to for spiritual guidance by a society whose members increasingly were unable to live without the aid of sacerdotal religion. The Oriental religions placed great importance on mysterious methods of purification, either through the performance of ceremonies or through mortification and penance. Belief in demon possession was common, and purification was sought to drive out evil spirits. Disease was widely regarded as being the result of demonic activity. Plotinus describes the teachings of the Gnostics, who asserted that diseases were spirit beings that could be expelled by magical formulas. From the second century A.D., attitudes much like those of Gnosticism became widespread in Greco-Roman culture (*Enneads* 2.9.14). In the late Empire magic came to play an increasing role in therapeutics. Roman traditional medicine, of course, contained elements of magic that had established themselves by long use. One finds these in many works of popular medicine. But the new influences were clearly of Oriental derivation and appealed to the increasingly superstitious attitudes that characterized the late Roman Empire. The population, oppressed by a growing autocracy and totalitarianism in government, faced with economic catastrophe, and characterized by a feeling of despondency and impotence, sought refuge in the irrational. Even philosophy turned to mystical and theurgic elements such as one finds in Neoplatonism. One form of magic that became popular was the belief that there were occult properties in certain animals, plants, and precious stones that could be manipulated to release magical forces through sympathy and antipathy. This belief came to be linked with alchemy and astrology and was widely employed in magical medicine. Astrology was also brought into the service of medicine and used by physicians and nonphysicians alike. One physician claimed on his tombstone that he had predicted by astrology his death at the age of ninety-three. Even Galen believed that the positions of the moon vis-à-vis the planets affected the condition of patients. Naturally, in the superstitious atmosphere that we see in the Roman Empire from the second century, it became increasingly difficult for rational medicine to flourish. The jurist Ulpian said that magicians and exorcists should not be considered physicians, though there are many who laud their efficacy in healing.

There were superstitious attitudes toward etiology and therapeutics throughout all periods of classical antiquity. Plutarch (ca. A.D. 50–ca. 120) wrote an essay entitled "On Superstition," which is included in his *Moralia*.[20] In it he compares the reactions to adversity of an atheist and a superstitious man. Although these two types (particularly the latter) are somewhat exaggerated, since they caricature opposite extremes, they provide an illuminating contrast of two attitudes that are probably found in most times and places. To Plutarch, atheism was an insensitivity to the divine, superstition an emotional slavery to a distorted concept of the divine. In times of adversity, an atheist, if he is a moderate man, takes his misfortune without a word and tries to procure help for himself. If he is immoderate, he is bitter and levels complaints against fate or chance. An atheist, when ill, attempts to recall an excess in eating or drinking or recent irregularities or vicissitudes, and seeks help. A superstitious man, however, when beset by misfortune, by even the slightest ill, loads himself with fears and suspicions, lamentations and moanings. He places the responsibility for his lot upon evil spirits or the gods, seeing himself as hateful in their sight, imagines that he is being punished by them, and acknowledges that his suffering is deserved because of his own conduct. Thus he makes no attempt to relieve the situation or undo its effects, lest he appear to be rebelling against his punishment. When ill he will not consult a physician, but may roll naked in the mire as he confesses his sins and mistakes. That these extremes existed and were often found in the classical world is beyond question.

Thus far in our survey of the relationship between religion and medicine in Greece and Rome we have had little to say about philosophical attitudes toward health and disease. To the Greeks, health was the *summum bonum*, the highest good. According to an old Attic drinking song, "health is the best thing" (Plato *Gorgias* 451E). Health guarantees long life, and without it nothing is worthwhile: "When health is absent," writes Herophilus, "wisdom cannot reveal itself, art cannot become manifest, strength cannot fight, wealth becomes useless, and intelligence cannot be made use of."[21] To be sick was to be less than fully a human being; to prolong life when only sickness and suffering could be anticipated was not regarded as desirable. The Christian idea that suffering could be redemptive was not part of the Greek and Roman understanding of disease. Health was regarded as a balance of constituent elements of the body, disease as a disturbance that upsets the harmony and symmetry of these elements. In order to maintain this balance, moderation and self-control (*sophrosyne*) were required. Hence there arose a dietetic medicine that tried to regulate the body as a whole by means of the control of one's regimen. Physicians attempted to heal their patients by arranging their way of life. In order to remain healthy one had to know how to live right. From its beginnings in the fifth century B.C., the importance of dietetics for the maintenance and restoration of health was recognized throughout antiquity. Since a life without health was a life not worth living, physicians encouraged people to live for their health; that is, to regulate their lives in the smallest detail to prevent sickness. "A sound mind in a sound body" was certainly a Greek ideal, and one that was passed on to the Romans. A body made healthy through moderation provided an analogy for soundness of mind that was the result of self-control. Philosophers generally rejected the Greek glorification of health, though they agreed that health is desirable and can be preserved through self-discipline. Rather, they made happiness depend upon virtue or some other intellectual or moral quality. But philosophers were much taken with the analogy between the care of the body and the cure of the soul. They taught that the soul may be sick like the body and require the aid of a philosopher, who is a physician of the soul. To medicine and regimen in the care of the body there corresponded discipline and instruction in the cure of the soul.

A well-known classical scholar has said of classical Greece that "the most far-reaching, and perhaps the most questionable, of all her gifts to human culture is the body-soul dichotomy."[22] (A dichotomous view of humanity, incidentally, was absent in Hebrew thought until Greek influence caused it to appear at least in some Jewish literature by the first century B.C.) This view, which held that the soul was the real self, was popular in many quarters and was particularly evidenced in various philosophical schools, manifesting itself sometimes in an asceticism or a contempt for the body that included an indifference to disease and suffering. There resulted a change from the classical emphasis on physical health to an emphasis on spiritual health, which might be acquired even at the expense of the body. This attitude can be seen in Stoicism and Cynicism.

Both Stoicism and Cynicism were agreed that virtue alone brings happiness. Virtue is the supreme Good, and conversely vice is the only evil. Only the wise person who knows the truth can be really virtuous. Everything in nature is rational and good, and a virtuous life is one that is lived in conformity to nature. Poverty, illness, pain, and death are all matters of indifference. Their presence or absence should not affect one's happiness. One should live in harmony with nature and therefore be independent of changes in fortune by cultivating the only real Good. Both the Stoics and the Cynics believed that people should be made self-sufficient and independent in order to meet the difficulties of life. Since no one can deprive wise people of their virtue, they always possess the real Good and therefore are happy. In the case of the Cynics this belief led to a renunciation of the conventions of society for a mendicant existence as beggar-philosophers. The Stoics, on the other hand, did not abandon society but sought to control the will, which they believed was the only thing that is always in our power, and to keep it unblemished. Hence they taught that one must train the soul to be indifferent to pain and illness, and even to the loss of one's family, since these things happen through divine providence, which is always good. Seneca wrote that one was healthy if one were content with oneself and did not depend upon things that people usually seek for happiness (*Moral Epistles* 72.7). Epictetus, an ex-slave who became a leading Stoic philosopher, summarized the Stoic view well in an essay titled "How One Should Bear Illnesses."[23] The purpose of studying philosophy, he wrote, is to prepare ourselves to face events in our lives like illness. "If now is the time for fever, take your fever in the right way; if for thirst, thirst in the right way, if for hunger, hunger aright. Is it not in your power?" The test of the philosopher is whether, even with a fever, one lives in conformity with nature. Being ill is a part of life, like walking or sailing or traveling. "What does bearing fever rightly mean? It means not to blame God or man, nor to be crushed by what happens, to await death in a right spirit, to do what you are bidden." It is not of concern to philosophers to worry about external things, like their wine or their oil or their bodies, but to look after their own ruling power. "For the two principles we must have ready at command are these: that outside the will there is nothing good or evil, and that we must not lead events but follow them." The attitude of submission and resignation enjoined by Stoicism in the face of pain and disease was as far as the classical world could go in its understanding of suffering. It remained for Christianity to endow it with a positive value, taken over from Judaism at least in its incipient form.

Pre-Christian Antiquity

NOTES

1. Henry Sigerist, *A History of Medicine*, vol. 1 (New York: Oxford University Press, 1951), p. 161.

2. There is extensive literature on primitive medicine, religion, and magic. Some examples from the last several decades: W. H. R. Rivers, *Medicine, Magic, and Religion* (London: G. Bell & Sons, 1924); Erwin H. Ackerknecht, "Problems of Primitive Medicine," *Bulletin of the History of Medicine* 11 (1942): 503–21, and "Psychopathology, Primitive Medicine, and Primitive Culture," *Bulletin of the History of Medicine* 14 (1943): 30–67; John Middleton, ed., *Magic, Witchcraft, and Curing*, 2 vols. (Garden City, N.Y.: Doubleday & Co., 1967).

3. See W. H. P. Römer, "Religion of Ancient Mesopotamia," in *Historia Religionum: A Handbook for the History of Religions*, ed. C. J. Bleeker and G. Widengren (Leiden, 1969), p. 155. It should not be thought that the Egyptians were unconcerned about moral failings, since they also produced penitential literature. Rather, the link between moral failing and retributive disease appears not to have been present in Egypt to the degree to which it seems to have been in Mesopotamia.

4. In *The Ancient Near East: Supplementary Texts and Pictures Relating to the Old Testament*, ed. James B. Pritchard (Princeton: Princeton University Press, 1969), pp. 589–91.

5. James H. Breasted, ed., *The Edwin Smith Surgical Papyrus* (Chicago: University of Chicago Press, 1930).

6. Some secondary literature on Egyptian medicine and religion: C. J. Bleeker, "The Religion of Ancient Egypt," in *Historia Religionum*, pp. 40–114; Paul Ghalioungui, *Magic and Medical Science in Ancient Egypt* (Mystic, Conn.: Lawrence Verry, 1963); John A. Wilson, "Medicine in Ancient Egypt," *Bulletin of the History of Medicine* 36 (1962): 114–23. On Mesopotamian medicine and religion: Robert Biggs, "Medicine in Ancient Mesopotamia," *History of Science* 8 (1969): 94–105; Edith K. Ritter, "Magical Expert (=Āšipu) and Physician (=Asû): Notes on Two Complementary Professions in Babylonian Medicine," in *Studies in Honor of Benno Landsberger on His Seventy-fifth Birthday* (Chicago: University of Chicago Press, 1965), pp. 299–321; W. H. P. Römer, "Religion of Ancient Mesopotamia."

7. The best treatment of medicine in ancient Persia is Dietrich Brandenburg, "Avesta und Medizin: Ein literaturgeschichtlicher Beitrag zur Heilkunde im alten Persien," *Janus* 59 (1972): 269–307.

8. There is a vast amount of literature on ancient Judaism, both from a later Jewish perspective and a Christian perspective. There are also many studies of medicine in the Bible (books, articles, and short treatments in Bible dictionaries), usually concerned with the identification of diseases, the significance of dietary laws, and so forth. Two books that may be profitably consulted on the subject under consideration (although both are concerned more with rabbinic than

biblical medical history) are: Julius Preuss, *Biblical and Talmudic Medicine,* trans. Fred Rosner (New York: Hebrew Publishing Co., 1978); Fred Rosner, *Medicine in Bible and the Talmud,* Library of Jewish Law and Ethics 5 (New York: Ktav Publishing Co., 1977).

9. Trans. H. G. Evelyn-White in the Loeb Classical Library (Cambridge, Mass.: Harvard University Press, 1936).

10. A. W. H. Adkins, "Greek Religion," in *Historia Religionum,* pp. 404–5.

11. Translations of Hippocratic works are taken from the Loeb Classical Library, edition of *Hippocrates,* trans. W. H. S. Jones and E. T. Withington (Cambridge, Mass.: Harvard University Press, 1923–31).

12. See Strabo 14.2.19 (657C) and Pliny *Natural History* 20.100.

13. Emma and Ludwig Edelstein, *Asclepius: A Collection and Interpretation of the Testimonies,* 2 vols. (Baltimore: Johns Hopkins Press, 1945); see esp. vol. 2, pp. 53–64.

14. Henry E. Sigerist, *History of Medicine,* vol. 2 (New York: Oxford University Press, 1961), pp. 65–66.

15. See Edelstein, *Asclepius,* 1:263–64, T. 458 and T. 459.

16. Ludwig Edelstein, *Ancient Medicine: Selected Papers of Ludwig Edelstein,* ed. Owsei and C. Lilian Temkin (Baltimore: Johns Hopkins Press, 1967), pp. 244–46.

17. Translations of Pliny the Elder are taken from the Loeb Classical Library edition of the *Natural History,* trans. W. H. S. Jones (Cambridge, Mass.: Harvard University Press, 1963).

18. Trans. Ian Scott-Kelvert in *Makers of Rome: Nine Lives by Plutarch* (Baltimore: Penguin Books, 1965).

19. See Pliny the Younger *Letters* 2.20.4–5.

20. Trans. F. C. Babbitt in the Loeb Classical Library, vol. 2 (1928).

21 Herophilus in Sextus Empiricus *Adv. Mathem.* 11.50. Quoted by Edelstein, *Ancient Medicine,* p. 358.

22. E. R. Dodds, *Pagan and Christian in an Age of Anxiety* (New York: Cambridge University Press, 1970), p. 29.

23. *Discourses* 3.10. Trans. P. E. Matheson in *The Stoic and Epicurean Philosophers,* ed. W. J. Oates (New York: Modern Library, 1957), pp. 361–62.

4

Medicine and Religion: Early Christianity Through the Middle Ages

DARREL W. AMUNDSEN
and
GARY B. FERNGREN

EARLY CHRISTIANITY

The relationship between health, disease, and medicine and early Christianity can best be understood by examining the place of suffering in the New Testament. The New Testament writers and early Christians held certain fundamental principles as axiomatic: (1) God is sovereign. (2) Man and all nature are fallen. (3) All conditions of human life are thus abnormal. (4) God's providential care can be seen in human history and particularly in the history of his people. (5) Salvation requires suffering—a vicarious and substitutionary suffering inherent in the typology of the Old Testament sacrificial system. (6) Nature itself will ultimately be redeemed in some eschatological sense. Central to all this is the thought that suffering is linked to evil, and evil to sin, and sin to the Fall.

It is against this background that we must see the Christian proclamation "Christ also died for sins once for all, the righteous for the unrighteous, that he might bring us to God, being put to death in the flesh but made alive in the spirit" (1 Pet. 3:18). The word translated "died" is *pascho*, a verb whose basic meaning is to experience something or to suffer. In the New Testament the word is often used to refer to Christ's sufferings or death. It is thus a word that describes his passion in the broadest sense. Christ's sufferings are regarded as an essential part of his atonement for sin.

While the sufferings that constituted Christ's passion are clearly seen as unique, he is nevertheless considered a participant in other levels of human suffering. His compassion for the sufferer is viewed as compassion for the human condition, for his mission was to deliver humanity from sin and the results of sin, that is, from suffering, corruption, and death. This deliverance is seen in New Testament terms as a consequence of salvation. While salvation is always presented with a view to eternity, it has implications for this world as well. But salvation does not relieve Christians from suffering here. On the contrary, they will never be free from suffering in this life. Indeed, Christians must expect to encounter more suffering as a direct result of their salvation than they would if they had remained in an unregenerate state. This especially involves suffering in the form of persecution. Enlarging on his statement that a slave is not greater than his master, Jesus says, "If they persecuted me, they will persecute you" (John 15:20). To suffer for Christ is a gift of grace, a privilege, even a joy (see Matt. 5:10–12; Acts 9:16; 1 Thess. 3:2–4; Phil. 1:29). Suffering is regarded not as the exclusive privilege of a select few but as the privilege of anyone who follows Christ in the manner described in 2 Timothy: "Indeed all who desire to live a godly life in Christ Jesus will be persecuted" (3:12).

The New Testament also teaches that a Christian must expect to suffer under God's discipline, God's training. According to the Epistle to the Hebrews, Christ, although he was God's own Son, "learned obedience through what he suffered" (5:8). Earlier he is said to have been made "perfect through suffering" (2:10). If Christ himself, although never deficient in obedience, can be taught obedience through suffering—if he, although incarnate God, can be edified and perfected through suffering—so also can suffering edify his followers.

Just as persecution for righteousness is a consequence of living a godly life in Christ Jesus, so also is suffering in other forms part of God's edification of God's children. The effect of discipline on the Christian's character, if the discipline is properly received, is considered salutary and more than sufficient compensation for the pain, since it bears a peaceful fruit of righteousness for those who have been trained by it (see Heb. 12:7–11). Many passages can be adduced from the New Testament where the edificatory aspects of suffering are stressed (e.g., Rom. 5:2–5; 1 Pet. 4:12; James 1:2–4). It seems that in New Testament terms suffering should be viewed by Christians as something in which they can rejoice for two reasons: (1) God uses suffering as a means of producing spiritual maturity, if there is a right response to the affliction; and (2) the very fact that Christians endure suffering, particularly in the form of persecution, is proof that they are children of God.

Although the Christian is to rejoice in afflictions, the New Testament clearly recognizes that suffering is not in itself pleasant. Thus believers are encouraged in their sufferings by such exhortations as the following, which appears in 2 Corinthians immediately after mention of the hope of the Christian's resurrection: "So we do not lose heart. Though our outer nature is wasting away, our inner nature is being renewed every day. For this slight momentary affliction is preparing for us an eternal weight of glory beyond all comparison" (4:16–17). These verses enunciate a theme dear to several New Testament writers: that the troubles which must be faced in this life are of small consequence in comparison with the joys of heaven. In several passages the correspondence between the sufferings and glory of Christ is stressed (e.g., Matt. 16:27; Phil. 2:9; Heb. 2:9). There is a sense in which the Christian participates in Christ's suffering by participating in the sufferings of the church, Christ's body (e.g., Acts 9:4–5; 1 Cor. 12:26–27).

Christians were also to engage actively in a direct ministry to their fellow sufferers, a ministry of consolation and encouragement. In Acts, Paul and Barnabas are described as "strengthening the souls of the disciples, exhorting them to continue in the faith, and saying that through many tribulations we must enter the kingdom of God" (14:22). The word translated "exhorting" also means to encourage, comfort, or console. This comfort or encouragement or consolation is not merely sympathy, the sharing of mutual woes and sorrows, but a spiritual dynamic whose activating source is God. God is the mediator through whom this spiritual dynamic comes, but it is to flow through the sufferer to other sufferers. Suffering is thus a training ground that enables the Christian, through participating in Christ's sufferings, to minister to the sufferings of fellow Christians. The relief that is provided is not removal of the suffering but a consolation that transforms the suffering into a positive force in the Christian's life.

Such a positive response to suffering is exemplified by Paul's handling of what is referred to as his "thorn in the flesh":

> And to keep me from being too elated by the abundance of revelations, a thorn was given me in the flesh, a messenger of Satan, to harass me. . . . Three times I besought the Lord about this, that it should leave me; but he said to me, "My grace is sufficient for you, for my power is made perfect in weakness." I will all the more gladly boast of my weaknesses, that the

power of Christ may rest upon me. For the sake of Christ, then, I am content with weaknesses, insults, hardships, persecutions, and calamities; for when I am weak, then I am strong (2 Cor. 12:7–10).

This attitude illustrates a central paradox in New Testament thought: Strength comes only through weakness. This strength is Christ's strength that comes only through dependence upon him. In the Gospel of John, Christ says: "I have said this to you, that in me you may have peace. In the world you have tribulation; but be of good cheer, I have overcome the world" (16:33). "In the world you have tribulation." It is simply to be expected and accepted. But for the New Testament Christian no suffering is meaningless. The ultimate purpose and meaning behind Christian suffering in the New Testament is spiritual maturity. And the ultimate goal in spiritual maturity is a close dependence upon Christ based upon a childlike trust. There can also be adduced from the New Testament numerous passages that encourage the Christian to trust in the heavenly Father (e.g., 1 Pet. 4:19; 2 Tim. 1:11–12; Phil. 4:6–7).

In contrast to Plutarch's superstitious man,[1] who is the victim of a god who hates him, whom he distrusts and hates in return, a Christian, as described in the New Testament, considers himself to be the child of a heavenly Father who loves him and, in spite of any appearance to the contrary, is causing all things to work together for the good. To New Testament Christians, God is a *person* to whom they may relate in a spiritual depth commensurate with the degree of their commitment to the person of Christ. It is the intimacy of this relationship, a relationship based upon love and trust, that gives meaning to suffering for the New Testament Christian and enables Paul to say of himself and of those of kindred spirits, "we exalt in afflictions."

Little is said in the New Testament about sickness as a form of suffering for the Christian. It is usually assumed that Paul's "thorn in the flesh" was a chronic illness that was transformed into a positive force in his life. Paul's statement that "in everything God works for good with those who love him, who are called according to his purpose" (Rom. 8:28) would surely not exclude sickness, nor would the assurance that occurs later in the same chapter: "Who shall separate us from the love of Christ? Shall tribulation, or distress, or persecution, or famine, or nakedness, or peril, or sword?" (8:35). Although Jesus promised his followers suffering and affliction in this life, he healed the sick who came to him, and the New Testament, or at least the Gospels, might appear to view sickness in a different light from other forms of suffering. In fact, however, they do not;

rather, the miracles of healing, which are variously described as wonders, signs, and mighty works, are presented as fulfilling Old Testament messianic prophecies (Matt. 8:16–17) and attesting to the validity of Jesus' claims to be the Messiah (Luke 7:22; John 10:37–38; Acts 2:22).

Paul called his "thorn in the flesh" a "messenger of Satan" sent to harass him, yet he did not link it directly to sin. That sickness came from Satan is expressed elsewhere in the New Testament; for instance, in Acts 10:38, where Jesus is described as having healed "all that were oppressed by the devil." In Luke 13 a woman is said to have "a spirit of infirmity," and Jesus refers to her as one "whom Satan bound" (13:11, 16). That sickness was popularly viewed as punishment for sin and that Jesus sought to deny a necessary connection is suggested by John 9:2–3. When Jesus' disciples encountered a person who had been born blind, they asked, "Who sinned, this man or his parents, that he was born blind?" Jesus answered, "It was not that this man sinned, or his parents, but that the works of God might be manifest in him" (cf. John 11:4). Yet in the same Gospel, Jesus is described as saying to a man whom he had just healed, "Sin no more, that nothing worse befall you" (5:14), thus allowing for a connection between a person's sin and a person's sickness, a connection that is maintained in 1 Cor. 11:30–32, where some sickness and death are said to have resulted from an abuse of the Lord's Supper.

Belief in demon possession and in disease that is caused by demons is encountered both in the New Testament and in late pre-Christian Judaism. We have already seen that disease was sometimes said to be from Satan. In such cases healing did not involve exorcism. Quite different was the case of disease thought to be caused by a demon, in which the healing was accomplished by driving out the demon, as in Matt. 9:32–33 and 12:22. But demon possession was yet a different matter, in which the demonic manifestation often took some form of mental derangement, including what was identified as epilepsy (e.g., Matt. 17:14–18; Luke 8:26–33). That the apostles distinguished between demon possession and disease generally is clear from Acts 5:16. Descriptions of demon possession in the early centuries of the Christian era cannot simply be dismissed as mythical Christian embellishment, since the phenomenon is commonly attested in secular sources throughout the Mediterranean area during that period. It is clear from the New Testament that most disease was not, however, attributed to a demonic causality.

Generally, three different sources of suffering are identified in the literature of the first several centuries of Christianity, namely, a divine source, an evil source, and a natural source.[2] More often than not, there was a hesitancy to attribute disease to God; rather, God was typically viewed as the regulator of disease whether it came from natural or evil sources. Tertullian (late in the second and early third centuries) held that any particular suffering was intended as a warning for Christians and as punishment for the heathen (*On Flight in Persecution* 1–2). Lactantius, writing in the early fourth century, described as divine retribution the excruciating agonies accompanying the death of Galerius, an emperor who had persecuted the Christians quite viciously (*On the Death of the Persecutors* 33).

Cyprian, in the third century, expressed the opinion that God sometimes uses sickness to convert the unbelieving (*On Psalm* 68.18), while the author of the second-century *Shepherd of Hermas* saw sickness and other misfortunes as punishment for those who have wandered from God (6.3). Irenaeus, writing in the second century, recognized in infirmities a schooling for endurance (*Against Heresies* 5.3.1). His contemporary Clement of Alexandria asserted in several places in his writings that by afflictions the Christian acquires moderation both in pain and pleasure and that he loses the fear of poverty, disease, and death (e.g., *Paedagogus* 1.8ff.). He said that "penury and disease, and such trials, are often sent for admonition, for the correction of the past, and for care for the future" (*Stromateis* 7.13).[3]

About the middle of the third century, the empire was afflicted by a series of plagues. After the city of Alexandria was visited by an especially devastating assault, the city's bishop, Dionysius, wrote that while the plague was an object of extreme fear to the pagans, "to us it was not so, but . . . a source of discipline and testing" (Eusebius *Ecclesiastical History* 7.22.6).[4] When the same plague was ravaging Carthage, Cyprian remarked that some of his fellow Christians were distressed that the pestilence did not strike only the pagans, "as if a Christian believes to this end, that, free from contact with evils, he may enjoy the world and this life." But the plague was a blessing because the things they were experiencing "are trying exercises for us, not deaths; they give to the mind the glory of fortitude; by contempt of death they prepare for the crown" (*Mortality* 8, 16).[5]

Somewhat later, during the first decade of the fourth century, Lactantius wrote that the relationship between the soul and the body is comparable to that between master and servant. The flesh must share in the campaign against evil and be ready to be despoiled or sacrificed in the service of its master (*The Divine Institutes* 5.22). Nevertheless, in spiritual warfare the soul can sometimes be refined through suffering, a point developed at some length by church fathers during the fourth century. Ambrose, writing to a friend suffering from a nonfatal illness, maintained that "this sickness was intended for your health and brought you more pain than peril. . . . He struck with illness; he healed you with faith. . . . He chose to admonish you in such a way as not to harm your health and yet to incite your devotion" (*Epistle* 66).[6] Gregory of Nazianzus, delivering his father's eulogy, ruminated on suffering: "But why should it be surprising that holy men suffer ills, either for the purification of some small stain, or for proving their virtue or testing their philosophy, or for the instruction of the weaker, who learn from their example to be brave instead of faint-hearted in misfortune?" (*On His Father* 28).[7] Gregory's close friend, Basil the Great of Caesarea, gave six reasons why Christians are afflicted with illness. First, some diseases are "for our correction." He includes as part of the corrective process both the suffering involved in the disease itself and the pain incurred in the treatment of the ailment. Our goal in such suffering "should be our spiritual benefit, inasmuch as the care of the soul is being taught in the guise of an analogy." Second, illness is often a punishment for sin and should be distinguished from a third category, namely, those infirmities that "arise from faulty diet or from any other physical origin." Fourth, some illness comes at the Evil One's request, for example, the case of Job, where God confounded Satan's boasts by the heroic patience of Job. Fifth, "God places those who are able to endure tribulation even unto death before the weak as their model." And last is the instance of any great saint, for example, the apostle Paul, who was afflicted with physical suffering "in order that he might not seem to exceed the limits of human nature and that no one might think him to possess anything exceptional in his nature."

Basil considered it extremely important that "when we suffer the blows of calamity at the hands of God, who directs our life with goodness and wisdom, we first ask of him understanding of the reason he has inflicted the blows; second, deliverance from our pains or patient endurance of them." This was important for a variety of reasons, but especially so that the afflicted would know whether or not to employ a physician. Only in two of the six categories should a physician be summoned: for illnesses arising from natural causes and for those which are for the Christian's correction. When we are ill as a punishment for sin and have "recognized our transgressions, we should bear in silence and without recourse to medicine all the afflictions which come to us." Of those in the three remaining categories Basil says, "What profit would there be for such men in having recourse to medicine? Would there not rather be danger that in their solicitude for the body they would be led astray from right reason?" (*The Long Rule* 55).[8]

Throughout the history of Christianity there has always been a degree of tension, often only latent, between theology and secular medicine, between the medicine of the soul and the medicine of the body. According to one view, if God sends disease either to punish or to test a person, it is to God that one must turn for care and healing. If God is both the source and healer of a person's ills, the use of human medicine would circumvent the spiritual framework by resorting to worldly wisdom. On another view, if God is the source of disease, or if God permits disease and is the ultimate healer, God's will can be fulfilled through human agents, who with divine help have acquired the ability to aid in the curative process. However, if it is not God but rather a diabolic force that causes suffering and disease in a person, the first, and to some minds the only, source of aid to which one may turn is God. Most Christians have asserted that the human agent of care, the physician, is an instrument of God, used by God in bringing succor to humankind. But in every age some have maintained that any use of human medicine is a manifestation of a lack of faith. This ambivalence in the Christian attitude, among both theologians and laity, has always been present to some degree.

In the second century Tatian spoke emphatically against the use of medicine as employing the bad to attain the good and warned that those who used it would be punished by God. He maintained that "if anyone is healed by matter, through trusting in it, much more will he be healed by having recourse to the power of God. . . . Why is he who trusts in the system of matter not willing to trust in God? . . . Why do you deify the objects of nature? And why, when you cure your neighbor, are you called a benefactor? Yield to the power of the Logos!" (*Address to the Greeks* 18).[9] Tatian's contemporary, Hippolytus, although not nearly as outspoken, seems to have shared his opinion (*Commentary on Song of Songs* 2), but this view certainly was not shared by all Christians of the second century. Clement of Alexandria writes that "health by medicine, and soundness of body through gymnastics . . . have their origin and existence in consequence of Divine Providence indeed, but in consequence, too, of human cooperation. Understanding also is from God" (*Stromateis* 6.17).[10] Clement's disciple Origen followed his teacher in his attitude toward medicine, maintaining that it is beneficial and essential for humankind. He held that a person seeking to recover from a disease had two alternatives, either to have recourse to the medical art, which he labels as the simple and more ordinary method, or to rise to the higher and better method, namely, to seek God's blessing through piety and prayers (*Against Celsus* 8.60). This either-or approach, which gives the higher places to divine healing, may not have been uncommon.

The two alternatives suggested by Origen have not always been regarded as mutually exclusive. They have often been viewed as complementary, sometimes employed separately, sometimes in conjunction with one another. Some Christians relied exclusively on prayer, others combined secular medicine with prayer. Some resorted to secular medicine only when prayer proved ineffective, while others turned to prayer only when secular medicine did not avail. Some sought a more dramatic approach to divine intervention than prayer (e.g., faith healing, involving a variety of procedures) and had no recourse to physicians. Others sought such religious means only as a last resort after physicians have despaired. These different attitudes still exist side by side within Christianity and cults peripheral to it. Except for those few who on religious grounds demonstrate complete hostility to secular medicine, even an exclusive resource to religious means does not necessarily imply a condemnation of medicine. It is not unusual today to encounter those who refuse medical treatment, relying on entirely religious means; when asked if they feel that seeking medical help would be wrong, they respond in the negative, but explain that in this particular case they are convinced they should rely only on God. Thus when we read accounts of those who relied on religious means for healing in the early centuries of Christianity, we must be cautious in seeing in them an implicit condemnation of secular medicine.

What evidence have we in early Christianity of these two approaches to healing—the use of medicine and the use of religious means? The history of miraculous healing in Christianity is rife with interpretive problems. Rationalists cannot reasonably discount all instances on record of phenomena that cannot be explained to their satisfaction, although they will approach the historical accounts with much skepticism. On the other hand, Christians who believe in the miraculous will likely differ with one another on several points that are of little or no importance to the rationalist historian. Did miraculous occurrences similar to those described in the New Testament continue in the succeeding centuries? Or if miracles in the New Testament sense ceased with the end of the apostolic age, did the charismata (divinely bestowed gifts such as tongues, prophecy, healing) continue? If God continues to perform miracles or if certain occurrences are attributed to Divine Providence, do they take place through individuals who have been divinely gifted or through ecclesiastical offices or through rites or sacraments?

It appears that during the early centuries of Christianity, prayer, either private or public, was often recommended for and employed in healing. A more formal process involving confession of sin, prayer by presbyters, and anointing with oil is mentioned in James 5:14–16. It is reasonable to assume that this practice was followed in the early church. It survived in the Eastern church as a rite for physical healing, but in Latin Christianity it evolved into the sacrament of extreme unction, which came to be used for anointing the terminally ill as an immediate preparation for death. Oil was commonly used, at least from the early third century, both in healing and in absolution from sin. We find in such works as the *Canones Ecclesiastici* and *Bishop Sarapion's Prayer Book* (mid-fourth century) prayers for the consecration of oil (and, in one instance, oil and water) to be used against every fever, demon, and sickness, as well as for the remission of sins. Consecrated oil could be taken home and used privately, a procedure that raised questions addressed by Pope Innocent I (early fifth century) in a letter (no. 28.5) in which he formally approved the practice. There is ample evidence that the anointing of the sick with oil, by both clergy and laity, was not uncommon in late antiquity and the early Middle Ages.

A variety of other means of healing is found in early Christian sources, at least beginning with the mid-second century, for example, healing by the laying on of hands and by the sacraments (baptism and the Eucharist). Some of the earliest sources to mention miraculous healing, including exorcism, are Justin Martyr, Theophilus of Antioch, and Irenaeus, all from the second century. In the latter part of that century and in the early third century, we find that Tertullian and Origen spoke of such occurrences. Origen said that he had personally witnessed many cases of exorcism, healing, and prophecy. He declined, however, to give any details, lest he give occasion to unbelievers to mock. Later in the third century Cyprian referred to healings that accompanied baptism.

In the early centuries of Christianity, then, references to miraculous healings and exorcisms occur. Beginning in the fourth century, however, accounts of exorcism and healing increased in both number and quality compared with those of the preceding centuries. Before the fourth century, Christian healing and exorcism were limited to the means indicated above; the incidences recounted were usually somewhat vague and lacking in sensationalism and detail. The majority of writers did not claim to have seen the events related; those through whom the healings or exorcisms were accomplished were not usually named. In the fourth century, however, we encounter literature full of marvels of a nature strikingly different from those of an earlier period. A wide variety of people, both alive and dead, are credited with miracles that in many instances must be labeled bizarre even by the most sympathetic reader. How can we account for this change?

Several factors converged to create an atmosphere conducive to credulity, common during the fourth century and even more pronounced in succeeding centuries. Late antiquity was not only an intensely religious age; it was also a superstitious one. Roman subjects of all religious persuasions, Christian or pagan, believed that they lived in a world inhabited by supernatural powers, both good and evil, which were active in every aspect of life. The belief in omnipresent and dangerous demons was widespread. Christians counted the pagan gods among the demons. Demons were active; charms, prayers, and exorcism were used to drive them away. The belief and practice of magic grew. The ordinary Roman had always believed in magic; indeed, a belief in some form of magic had been common among the lower levels of society at nearly all times. Although magic was prohibited by law in the early empire, its use was widespread. But by the late third century, the old Roman religious institutions had lost their appeal for all social levels. There existed a spiritual void that was soon filled by a variety of religious manifestations, including a deepening influence of magical practices. This influence was even felt in the highest intellectual circles; it was seen, for example, in the debased Neoplatonism of Iamblichus.

Pagans believed in magic, employing it increasingly for a variety of purposes. Most Christians did not doubt its reality, although Christian leaders regarded it as being the result of demonic activity and condemned its use. While at first Christians thought the employment of traditional magic to be sinful, in many forms it was also regarded as efficacious; it was only a matter of time before some magical practices began to be adopted by Christians. In the late fourth or early fifth century, John Chrysostom commended a hypothetical Christian woman who would rather have had her sick child die than use amulets. He said that amulets are "unavailing, and a mere cheat and mockery," although the woman herself believed that they would be effective; she therefore chose "rather to see her child dead than to put up with idolatry." She was, however, beset by fellow Christians who urged her to use these means since, in their opinion, there was nothing wrong with them (Homily 8 on Col.).[11] Many Christians probably wore amulets of some kind and engaged in whatever white magic they considered consistent with their conception of Christianity. Yet magical practices were condemned by church fathers (including both those who believed in their efficacy, as most probably did, and those who, like Chrysostom, denied it), by church councils (e.g., the Synod of Laodicea, can. 36, in the mid-fourth century), and by civil law (for example, see entries under "Magic" in the index to the *Codex Theodosianus*). Some types of magical procedures continued to be employed by superstitious Christians even though they were denounced by religious authorities. Other practices eventually came to be approved by the church and constituted a form of "Christian magic" (though its connection with magic would have been vigorously denied). For many the cross became an all-powerful charm and the name of Jesus an irresistible spell.

Even more significant for its impact on popular Christianity was the rapid development in the fourth century of the veneration of martyrs and saints ("holy men"). The remains of saints and martyrs were thought to have supernatural power. Relics, whether the remains of a martyr or some object that had an association with that martyr, were in demand. An insatiable appetite for relics grew up, with the result that they were zealously sought and jealously guarded. While some, like Augustine, were alarmed by the traffic in relics and the abuses that it produced, nearly all Christians believed in their miraculous efficacy. The cult of saints, particularly the hero cults, which came in time to replace pagan gods, satisfied the deep craving for wonderworking that was endemic in late classical antiquity.

Early Christianity Through the Middle Ages

Belief in the miraculous practices of relics was so much a part of the spirit of the age that even the deepest Christian thinkers (e.g., Gregory of Nyssa, Basil the Great, Hilary, Jerome, Gregory of Nazianzus, Cyril of Alexandria, Ambros, Chrysostom, Athanasius, and Augustine) believed in their efficacy and supported the founding of shrines in which to house relics. A. H. M. Jones writes:

> Like the old gods, they cured the sick, gave children to barren women, protected travellers from perils of sea and land, detected perjurors and foretold the future. Some acquired widespread fame for special power. SS. Cyrus and John, the physicians who charged no fee, were celebrated for their cures, and their shrine at Canopus, near Alexandria, was thronged by sufferers from all the provinces, as in the old days had been the temple of Asclepius at Aegae. But the main function of the saints and martyrs in the popular religion of the day was to replace the old gods as local patrons and protectors.[12]

The veneration of saints and martyrs, the traffic in relics, Christian magic, an excessive preoccupation with demonism, and miracle-mongering—all represented an infusion of pagan modes of thinking into Christianity.

With the legalization of Christianity by Constantine in 313 and the increasing favoritism shown to it by subsequent Christian emperors, a large number of proselytes entered the church who had only partially renounced paganism. Concessions were made within the church that permitted the nominally or half-converted to retain pagan practices, while at the same time the generally superstitious outlook of the age influenced Christian practices. A vast literature grew up to appeal to the appetite for wonderworking: lives of hermits, monks, and martyrs that are essentially Christian romances full of legendary miracles. These miracle-narratives or teratologies, as they are called, owed their inspiration to the earlier apocryphal writings that attempted to satisfy popular Christian curiosity about the lives of Jesus and the apostles by describing legendary anecdotes and bizarre and fantastic miracles attributed to them. Miracles had an apologetic value for both Christians and pagans. Teratologies had always played a vital propagandistic role in cults like those of Isis, Serapis, Mithra, and Asclepius. During the second and third centuries Asclepius was the chief rival of Christianity; it was against him that Christians leveled some of their strongest attacks. During the fourth century their attention was directed to the more sensational oriental cults of Isis, Serapis, and Mithra. It was important that Christians be able to cite examples of miracles to support the claims of their religion, just as the pagan cults for centuries had advertised miracles in support of theirs.

Augustine illustrates this appropriation of miracles. In his early years he was little concerned with miracles, although he believed that they had occurred both in the past and in his own day. His emphasis was almost entirely on "healing the eyes of the heart" rather than on healing bodily ills. He had witnessed a few healing miracles but spoke little of them until his later years, when his attention was focused much more than before on human suffering and the utility of miracles both for alleviating the ills of Christians and for converting pagans. He began systematically to record reports of local miracles—seventy in less than two years in Hippo. He also had first-person accounts composed by the beneficiaries of the miracles and had these read in church. A brief sketch of the first ten miracles recounted in the *City of God* (22.8) should suffice to give the reader an appreciation of their nature. In the first, a blind man was cured by saints' relics. In the second, painful surgical intervention was made unnecessary by fervent prayer. In the third, a woman was cured of breast cancer by following advice received in a dream to have a newly baptized woman make the sign of the cross on the affected breast. In the fourth, a physician was healed of gout by baptism. In the fifth, a man suffering from paralysis and hernia was healed by the same sacrament. The sixth instance recorded that demons, who were causing sickness among both cattle and slaves on a farm, were driven out by a priest who celebrated the Eucharist there and offered prayers. In the seventh, a paralytic was healed at a shrine built over a deposit of "holy soil" brought from the vicinity of Christ's tomb. The eighth involved two miracles: a demon was driven from a youth at a shrine, and the injury done to the youth's eye by the departing demon was miraculously healed. In the ninth, a young female demoniac was freed from possession when she anointed herself with some oil into which had fallen the tears of a priest who was praying for her. In the tenth, a demon was driven out of a young man by the prayers of a bishop. The "miracle section" of the *City of God* contains the assertion that "even today miracles are being wrought in the name of Christ, sometimes through His sacraments and sometimes through the intercession of the relics of His saints."[13] These examples reveal the essentially magical nature of many of the cures. Some means used to effect healing do not differ appreciably from those of the pagan healing cults.

It was in the fourth century too that asceticism, particularly monasticism, began to influence Christian thinking. Life for many Christians during the early centuries had been difficult because of persecution. In the fourth century, when nominal converts and government patronage that followed recognition made the church seem more worldly, some Christians began to seek a deeper form of religion through asceticism. Insofar as Christian piety stressed denial of the flesh, asceticism had always existed within Christianity. But the new asceticism that spawned monasticism arose not from within Christian belief and practice but from older cultures, particularly those of the East.[14]

Monasticism, then, originated in the deserts of Egypt, Palestine, and Syria and may owe something to groups like the Essenes and the Oriental cults. But the denial of the body that it taught fit well with a similar strain of classical thought, for the same theme is found as well among the Pythagoreans, in Socrates, and in the Neoplatonists. The earliest monks were hermits or "anchorites" who went into the deserts and other desolate regions where they practiced extreme forms of mortification—rigorous fasts, long vigils in prayer, and the like. Some hid themselves in tombs and caves, lived celibate lives and avoided any human companionship, refused to wash, and spent their time in some dull and mechanical operation. Ascetics began to replace martyrs as heroes of the faith and models of Christian emulation. Among the "desert fathers," renunciation of the world and self-mortification often went to bizarre extremes. One monk, the younger Macarius, is said to have exposed his naked body to be stung by poisonous flies for six months in penance for having crushed a fly in anger. Simeon Stylites, who lived for over thirty years on a tiny platform atop a pole whose height he increased to sixty feet, is said for a time to have allowed vermin to eat into his body. Such perverse examples of self-torture gained popular admiration; spiritual biographies of monks were widely read.

Anchoritic monasticism had serious dangers, however, not the least of which were self-delusion, pride, and mental instability. By the fourth and fifth centuries it had begun to give way to cenobitic monasticism, an ordered community life for monks and nuns. This form of monasticism was popularized in the East by Basil the Great. Athanasius, Jerome, and John Cassian introduced monasticism into the West in the fourth century. Although Western monasticism was influenced by Eastern practices, it developed its own distinct character. It tended to be more practical, less austere, and more concerned with charity. The form of monastic life that eventually became dominant in the West was imported into Italy by Benedict in the sixth century. His *Rule* set the pattern for the communities he established. It became popular largely because it avoided extreme forms of asceticism and stressed contemplation, prayer, and manual labor. The extreme contempt of the world and exaggerated degradation of the body, imported into Christian piety and practice by asceticism, also introduced subtle changes in concepts of salvation and suffering. There was a tendency to see Christian suffering as contributing to salvation and to pursue suffering for expiatory ends. Although asceticism was to play an important role in Western culture through monasticism, the charitable and philanthropic impulse of the movement was to play a far more significant role in Christian attitudes toward sickness and suffering. There were still occasional voices in the fourth century that condemned the use of medicine, but this attitude lessened increasingly. As the church came to recognize the importance of secular medicine in caring for the needs of those who suffered, it was the monastic clergy who took the lead in administering medical care to those who required it by establishing hospitals as well as orphanages and homes for the poor and the aged. This brings us to a consideration of the second approach to healing in early Christianity: the use of secular medicine.

We have already seen the caution with which Basil the Great approached secular medicine, advising its employment only in two of his six categories of illness. But when writing to his physician he says, "It seems to me that he who would prefer your profession to all other of life's pursuits would make a proper choice" (*Epistle* 189).[15] With regard to medicine, two considerations were most important in Basil's mind: (1) God created the medical art to provide an analogy for Christians, "a model for the cure of the soul," "a parallel to the care given the soul," "an example for the proper care of the soul." That, in his opinion, is medicine's chief end and purpose. (2) Medicine should be employed in only two of his six categories of physical afflictions. Yet he writes that since "each of the arts is God's gift to us, remedying the deficiencies of nature . . . to reject entirely the benefits to be derived from this art is the sign of a pettish nature" (*The Long Rule* 55).[16]

Basil's nature was not pettish, nor was he as reluctant to provide medical care for the sick as it might appear. Indeed, he is often lauded as an exemplar of Christian charity for his founding in 372 of a vast charitable institution, the Basileias, which became the prototype of Christian hospitals and included, among other facilities, separate hospitals for those afflicted by contagious and noncontagious diseases. Gregory of Nazianzus refers to this institution as a place where illness became a school of wisdom, where disease is regarded in a religious light, where misery is changed to happiness, and where Christian charity shows its most striking proof (*On St. Basil* 63). Medical facilities were amply staffed by priests, physicians, and nurses.

It would be easy to be diverted into a discussion of the history of the foundation and development of Christian hospitals. Jerome's late-fourth-century account of his friend, a lady named Fabiola, establishing a hospital or infirmary in Rome, is well known. He tells in much detail of the devotion with which she gathered the sick from the public squares of the city and nursed the most wretched cases with her own hands (*Epistle* 77.6.1–2). The founding of Christian hospitals was a logical development of Christian charity. Christ's commandment to love your neighbor as yourself (Matt. 19:19; 22:39; Mark 12:31–33) was not simply a piece of advice, it was a categorical imperative. Love for one's neighbor can manifest itself in a variety of ways. But spiritual concern was never to take precedence over immediate material or physical help for those in need. This is bluntly stated in the Epistle of James: "Religion that is pure and undefiled before God and the Father is this: to visit orphans and widows in their afflictions" (1:27). Indeed, Christ's examples of charity include the following: "I was hungry and you gave me food, I was thirsty and you gave me drink, I was a stranger and you welcomed me, I was naked and you clothed me, I was sick and you visited me, I was in prison and you came to me. . . . As you did it to one of the least of these my brethren, you did it to me" (Matt. 25:35–40). "I was sick and you visited me." The verb here rendered "visited" also yields the meanings "to care for," "to be concerned about," and "to succor" and was sometimes used to refer to a physician's medical visitation of a patient.

That the visitation, care, and comfort of the sick became a duty incumbent upon all believers is repeatedly stressed in early Christian literature. Although it was urged upon all believers, in the course of time it became more and more the specific duty of deacons, deaconesses, and widows, and eventually came directly under the bishops' supervision as part of their responsibility. It was especially the mark of the very devout. In the words of Henry Sigerist, Christianity introduced

> the most revolutionary and decisive change in the attitude of society toward the sick. Christianity came into the world as the religion of healing, as the joyful Gospel of the Redeemer and of Redemption. It addressed itself to the disinherited, to the sick and afflicted, and promised them healing, a restoration both spiritual and physical. . . . It became the duty of the Christian to attend to the sick and poor of the community. . . . The social position of the sick man thus became fundamentally different from what it had been before. He assumed a preferential position which has been his ever since.[17]

During the outbreaks of plague in the mid-third century, Christians responded with a spectacular degree of activity on behalf of fellow Christians and pagans alike suffering from the pestilence. Their zeal was nearly suicidal, since death incurred in such a fashion was considered to rank with martyrdom (see Eusebius *Ecclesiastical History* 7.22.7–8). Dionysius, bishop of Alexandria, describes his flock's activities as "visiting the sick without a thought as to the danger, assiduously ministering to them, tending them in Christ, and so most gladly departing this life along with them" (ibid. 7.22.7).[18] Their activity stood in stark contrast to that of the pagans, who deserted the sick or threw the bodies of the afflicted out into the streets. Cyprian, in Carthage, saw the plague as beneficial because it "searches out the justice of each and every one and examines the minds of the human race, whether the well care for the sick . . . whether physicians do not desert the afflicted begging for help . . . whether the proud bend their necks, whether the shameless soften their affrontry . . ." (*Mortality* 16).[19] Mention should also be made of the Parabolani, a little-known group in the fourth century whose name means "the reckless ones" because of their primary duty of assisting the ill during epidemics.

On the one hand there was an imperative to extend care to the ill, while on the other hand there was a desire to leave the afflictions of this life and be with the Lord. Some Christians actively courted martyrdom, but more balanced minds condemned such activity as tantamount to suicide. It is sometimes suggested that early Christians were, if not sympathetic, at least neutral toward suicide and that it was Augustine who introduced a negative attitude toward it. But Clement of Alexandria in the second century flatly stated that the Christian "does not withdraw himself from life. For that is not permitted him" (*Stromateis* 6.9).[20] In the same century, Justin Martyr anticipated the hypothetical suggestion of the enemies of Christianity: "Go then all of you and kill yourselves, and pass even now to God, and do not trouble us." To this he responds, "If we do act thus, we ourselves will be opposing the will of God" (*Second Apology* 4).[21] Augustine was merely following this tradition when he wrote, "We are surrounded by evils which patience must endure until we come to where all good things are sources of inexpressible happiness and where there will be no longer anything to endure" (*City of God* 19.40).[22] Augustine's contrast of the inexpressible happiness of heaven with the evils of this world partakes of a common theme in early Christian authors who juxtaposed the Christian with the pagan on the question of attitude toward death. While pagans are thought of as fearing death, the Christian rejoices at the death of his loved ones and anticipates with eagerness his own day of "homegoing." The joys of heaven are often emphasized to show the folly of clinging to this life.

Augustine pointed to the irony that so many, when faced with troubles, cry out, "'Oh God, send me death; hasten my days.' Yet when sickness comes they run about, physicians are fetched, and money and rewards are promised" (*Sermon* 34.1).[23] Elsewhere he lamented at the things people will do to live a few days. When they are ill and the physicians have despaired of helping them, if some physician is able to cure them, they will give up the very sustenance of life to live a little longer (ibid. 344.5). But this was not what the Christians were to do. They were to put their faith in God, leave the results in God's hands, and not cling to life with desperation. Writing in a similar vein, Basil expressed succinctly what seems to be a quite balanced position, probably representing the mainstream of Christian thought of his time.

> Whatever requires an undue amount of thought or trouble or involves a large expenditure of effort and causes our whole life to revolve, as it were, around solicitude for the flesh must be avoided by Christians. Consequently, we must take great care to employ this medical art, if it should be necessary, not as making it wholly accountable for our state of health or illness, but as redounding to the glory of God (*The Long Rule* 55).[24]

Few references to Christian physicians are found in the period when Christians were a persecuted minority. Luke is said to have been a physician (Col. 4:14), and martyred Christian physicians are occasionally mentioned. In the fourth century Christianity displaced paganism, becoming first the favored and then the only tolerated religion. While Christianity remained a religion of conviction for some, it became a religion of convenience for many, and in the late empire there was a not entirely harmonious marriage of the new religion with the extremely varied cultural and intellectual strains of classical Mediterranean society, including that of medicine.

We know next to nothing about the effect of Christianity on actual medical practice. Christians who were also physicians may well have felt bound to apply to their practice the philanthropic and moral precepts of their religion. On the other hand, physicians who also happened to be Christians may have found their principles of conduct and responsibility less tempered by their religion. The extent of a physician's conformity to Christian ideals probably reflected the degree of his Christian conviction. We cannot expect the average physician of the period after the Christianization of the Empire to have acted much differently from the pagan counterpart of a few generations earlier, except that the religious pressures against abortion and active euthanasia may have deterred many nominally Christian physicians from such practices. But in late antiquity the physician who was also a fervent Christian might well have found his primary commitment to be to Christ and his secondary commitment to be to the medical art, the practice of the latter being a vehicle for presenting the former. Such were Zenobius and Hypatios, the former a priest and the latter a monk, physicians whose spiritual and medical interests blended into a common concern for the spiritually and physically ill. Around 375, Basil wrote a letter to the secular (but Christian) physician Eustathius, extolling him for his combination of the medical and spiritual: "And your profession is the supply vein of health. But, in your case especially, the science is ambidextrous, and you set for yourself higher standards of humanity, not limiting the benefit of your profession to bodily ills, but also contriving the correction of spiritual ills" (*Epistles* 189).[25] The extent to which secular physicians set for themselves these "higher standards of humanity" simply cannot be determined. But there is ample evidence that a growing number of priests or monks in late antiquity were also physicians.

THE MIDDLE AGES

During the thousand-year period called the Middle Ages, the relationship of Christianity and health, disease, and medicine was varied and complex. Christian attitudes and practices that prevailed at the end of classical antiquity did not change significantly. This continuity can be seen from three perspectives. First, throughout the Middle Ages either open or hidden tension between religion and medical practice remained. Second, several specific practices continued. Third, there was continuity between late antiquity and the early Middle Ages in some practices that, by the end of the period under consideration, were to change markedly, particularly as these practices were linked with facets of a society that was to undergo drastic social, cultural, economic, and political changes. Claims of miraculous healing continued throughout the Middle Ages. The clerical and especially the monastic medical practitioners of late antiquity grew in number and significance during the early Middle Ages, though these had diminished by the Reformation. There were secular physicians, at least nominally Christian, during the early Middle Ages, but we know little about them. During the later Middle Ages secular physicians began to increase in number and importance, and the practice of medicine emerged as a profession in a sense that it had never been before. The reaction of Roman Catholicism to the burgeoning secular medical profession during the late Middle Ages was without precedent in the church's attempts to limit and regulate practice, to influence and dictate medical ethics and moral responsibility, and to employ coercive measures to ensure compliance.

Gregory the Great (late sixth century), one of the most significant figures of the early Middle Ages, contributed much to the formation of the distinct character of early medieval Catholicism. He regarded sin as sometimes the immediate cause of illness and also recognized demonic activity. But he saw illness primarily as a form of training for the Christian. In his *Book of Pastoral Rule* (2.13) he instructed the clergy to encourage the sick with the comfort that in their affliction they should see proof of their being children of God, advice fully consistent with Heb. 12:5-8. He also stressed ascetic virtues and displayed belief in miracles associated with the veneration of saints and relics. He recommended to Augustine of Canterbury that he should exploit to the fullest the cult of saints and relics, since in its affinity with pagan pantheism it had great potential for helping to convert the English. Particularly because of its utility in missionary activity among the barbarians of northern Europe, the veneration of saints and relics expanded and remained vital north of the Alps, where the credulity of the barbarians was as strong as that of the Romans.

It is difficult to define the miraculous when one considers an environment in which miracles were thought to occur with such frequency that they were part of ordinary life. This did not lessen miracles being remarkable occurrences which evoked great excitement and joy; usually the miracles recorded (their number is astronomical) involved the relief of human suffering by the healing of disease or defect. Throughout the Middle Ages a thriving practice of and fervent belief in miraculous healings associated with the veneration of saints and relics continued. A well-known medievalist writes of the twelfth century: "In a society dependent on miracles for much that made life tolerable, it was hard to be a skeptic for long. Miracles were the main arguments in establishing truth in the pre-scholastic age."[26] But even in the epistemologically more refined climate of the later, scholastic Middle Ages, the belief in and recording of miracles was as great as, if not greater than, ever before. Closely related to the veneration of saints and relics was the popularity of pilgrimages, a practice which, having begun in late antiquity, maintained its strong appeal beyond the close of the Middle Ages. Pilgrimages involved travel to one of the great shrines, often in hope of either being healed or witnessing a miracle. Particularly during the late Middle Ages, much fraud was involved in many of the smaller and less famous shrines where mechanical devices were sometimes quite ingeniously contrived to deceive the pious.

Occasionally, voices of skepticism were raised against some practices. These varied from a specific skepticism about a particular shrine to a more general skepticism about the whole range of reported miraculous occurrences. In the former category are many of those voices within medieval Catholicism that yearned for the *renovatio*, reform within the bounds of accepted orthodoxy. In the latter category are those such as Jan Hus (1374–1415), whose attempts at reform struck so deeply at the core of contemporary Catholicism that he appeared heretical in his denunciation of what he regarded as gross abuses, including allegedly miraculous performances under the auspices of corrupt clergy. Some people, little concerned about reform, were simply skeptical about a particular saint or relic or shrine. Many tales record that for their sometimes outspoken contempt for a specific miraculous power, skeptics would be quite spectacularly converted by a retributive miracle that afflicted them with disease, deformity, blindness, dumbness, crippling, madness, or death. After sufficient time for contrition, the saint or relic responsible for the affliction would perform a healing miracle to undo the effects of the retributive miracle, except for those smitten with death (although there were undoubtedly exceptions here too).

Early Christianity Through the Middle Ages

Not every skeptic was struck; many, of course, were not. For example, a local chronicler in the thirteenth century who recorded Saint Wulfstan's miracles mentioned a parish priest of Worcestershire, whom he describes as being "of frivolous turn of mind . . . and quite unlike other men"[27] because he did not believe in Saint Wulfstan's miracles, but would recommend to his sick parishioners medical treatment such as herbs and phlebotomy. To this chronicler, the priest's actions simply betrayed his skepticism. It was not uncommon, however, to have some medical treatment administered by the clergy at major shrines, particularly at pilgrimage centers, many of which possessed excellent medical libraries. These pilgrimage shrines must have presented pathetic sights. Crowds of the crippled, ill, and dying filled these great centers; many remained until they either died or recovered. The fact that in some instances medical aid was given by clergy who had some knowledge of medicine is completely in accord with the New Testament injunction to minister to the sick as an act of Christian charity, an imperative that led some clergy in late antiquity to practice medicine gratis for the destitute, as we have already seen. The medical charity of the clergy both in late antiquity and throughout the Middle Ages may well have been connected with shrines devoted to miraculous occurrences.

By the early Middle Ages, our sources, which are by then almost entirely clerical, reveal a strong emphasis on the practice of medical charity by the clergy, especially by monks. A clear distinction must be made here between monastic medical care for monks and that for the laity. A chapter from the *Rule of Saint Benedict* (sixth century) is often cited by scholars as evidence for an obligation to care for those among the laity who are sick. The passage reads in part:

> Before all things and above all things care must be taken of the sick, so that they may be served in very deed as Christ himself; for he said: "I was sick and ye visited me;" and "what you did to one of these least ones, ye did unto me." But let the sick on their part consider that they are being served for the honour of God, and not provoke their brethren who are serving them by their unreasonable demands. Yet they should be patiently borne with, because from such as these is gained a more abundant reward. Therefore let the abbot take the greatest care that they suffer no neglect. For these sick brethren let there be assigned a special room and an attendant who is God-fearing, diligent, and careful. . . . Let the abbot take the greatest care that the sick be not neglected by the cellarers and attendants; for he must answer for all the misdeeds of his disciples (chap. 36).

The Historical Setting

The concern here is clearly with the care of sick monks; nothing is said or even implied about any obligation to the general populace. However, the cellarer, who is made largely responsible in the above passage for the care of his sick brothers, is admonished elsewhere in the *Rule* to "take the greatest care of the sick, of children, or guests, and of the poor, knowing without doubt that he will have to render an account for all these on the Day of Judgement" (chap. 31).[28] The "children, guests, and poor" in this context certainly are not monks, nor is care for "the sick" limited to them. Still this is far from a concise articulation of a monastic obligation to succor the ill of the lay community at large.

A more general obligation to treat the sick is recommended by Cassiodorus, also in the sixth century. After leaving the court of the Ostrogothic kings of Italy to pursue a religious life, Cassiodorus founded a monastery. In his *Introduction to Divine and Human Readings*, he wrote to those of his monks who were also physicians:

> I salute you, distinguished brothers, who with sedulous care look after the health of the human body and perform the functions of blessed piety for those who flee to the shrines of holy men—you who are sad at the sufferings of others, sorrowful for those who are in danger, grieved at the pain of those who are received, and always distressed with personal sorrow at the misfortunes of others, so that, as experiences of your art teaches, you help the sick with genuine zeal; you will receive your reward from him by whom eternal rewards may be paid for temporal acts. Learn, therefore, the properties of herbs and perform the compounding of drugs punctiliously; but do not place your hope in herbs and do not trust health to human counsels. For although the art of medicine is found to be established by the Lord, he who without doubt grants life to men makes them sound. For it is written: "And whatsoever you do in word or deed, do all in the name of the Lord Jesus, giving thanks to God and the Father by Him."

He then pointed out various medical authors whose works he had "stored away in the recesses of our library" (1.31).[29]

There is abundant and irrefutable evidence that in the early Middle Ages, both in the Latin West and in contemporary Byzantine society, monasteries became the refuge of the sick, the poor, and the persecuted. Our primary sources supply many examples of monastic medical care of the laity. Although the monastic clergy undoubtedly took the lead in giving medical assistance and establishing and maintaining charitable institutions such as *xenodochia* and hospices, the secular clergy sometimes knew medicine and extended medical care to the destitute as a good work.[30] A commonly cited example is Bishop Masona of Merida, who in the sixth century founded a *xenodochium*, staffed it with physicians, and sent his clergy out to find patients, making no distinction between Christian and Jew, slave and free (*De vitis patrum Emeritensium* 4). Numerous similar illustrations attest to the underlying philanthropic basis of monastic and clerical medicine.

Medical practice by the clergy continued throughout the Middle Ages. In addition, many medical treatises were written by priests or monks in order to help the poor. One of the most famous is the *Thesaurus pauperum* (A Treasury for the Poor), which listed simple but salubrious herbs that could be gathered in the fields. The probable author, Peter Hispanus, became pope in 1276 under the name John XXI. A medical treatise from the thirteenth century was written by "a sinner, but by the grace of God, a member of a religious order" to instruct his fellow clerics so that they could treat the poor gratis. They could receive fees from the rich.[31]

The latter stipulation raised problems that precipitated ecclesiastical legislation often misinterpreted by modern scholars as forbidding medical or surgical practice to the clergy in the later Middle Ages. A recent study has demonstrated that at no time during the Middle Ages were clergy generally forbidden to practice medicine; the practice of surgery was forbidden only to clergy in major orders.[32] The first piece of conciliar legislation incorporated into officially codified canon law concerned those clergy who lived under a rule; they were called regular clergy or religious, that is, monks and canons regular. These clergy were bound by a vow of stability; that is, they had an obligation of residence. They were merely forbidden to leave their cloisters to *study* medicine or secular law. The second piece of legislation extended these prohibitions to clergy having specific spiritual functions and to those possessing benefices. The third removed the prohibition from clergy having parochial churches, while the fourth, addressed only to regular clergy, permitted their departure for study if permission was first obtained from their prelates with the consent of the majority of the members of their religious house.[33] The practice of surgery was forbidden by the Fourth Lateran Council in 1215 (canon 18 = *Decretales* 3.50.9) only to clergy in major orders but not minor orders, probably because those in major orders would have been most severely affected by incurring a canonical irregularity, a likely possibility when a patient might die following surgery.

This is not to suggest that ecclesiastical authorities were unconcerned about clerics practicing medicine and surgery. They were troubled about two matters in particular, the first being relatively minor, the second more significant. Both are mentioned in the text of a canon from the Second Lateran Council of 1139 (canon 9). The first is that in medical practice it is likely that a clergyman will encounter sights not proper for him. "Since an impure eye is the messenger of an impure heart, those things about which good people blush to speak, religion ought not to treat." But more important, "the care of souls being neglected and the purposes of their order being set aside, they promise health in return for detestable money and thus make themselves physicians of human bodies."[34] This canon actually forbad the *practice* of medicine by regular clergy, but was of little consequence since it was never incorporated into medieval canon law. It does, however, show an uneasiness that those religious who practice medicine might encounter inappropriate and unseemly things. Yet the great concern was the possibility of an avaricious motive for practicing medicine. This was an era of great social change, one in which there was a significant increase in a wide variety of commercial and professional activities. The church was greatly concerned about the spiritual aspects of commercial activity in general and the involvement of clergy in secular matters in particular.

In the twelfth century a change within the traditional order of the cardinal vices occurred. In both theological and popular conceptions, the sin of avarice was displacing pride as the supreme vice. This change affected attitudes toward the secular activities of the clergy. From the earliest period of the church, the clergy had engaged in secular pursuits. Gradually one criterion came to be applied in determining whether any activity was within the bounds of propriety: Was it undertaken for service or for selfish gain? Small wonder that the clergy's involvement in many walks of life, including medicine, diminished in a society that was rapidly changing from a primarily rural to a much more urbanized economy, in a climate in which commercial and economic activities were increasing in variety and intensity, in an environment in which professions in a relatively modern rather than an ancient sense were burgeoning, in which guilds contributed much to the regulation and universities to the outlook of society, and in which life generally was marked by an increasing laicization and secularization. The same conditions that contributed to a decrease in the clergy's practice of medicine in the late Middle Ages also caused the church to look afresh at secular medical practice.

Contrary to what is sometimes directly asserted about the relationship between medieval Catholicism and science, at no time has the church or any of its leading dignitaries evinced an openly hostile attitude toward (much less an official condemnation of) the practice of medicine per se. The number within the church who have expressed absolute and unequivocal contempt for secular medicine under any circumstance have been small. Of somewhat larger number are those who have made statements that can be interpreted as condemning medical practice. A good example is Gregory of Tours (sixth century), whose enthusiasm for the miracles wrought at the shrine of Saint Martin knew no bounds. He was often delighted to heighten his audience's appreciation of the spectacular nature of a particular healing by describing in detail the sorry attempts of physicians and their abysmal failure and despair in contrast with the efficacy of Saint Martin's miraculous intervention. But when his tales of the failure of physicians, used as a foil to Saint Martin's miracles, are culled from his writings to illustrate early medieval attitudes toward medicine, they do not give a balanced picture even of Gregory's attitude. He himself enlisted the help of physicians and recommended to others that under certain circumstances they do likewise.

Nevertheless, that tension between Christianity and medicine did exist and must be emphasized. The relationship between the cure of the soul and the care of the body was too close for the most active adherents of Christianity to remain neutral to the potential of medicine for good or for ill. During the Middle Ages, even when a physician was not a particularly committed Christian, the expectations of a predominantly Christian society tempered his conduct.

The medical literature that has survived from the early Middle Ages is extensive and diverse and ranges from general surveys of medical knowledge to treatises dealing with specific areas of medicine. Some manuscripts contain treatises dealing with medical etiquette and ethics. While it is impossible to determine the audience for which these were intended, it is highly probable that they were composed by monks in an attempt to articulate ideals of character and conduct for medical practitioners, whether clerical or secular.[35] One manuscript from the eighth century exhorted physicians to serve the rich and the poor alike, looking for eternal rather than material rewards. This treatise ended with the exhortation: "Aid the sick, your reward coming from Christ, for whoever gives a cup of cold water in his name is assured of the eternal kingdom. . . ." Another manuscript, this one from the ninth century, urged the physician to "take care of rich and poor, slave and free equally, for among all such people medicines are needed." By the twelfth century deontological treatises were being written by secular physicians. While their tone is eminently practical, they are not without Christian sentiment. The area in which secular physicians probably felt the most pressure was in the practice of medical charity, a matter discussed at length in the deonto-logical treatises.

The imperative to charity is strongly expressed in the theological litera-ture, and frequent discussions of it are found in the medico-ethical treatises of the late Middle Ages. The charge that physicians are greedy is an extremely durable prejudice, and medieval practitioners were quite sensitive to it, at least in their writings. That physicians were also unreligious was a common belief in the late Middle Ages and was often expressed by the adage *"Tres medici, duo athei"* (Out of three physicians, two will be atheists). Thus Juhn Mirfield, an English cleric who wrote about but did not practice medicine, commented in 1404:

> The physician, if he should happen to be a good Christian (which rarely chances, for by their works they show themselves to be disciples, not of Christ, but of Avicenna and of Galen), ought to cure a Christian patient without making even the slightest charge if the man is poor; for the life of such a man ought to be of more value to the physician than his money.[36]

The surgeon Henri de Mondeville (late thirteenth and early fourteenth centuries) complained that when the sick come to the surgeon mas-querading as paupers,

> they claim that charity is a flower when they find someone else who will help the poor, and thus think that a surgeon should help the unfortunate; they, however, would never be bound by this rule. . . . I tell these people, then pay me for yourself and for three paupers and I will help them as well as you. But they never answer me, and I have never found a person in any position, whether clerk or layman, who was rich enough, or honest enough to pay what he had promised until I made him do so.[37]

Mondeville advised that surgeons should be medical Robin Hoods: ". . . The surgeon ought to charge the rich man as much as possible and get all he can out of them, provided that he does all that he can to cure the poor."[38] His motive for extending charity to the poor was more than the advantage that might accrue to his reputation and to the honor of the profession. Enlightened self-interest combined with an appreciation of eternal perspectives for a result fully compatible with the theology of his time:

> You, then, surgeons, if you operate conscientiously upon the rich for a sufficient fee and upon the poor for charity, you ought not to fear the

ravages of fire, nor of rain nor of wind; you need not take holy orders or make pilgrimages nor undertake any work of that kind, because by your science you can save your souls alive, live without poverty, and die in your house.[39]

During the last two centuries of the Middle Ages, Europe was devastated by various attacks of plague. In response, many physicians wrote tractates that were usually concerned with prophylaxis, although some dealt with treatment. Several of these appear to have been written as a genuine expression of Christian charity. For example, John of Burgundy (fourteenth century) closed his tractate with the following words: "Moved by piety and anguished by and feeling sorrow because of this calamity . . . I have composed and compiled this work not for a price but for your prayers, so that when anyone recovers from the diseases discussed above, he will effectively pray for me to our Lord God. . . ." Francischino de Collignano (fourteenth century) wrote that he was moved "by pure love, by affection and charity for all the citizens and especially for friends," while Michael Boeti (fifteenth century) wrote his tractate "in response to the requests of certain of my friends, for the service of God and for the common good." Not only did the authors of the plague tractates write them generally without thought of profit, but they attempted to make their advice employable by the poor as well as the well-to-do. Many of the tractates listed for the various recommended substances, both prophylactic and curative, alternatives readily available to the poor.[40]

Guilds or colleges of physicians and surgeons also performed acts of medical charity in the late Middle Ages as a part of their obligation to the community. In this regard it is important to be aware of a significant change in the very basis for the practice of medicine. If one development were to be identified as the single most important element in the social history of medicine, it might well be the change from the practice of medicine as a right to a privilege. This change occurred in the late Middle Ages, brought about by movements from both outside and within the medical profession. It involved the imposition of licensure requirements by secular or ecclesiastical authorities in an attempt to protect the public from charlatans, and the organization of medical and surgical guilds (including universities) by practitioners in an effort to secure and protect a monopoly in providing medical and surgical service. The latter is also a form of licensure. The earliest instance of medical licensure was that imposed by Roger II of Sicily in 1140 and strengthened in 1231 by his grandson, Frederick II. This was unlike developments elsewhere in

The Historical Setting

Europe, where tradesmen (artisans, merchants, physicians, and professors) were organizing themselves into guilds, gaining charters from municipal, royal, or ecclesiastical authorities, and guaranteeing standards of quality of goods or services in exchange for the privilege of holding a monopoly in their particular service or commodity. Whether imposed from above, as was the case in Sicily, or sought by the physicians or surgeons themselves, as was happening elsewhere, the limiting of practice to a group who could ensure competence was, as the original documents indicate, always claimed to be for the public good.

The church was often involved in both granting and protecting medical or surgical guild monopolies. In this regard it must be borne in mind that medieval society was, with the exception of a small number of Jews and heretics, exclusively Roman Catholic. Since there was only one church of which everyone was a member, it was thus both able and, from a medieval perspective, obliged to exercise coercive jurisdiction over areas of life that now would be the concern of either secular authority or individual conscience. Although we shall later discuss the church's efforts in the second category, it is the first that concerns us here. Not only was the church involved in the granting of charters of monopoly to medical and surgical guilds or *collegia* or universities, as was the case, for instance, at Montpellier, but it was also the authority to which appeal was often made in the enforcement of monopoly privileges, whether the original charter had been granted by secular authority or by ecclesiastical authority. An example of the church's involvement in enforcement is Paris, where both the medical and surgical corporations maintained a constant struggle against practice by unlicensed practitioners.[41] They frequently appealed to ecclesiastical courts, which would hear the case and either excommunicate the defendant or threaten excommunication for a second offense. Often the alleged charlatans were women: the court records make interesting reading, as witness after witness testifies that the "quack" in question treated and cured them and provided them with comfort when the licensed physicians had failed. Since the cases never involved efficacy of treatment but rather legal right to practice, the accused were invariably found guilty and either excommunicated or threatened with excommunication in the event of a second offense. (It must be remembered that in medieval society excommunication affected every area of one's life and was a much more serious affair than in a pluralistic society.) The unlicensed practitioners and their erstwhile patients may well evoke our sympathies, especially given the generally ineffective nature of the licensed physicians' highly academic and, from a modern perspective, fatuous methods of treatment. Nevertheless, ecclesiastical authorities were legitimately concerned with the danger to the public that would ensue if there were no restrictions on medical and surgical practice. Licensure guaranteed competence if, and only if, competence was measured by standards of education rather than efficacy of treatment. And the church clearly supported the former criterion.

The church also attempted through a variety of means to prevent Christians from obtaining medical or surgical services from Jews and Muslims. While this might strike the reader as reprehensible, in light of the concern of medieval Catholicism with the potential for spiritual harm in medical practice and because a greater importance was given to the cure of the soul than to the care of the body, restriction of medical practice on Christians to Christians is understandable. Indeed, failure to attempt to institute and enforce such a policy would have been irresponsible, since the spiritual obligations of the physician to patients were of central importance to ecclesiastical authorities. Not that the church wished for physicians of the body to minister to the spiritual needs of patients; this was a responsibility of the physicians of the soul such as the pastoral clergy. Rather, the church was concerned that medical practitioners do nothing by commission or omission to harm the spiritual state of their patients.

We have mentioned above that in the late Middle Ages the church was involved in areas now exclusively under secular authority or in the realm of individual conscience. In the latter category there were concerns that during the early Middle Ages had been covered by penitential literature and procedures. The Penitentials were stark lists of sins with the appropriate penance specified for each offense. By the late twelfth century they appeared outdated and inconsistent with a society that was becoming significantly different from that of the early Middle Ages. In addition, at the Fourth Lateran Council (1215) there a canon was adopted (canon 21) which became part of canon law (*Decretales* 5.38.12). It required, under pain of excommunication, annual confession to one's own priest. This canon, along with slightly earlier concerns of moral theologians, gave rise to a large quantity of literature: confessional manuals and more extensive casuistic discussions generally called *Summae confessorum*, dating from the early fourteenth century to well beyond the end of the Middle Ages. Confessional examination penetrated every area of domestic, social, and economic life. Many of the sins peculiar to various occupations are included in the latter category. Earlier moral theologians had been concerned with the moral implications of various occupations, including medical practice. In this section we shall give a brief synthesis of the discussion of the sins of physicians and surgeons contained in several of the *Summae confessorum* of the last two centuries of the Middle Ages.[42] It should be borne in mind that these *summae* were intended as tools to aid the priest in interrogation of penitents by providing questions designed to uncover and deal with specific sins.

Several *summae* stressed the responsibility not to practice unless one is competent. One *summa* asserted that physicians must be expert in the art by accepted standards of expertness and that simply having a doctorate is not sufficient. Practicing without the necessary competence, even if one were licensed, was a sin. If a physician harmed a patient from ignorance, whether by omission or commission, it was a sin. Harming a patient by negligence was defined as a sin, as was experimenting on patients, particularly on the poor or religious. Keeping abreast of medical literature and techniques was a physician's responsibility, as was consulting with colleagues when in doubt. Rash treatment was condemned. Physicians in doubt about the effects of a particular medicine should leave the patient in God's hands rather than expose him or her to the danger of the medicine. Surgeons in doubt about the need for an operation or about their own ability to perform it should leave the patient in God's hands also. The physician sinned who intentionally failed to administer an effective medicine that cured quickly in order to prolong the illness and make more money.

A small number of the *summae* discussed relations with colleagues only with regard to mutual envy and disparagement as well as pride. Relations with paramedical groups such as apothecaries were described. They were not to include partnerships for profit, and a physician was not to receive commissions from apothecaries or send patients to those whose competence was doubtful.

The *summae* were very concerned with fees. Physicians sinned who demanded excessive fees, especially from the poor. Further, the physician's obligations to care were clearly delineated. That the physician was not to desert patients, even if there were virtually no hope of recovery, was stressed. It was a sin, however, for physicians to cause unnecessary expenses or promise to cure when they could not. The question of treating the poor gratis arose and was resolved generally by following a principle enunciated by Thomas Aquinas: Since "no man is sufficient to bestow a work of mercy on all those who need it," charity ought first to be given to those with whom one is united in any way. Otherwise, if a person "stands in such a need that it is not easy to see how he can be succored otherwise, then one is bound to bestow the work of mercy on him." Accordingly, a physician was not obligated always to treat the destitute, "or else he would have to put aside all other business and occupy himself entirely" with treating the poor (*Summa Theologica* 2–2.71.1). Most *summae*, following Aquinas, indicated that the physician must treat the poor gratis if it were clearly seen that they would otherwise die. A more difficult case involved the question whether to treat a sick man who was not willing to pay, rather than let him die. The physician sinned who did not undertake his care, even paying for the medicines. If the miser recovered, the physician had the legal right to demand a fee from him; if he died then from his heirs. To refrain from treating such a person was a sin, even if the sick person positively refused treatment, since insanity could then be assumed.

Several matters are subsumed under the rubric of spiritual obligations, matters in which the physician's interest in the health of the body could differ from the church's interest in the health of the soul. A canon promulgated at the Fourth Lateran Council (1215; canon 22 = *Decretales* 5.38.13) stated:

> Since bodily infirmity is sometimes caused by sin, the Lord saying to the sick man whom he had healed: "Go and sin no more, lest some worse thing happen to thee" (John 5:14), we declare in the present decree and strictly command that when physicians of the body are called to the bedside of the sick, before all else they admonish them to call for the physician of souls, so that after spiritual health has been restored to them, the application of bodily medicine may be of greater benefit, for the cause being removed the effect will pass away. We publish this decree for the reason that some, when they are sick and are advised by the physician in the course of the sickness to attend to the salvation of their soul, give up all hope and yield more easily to the danger of death. If any physician shall transgress this decree after it has been published by the bishops, let him be cut off from the church till he has made suitable satisfaction for his transgression. And since the soul is far more precious than the body, we forbid under penalty of anathema that a physician advise a patient to have recourse to sinful means for the recovery of bodily health.[43]

Two important points are raised here, the first involving the physician's obligation to call a confessor for a patient before undertaking treatment, the second prohibiting a physician from recommending for bodily health recourse to sinful means. In the case of the second, the *summae* specified as sin a physician's advising fornication, masturbation, incantation, consumption of intoxicating beverages, breaking the church's fasts, or eating meat on forbidden days. Recommending or practicing abortion and active euthanasia received little attention in the *summae* under "sins of physicians," probably because during the period under consideration a woman seeking an abortion would likely have turned to another woman such as a midwife rather than to a male physician, and active euthanasia would have been regarded simply and obviously as homicide. In connection with the canon from Lateran IV quoted above, the *summae* stated that if physicians did not inform a terminally ill patient of his condition they sinned for two reasons: (1) patients, if informed of impending death, regardless of their spiritual state, would be able to improve it in the face of death; (2) patients may also then make wills, thus saving their heirs from undue strife.

The stipulation that the physician must "before all else," when called to the bedside of the sick, "admonish them to call for the physicians of souls" creates the most problematic area in the relationship of medical practitioners with the Catholic church during the late Middle Ages. Two reasons are given for this requirement. The first is that confession has a curative effect and thus will sometimes make the physicians' attendance unnecessary and otherwise more effective. Secondly, if it is commonly assumed that physicians advise the calling of a confessor only when they despair of their patients' recovery, patients thus advised will give up all hope. In their attempts to interpret this canon so that the confessor could intelligently interrogate a physician penitent, the authors of the *summae* raised and discussed a variety of questions, including: (1) Does this provision that the physician recommend the calling of a confessor for each new patient apply to every new case a physician undertakes? (2) Is the physician responsible to ensure a patient's compliance? (3) If the patient is unwilling to call a confessor, must the physician withdraw from treatment? Some *summae* stated that this canon applied only in the case of serious illness or injury, and some even specified or gave examples of illnesses in which it would apply and those in which it would not. Others stipulated simply that it must be done in all cases; if the patient refused to comply with the advice, the physician must withdraw from the case. One writes that since the Christian is bound to do good even to the bad and to the unjust, the physician was obligated to treat the patient even if he or she refused to comply with the admonition.

Physicians undoubtedly had strong opinions on the question of having their patients call a confessor, but relatively little record of their attitudes appears to have survived. Some, however, are known. Even before this canon was promulgated, one anonymous deontological treatise, written in the twelfth century (probably by an Italian physician), suggested the following to fellow physicians:

> When you reach his house and before you see him, ask if he has seen his confessor. If he has not done so, have him either do it or promise to do it. For if he hears mention of this after you have examined him and have considered the signs of the disease, he will begin to despair of recovery, because he will think that you despair of it too.[44]

The author, of course, was a member of a society in which belief in the necessity of confession before death was deeply ingrained. While he may not have considered it especially his own spiritual duty to look after his patient's spiritual as well as physical health, he must have considered the alternative, that is, advising the patient to confess only when in dire straits, to be potentially dangerous to the patient. The action recommended by this physician and the motivation behind it are identical to those of the canon of Lateran IV, except that the latter includes an additional motivation: Since sickness is often caused by sin, the act of confession will itself have a curative effect that will either render the physician's care unnecessary or make it more effective.

The advice on confession that appeared in a treatise attributed to the physician Arnold of Villanova (late thirteenth and early fourteenth centuries) significantly differed in emphasis from that in the anonymous twelfth-century piece just quoted:

> When you come to a house, inquire before you go to the sick whether he has confessed, and if he has not, he should immediately or promise you that he will confess immediately, and this must not be neglected because many illnesses originate on account of sin and are cured by the Supreme Physician after having been purified from squalor by the tears of contrition, according to what is said in the Gospel: "Go, and sin no more, lest something worse happens to you."[45]

This version, written after Lateran IV, strikingly resembles part of the canon, even quoting the same Scripture verse; it demonstrates the direct influence of a constitution of canon law on a strictly secular piece of deontological literature. Whether this is simply lip service to ecclesiastical authority or whether this reflects genuine approbation of the underlying principle upon which the legislation was based must remain an open question. The surgeon Henri de Mondeville (late thirteenth and early fourteenth centuries) wrote: "Do not let the patient be concerned about any business except about spiritual matters only, such as confession and his will and arranging similar affairs in accordance with the rules (*documenta*) of the catholic faith."[46] It should be observed that Mondeville mentions, along with confession, the matter of a will, a requirement included in the *summae* but not in the canon under consideration from Lateran IV. The author of an anonymous plague tractate composed in 1411 gave some advice that demonstrated that he was familiar with and faithful to the provisions of this canon:

> If it is certain from the symptoms that it is actually pestilence that has afflicted the patient, the physician first must advise the patient to set himself right with God by making a will and by making a confession of his sins, as is set forth according to the Decretals: since a corporal illness comes not only from a fault of the body but also from a spiritual failing as the Lord declares in the gospel and the priests also tell us.[47]

Returning to the *summae*, the diversity of opinions that they expressed about the canon under consideration showed that by the early sixteenth century there was no uniformity either of practice or interpretation of this canon. In 1566, incidentally, Pope Pius V promulgated his constitution *Super gregem*, which specified that physicians were to discontinue their treatment of a patient after the third day if he or she failed to produce a document signed by a confessor certifying that the patient had duly confessed. Physicians violating this rule were to be declared in disgrace, denied the privilege of practicing, and ejected from their university or medical and surgical associations. This tightening of the requirement took place after the Reformation, and thus is beyond the purview of the present chapter; hence only those physicians and surgeons who were Roman Catholics were affected.

What effect might the concerns of the church, expressed in the *Summae Confessorum*, have had on medical practice? We must bear in mind that during the period under consideration there was, in the Latin West, only one church. The willing or unwilling allegiance of nearly the entire population of Western Europe, combined with the universal prestige of the church's institutions, enabled it to exercise coercive authority by promulgating laws that were expected to be obeyed. The extent to which the confessional influenced conduct cannot be gauged with certainty. There was an absolute necessity of annual confession. The church had and duly exercised the authority "to loose and to bind." Forgiveness and certification of confession were given only to those who satisfied the requirements of the confessional. We may tend to think that the primary threat to the recalcitrant was the danger of eternal consequences, but at that time excommunication affected everyday life. Excommunication was especially important to anyone in a licensed profession since it caused the privilege of exercising the vocation granted by the license to be revoked and thus deprived one of a livelihood. Annual confession must also have been a powerful means of social control. The stated goal of confession was not only the forgiveness of known sins but also the correction of sinful practices and education of the laity to increase their sensitivity to previously unknown sins, both of commission and omission. The best confession was regarded as one that produced a life altered to conform as closely as possible to the expectations and standards of the church.

NOTES

1. Discussed in Chapter 3, p. 88.

2. See Evelyn Frost, *Christian Healing: A Consideration of the Place of Spiritual Healing in the Church of Today in the Light of the Doctrine and Practice of the Ante-Nicene Church*, 2d ed. (London: A. R. Mowbray, 1954), pp. 204–5; and Victor G. Dawe, "The Attitude of the Ancient Church Toward Sickness and Healing" (Ph.D. diss., Boston University School of Theology, 1955), p. 130.

3. Alexander Roberts and James Donaldson, eds., *The Ante-Nicene Fathers* (Buffalo: Christian Literature Publishing Co., 1885–96).

4. From the Loeb Classical Library translation by Krisopp Lake and J. E. L. Oulton (Cambridge, Mass.: Harvard University Press, 1926–32).

5. *The Fathers of the Church: A New Translation* (Washington, D.C.: Catholic University of America Press, 1947–).

6. Ibid.

7. Ibid.

8. Ibid.

9. In *Ante-Nicene Fathers*.

10. Ibid.

11. *A Select Library of the Nicene and Post-Nicene Fathers of the Christian Church* (various publishers, 1887–1900).

12. A. H. M. Jones, *The Later Roman Empire, 284–602: A Social, Economic, and Administrative Survey*, 2 vols. (Norman: University of Oklahoma Press, 1964).

13. In *Fathers of the Church*.

14. I. G. Smith, "Monastery," in *A Dictionary of Christian Antiquities*, ed. William Smith and Samuel Cheetham (London, 1880), p. 1219.

15. In *Fathers of the Church*.

16. Ibid.

17. Henry Sigerist, *Civilization and Disease* (Ithaca: Cornell University Press, 1943), pp. 69–70.

18. Loeb Classical Library translation.

19. In *Fathers of the Church*.

20. In *Ante-Nicene Fathers*.

21. In *Fathers of the Church*.

22. Ibid.

23. In *Nicene and Post-Nicene Fathers*.

24. In *Fathers of the Church*.

25. Ibid.

26. R. W. Southern, *Medieval Humanism* (New York: Harper & Row, 1970), p. 137.

27. Quoted by Jonathan Sumption, *Pilgrimage: An Image of Mediaeval Religion* (Totowa, N.J.: Rowman & Littlefield, 1975), p. 61.

28. Translation by Justin McCann, *Saint Benedict* (New York: Sheed & Ward, 1937).

29. Translation by Leslie Webber Jones, in *An Introduction to Divine and Human Readings* (New York: Columbia University Press, 1946).

30. To avoid any semantic confusion, one should note that secular clergy were those who were in orders but not living under a rule, thus not monks. A member of the secular clergy who practiced medicine would not be a secular physician (i.e., a physician who was not a member of the clergy) but rather a clerical physician who was a cleric but not a monk.

31. C. H. Talbot, *Medicine in Medieval England* (New York: American Elsevier, 1968), p. 96.

32. Darrel W. Amundsen, "Medieval Canon Law on Medical and Surgical Practice by the Clergy," *Bulletin of the History of Medicine* 52 (1978): 22–44. In major or holy orders were subdeacons, deacons, and priests; in minor orders were porters, acolytes, exorcists, and lectors.

33. The first two are included in the *Decretales* of Gregory IX, promulgated in 1234 (3.50.3 and 3.50.10); the third and fourth are in the *Liber Sextus* of Boniface VIII, promulgated in 1298 (3.24.1 and 3.24.2).

34. H. J. Schroeder, trans., *Disciplinary Decrees of the General Councils* (St. Louis: B. Herder Book Co., 1937), pp. 201–2.

35. Translation in Loren C. MacKinney, "Medical Ethics and Etiquette in the Early Middle Ages: The Persistence of Hippocratic Ideals," *Bulletin of the History of Medicine* 26 (1952): 1–31.

36. P. H. S. Hartley and H. R. Aldridge, *Johannes de Mirfeld of St. Bartholomew's, Smithfield: His Life and Works* (London, 1936), p. 132.

37. Translation in Mary Catherine Welborn, "The Long Tradition: A Study in Fourteenth-Century Medical Deontology," in *Medieval and Historiographical Essays in Honor of James Westfall Thompson*, ed. J. L. Cate and E. N. Anderson (Chicago: University of Chicago Press, 1938), p. 356.

38. Translation in E. A. Hammond, "Incomes of Medieval English Doctors," *Journal of the History of Medicine and Allied Sciences* 15 (1960): 156.

39. Ibid.

40. Darrel W. Amundsen, "Medical Deontology and Pestilential Disease in the Late Middle Ages," *Journal of the History of Medicine and Allied Sciences* 32 (1977): 418–19.

41. See the discussion by Pearl Kibre, "The Faculty of Medicine at Paris, Charlatanism and Unlicensed Medical Practices in the Later Middle Ages," *Bulletin of the History of Medicine* 27 (1953): 1–20.

42. For a more thorough analysis, see Darrel W. Amundsen, "Casuistry and Professional Obligations: The Regulation of Physicians by the Court of Conscience in the Late Middle Ages," *Transactions and Studies of the College of Physicians of Philadelphia* 3 (1982): 22–39, 93–112.

43. Translated by Schroeder, *Disciplinary Decrees*, p. 236.

44. Latin text in S. DeRenzi, *Collectio Salernitana* (Naples, 1852–57), 2:74.

45. Translation in Henry E. Sigerist, "Bedside Manners in the Middle Ages: The Treatise *De Cautelis Medicorum* Attributed to Arnald of Villanova," *Quarterly Bulletin of the Northwestern University Medical School* 20 (1946): 141.

46. Latin text in Paul Diepgen, *Die Theologie und der ärztliche Stand* (Berlin: Grunewald, 1922), p. 51, n. 287.

47. Translation in Amundsen, "Medical Deontology," p. 416.

5

Medicine and Christianity in the Modern World

RONALD L. NUMBERS
and
RONALD C. SAWYER

The medical world of the early sixteenth century, at the dawn of the modern era, bore greater resemblance to that of antiquity than to what we know today. Physicians understood little about the cure of disease and even less about its cause. Hospitals provided solace and shelter but scarcely any therapy. Medical science remained firmly in the grasp of ancient authorities. Christianity permeated all aspects of medical life: theories, institutions, and practices, but above all, the beliefs of the people. Nearly five centuries later the situation had changed dramatically. Physicians not only understood the cause of much disease but possessed the knowledge and skill to treat it. Hospitals had evolved into technological centers where machines played as vital a role as humans. Medical scientists looked with hope toward the future rather than with respect toward the past. Many medical institutions retained a nominal connection with organized religions, and Christian beliefs continued to influence the health practices of countless individuals, but the dominant motif in medicine was clearly science, not Christianity.

In this essay we hope to illuminate the changing relationship between these two cultural forces during this span of nearly half a millennium. Of necessity we shall fly far over the historical landscape, observing the mountains and valleys but catching few glimpses of topographical detail. We shall pass in silence over many issues of significance such as medical ethics, attitudes toward life and death, and ideas about mental illness, choosing instead to devote our limited space to what we consider to be the main shifts in the relationship between Christianity and medicine, an

133

interaction that was often positive, sometimes negative, but always important.

ENEMIES OR ALLIES?

In *The History of the Warfare of Science with Theology in Christendom* (1896), the most influential book ever written on the subject, Andrew Dickson White alleged that "theological dogmas," particularly but not solely those associated with the Roman Catholic church, were among the greatest stumbling blocks to the growth of modern medical science. According to his interpretation of the historical record, the church thwarted medical progress all through the Middle Ages and opposed the revival of human dissection during the Renaissance on the grounds that it was sacrilege to desecrate the dead. Andreas Vesalius, whose work in the sixteenth century set a new standard for human anatomy, is described as incurring "ecclesiastical censure," braving "the most terrible dangers," and finally being "hunted to death by men who conscientiously supposed he was injuring religion." In the eighteenth and early nineteenth centuries, argued White, the battleground shifted from anatomy to immunology, as churchmen tried to suppress the introduction of inoculation and vaccination against smallpox by linking these measures with "sorcery and atheism." In his own time the conflict had come to focus on the use of anesthetics in childbirth. "Pulpit after pulpit," he wrote, denounced the practice "as impious and contrary to Holy Writ" because it sought "to avoid one part of the primeval curse on woman."[1]

Although it is undeniably true that some individuals used theological arguments to oppose certain medical developments, it is also true that such contentions never represented more than a minority opinion and were always far less significant than the criticism from conservatives within the medical community who, for whatever reasons, feared change. Given our current knowledge of medical history, it would be easier to make a case for Christianity's being an ally of medical science than its enemy. This becomes readily apparent when we look at the three examples White marshaled from the history of anatomy, immunology, and obstetrics.

The most cited evidence for the church's opposition to human dissection is a bull promulgated by Pope Boniface VIII in 1300 prohibiting the boiling of bodies, a technique used by Crusaders to separate the flesh from bones of their fallen comrades before shipping the remains back home. Since anatomical investigators sometimes employed the same method, they may have believed that the papal ban applied to scientific work as well as to the Crusaders. Yet even in the late Middle Ages infrequent dissections met with little interference from the church. By the time Vesalius assumed his position as *explicator chirurgiae* at the University of Padua in 1537, human dissection had become a routine part of the medical curriculum. At no time did the church restrict his activities or threaten him with harm. And on occasions when he could not locate facilities large enough to accommodate the great number of spectators who came to watch him, religious authorities even permitted him to use churches as anatomical theaters.[2]

Contrary to White's allegation, the Roman Catholic church actively supported anatomical research during the sixteenth and seventeenth centuries. Many of the greatest anatomists of the time taught at the Sapienza, the papal medical school in Rome, and simultaneously served as papal physicians: Realdo Colombo, who discovered the pulmonary circulation of the blood; Bartolommeo Eustachio, who described the tube connecting the middle ear with the nasal passages; Andrea Cesalpino, who antedated William Harvey in postulating the circulation of the blood; and Marcello Malpighi, who first observed capillaries. Working in the shadow of the Vatican, Colombo, a contemporary and rival of Vesalius, in one year alone dissected fourteen cadavers, and high church officials often witnessed his public demonstrations.[3]

We do not mean to suggest that there was never any religious opposition to the dissection of human bodies, only that the church never formally disapproved of the practice. Thus instead of focusing on the occasional instances when churchmen may have protested the robbing of bodies from consecrated ground or expressed other objections, we would be more accurate to emphasize that, except in ancient Alexandria, human dissection first flourished in Catholic Italy—and with the church's blessing.

The history of the religious response to inoculation and vaccination against smallpox presents a similar story. Although some clerics did view such measures as evidencing "a distrust of God's overruling care," many more actively promoted them. In fact, it was a Puritan divine, Cotton Mather, who in 1721 initiated the first American trials of inoculation. When a leading Boston physician argued that the procedure was not only unsafe (which it was) but irreligious because it interfered with God's will, Mather and five other prominent ministers countered that such reasoning would rule out all medical intervention. Cannot pious persons, they asked,

> give into the method or practice without having their devotion and subjection to the All-wise Providence of God Almighty call'd in question? . . . Do we not in the use of all means depend on GOD's blessing? . . . For, what hand or art of Man is there in this Operation more than in bleeding, blistering and a Score more things in Medical use? which are all consistent with a humble trust in our Great preserver, and a due Subjection to His All-wise Providence.[4]

In Europe, too, clergy often led efforts to immunize the population against smallpox. This was especially true in rural areas, which often lacked trained medical personnel. In Dauphiné, France, for example, the local curé in 1786 administered the first smallpox inoculation ever given in the parish. During the nineteenth century, after vaccination replaced inoculation, the church continued to play a positive role. When a smallpox epidemic broke out in 1822, the archbishop of Paris sent a letter to the priests of his diocese reiterating the church's commitment to the prevention of disease and urging them to cooperate with civil authorities in a vaccination campaign. He authorized his subordinates to promote vaccination both publicly and privately, even during the administration of the sacraments.[5]

Theological criticism of the use of chloroform during childbirth, introduced by the Edinburgh physician James Young Simpson in the late 1840s, proved more of a nuisance than an obstacle to its adoption. Both sides in the debate claimed biblical support. When Simpson's critics cited God's curse upon Eve—"in pain you shall bring forth children" (Gen. 3:16)—as a reason for not anesthetizing parturient women, he reminded them that God had mercifully "caused a deep sleep to fall upon Adam" (Gen. 2:21) before removing his rib. Prominent clerics rallied to his cause, and even White credits the Scottish divine Thomas Chalmers with using his pulpit to turn the tide of public opinion in Simpson's favor. The recent judgment of a historian places this skirmish in its proper perspective. "Although a few clergymen and theologians opposed obstetrical anesthesia on religious grounds, the attack from this front was never too serious," writes John Duffy. "Surprisingly enough, the real threat to obstetrical anesthesia came from within the ranks of the medical profession itself."[6]

In contrast to the purported instances when religious belief clashed with medical science, there are numerous examples of positive relationships between medicine and Christianity. During the early modern period, when medical science was in its infancy, Christian theology frequently influenced medical theory. Physician-reformers like the Swiss-born Paracelsus and the Fleming John Baptist van Helmont drew heavily on religious themes in formulating their chemical explanations of disease, as did the Spanish physician-theologian Michael Servetus in arguing for the pulmonary circulation of the blood. In an antitrinitarian work entitled *The Restoration of Christianity* (1553), Servetus contended that there was only one basic fluid in the body—not three as ancient authorities taught—and that this substance, blood, circulated from the heart through the lungs and back to the heart again. His physiological speculations went largely unnoticed, but his theological heresies so aroused the enmity of John Calvin that he ordered Servetus and his book burned together at the stake.[7]

During the nineteenth and twentieth centuries, as medicine grew less speculative and more empirical, Christian doctrines ceased to influence the content of medical science in any obvious way. At the same time, however, Christian principles often determined how medical knowledge would be applied. The Victorian movement to clean up filthy and disease-ridden cities drew much of its strength on both sides of the Atlantic from religiously motivated individuals, who saw an intimate connection among dirt, disease, and moral degradation. John H. Griscom, the Quaker physician who led the fight in New York City to improve the health of the working classes, sought nothing less than a *"sanatory* regeneration of society." "Cleanliness," he wrote in characteristic fashion, "is said to be 'next to godliness,' and if, after admitting this, we reflect that cleanliness cannot exist without ventilation, we must then look upon the latter as not only a *moral* but *religious* duty." Such religiously based commitment to a healthful environment may, as it has been argued, have induced some of the sanitarians to resist the germ theory of disease when it came along in the late nineteenth century, but this should not obscure the fact that the reforms prompted by Christian piety improved the health, if not the morals, of millions of people.[8]

THE NATURAL AND THE DIVINE

Throughout the modern period, theologians and physicians alike wrestled with the question of whether disease arose naturally or resulted from divine displeasure or satanic perversity. This issue was potentially disruptive because, as one historian has noted, physicians needed "an idea of regularity in nature as a basis for science" while theologians needed "an idea of irregularity as expressive of transcendent manipulation by God."[9] Nevertheless, conflict rarely occurred. Instead, each community displayed a remarkable degree of toleration for the views of the other. Perhaps this is not surprising when we recall that most physicians were also Christians and that theologians shared the desire of all humans to understand and control disease.

Already by the sixteenth century, supernatural explanations of disease had largely disappeared from medical literature except in discussions of epidemics and insanity, which remained etiological mysteries, and venereal diseases, which were attributed to sin. In writing about the common afflictions of humanity—fractures, tumors, endemic diseases, and such—physicians seldom mentioned religion. Even when discussing the plague, the most feared disease of all, they tended merely to acknowledge its supernatural origin before passing quickly to more mundane subjects. The French surgeon Ambroise Paré, for example, explicitly confined himself to "the natural causes of the plague," saying that he would let divines deal with its ultimate causes. It is significant that neither Paré nor most of his colleagues denied a supernatural component to disease.[10]

Theologians for their part generally placed greater emphasis on supernatural causes and cures but accommodated medical knowledge by maintaining that God usually effected his will through natural agencies rather than by direct intervention. Theology thus seldom precluded searching for natural causes or using natural therapies. Martin Luther, though skeptical about the efficacy of medicine, nevertheless described a physician as "our Lord God's mender of the body, as we theologians are his healers of the spirit." And when some radical Protestants attempted to justify their refusal to seek protection from the plague in terms of the doctrine of predestination, Théodore de Bèze, Calvin's successor at Geneva, argued that "we must use those things which God himself going before, nature telleth us to be ordained by him to prolong our life so long as shall please him." Such logic provided physicians ample freedom to continue their quest for natural explanations and therapies.[11]

If significant disagreement failed to arise over medical theory, there remained the possibility of conflict over medical practice. During times of epidemics, for instance, physicians prescribed natural remedies while the clergy encouraged the sick to fast and pray. As one English cleric put it, "In the time of Pestilence, Penitencie and Confession are to be preferred before all other medicaments." Such religious acts rarely interfered with secular therapy, but when Catholic priests ordered public processions in order to seek divine aid, they occasionally clashed with public-health authorities. When the plague struck the small Italian town of Monte Lupo in 1631, for example, the local priest defied the quarantine imposed by the public health magistracy and led his parishioners through the streets. How often such incidents occurred is impossible to tell.[12]

The secularization of medical theory occurred first among physicians and then spread to other segments of society at a pace that varied with the progress of medical knowledge. As soon as diseases could be assigned to specific natural causes, religious explanations became almost superfluous. Thus theological interpretations of smallpox declined in the eighteenth century with the advent of inoculation, while outbreaks of diphtheria, yellow fever, and cholera continued to elicit theological responses into the nineteenth century. The pattern of change can be seen clearly by contrasting the American response to cholera in 1832 and 1849, when the origin of the disease remained obscure, with that of 1866, when its cause was known.[13]

By the 1830s and 1840s physicians had already ceased to air their theological views, even those pertaining to epidemics, in medical publications. Whatever their private religious beliefs, they now kept them to themselves; as physicians, they dealt only with natural causes. No physician should "be satisfied with the reflection that the result was one of God's providences," advised the president of the State Medical Society of Wisconsin following the 1849 epidemic, but should seek its natural cause until he has "fully unravelled the mystery." However, as long as cholera remained a mystery, religious persons felt free to regard it as a miracle, "a *scourge,* a *rod* in the hand of God."[14]

By 1866 this attitude had changed. During the previous decade a London physician, John Snow, had succeeded in tracing the cause of cholera to contaminated water supplies and in showing how the disease could be prevented by disinfection. Thus, when cholera threatened to return in 1866, Americans devoted their energies to improving sanitation rather than to discussing the theological meaning of the event. "Cholera, a scourge of the sinful to many Americans in 1832, had, by 1866, become the consequence of remediable faults in sanitation," writes the historian Charles Rosenberg. "Whereas ministers in 1832 urged morality upon their congregations as a guarantor of health, their forward-looking counterparts in 1866 endorsed sanitary reform as a necessary prerequisite to moral improvement." God's role in causing epidemics had nearly vanished.[15] And during the next few decades, as medical scientists led by Robert Koch and Louis Pasteur discovered the specific microorganisms responsible for various diseases, God's role would, for many, disappear altogether.

THE ANGELICAL CONJUNCTION

The Puritan preacher Cotton Mather, who knew more about medicine than many physicians, once described the combined practice of spiritual and physical healing as the "angelical conjunction." Indeed, so complementary were the roles of physician and priest that throughout much of the Middle Ages clerics often provided medical care, even though the ministerial and medical professions were formally distinct.[16]

The segregation of preaching and healing resulted from a variety of factors. Although the Roman Catholic church did not, during the Middle Ages, formally forbid the practice of medicine by clerics generally, it did question the appropriateness of clergy engaging in medical practice. During the late Middle Ages and Renaissance, guilds of physicians, surgeons, and apothecaries all sought legal monopolies over the healing arts. Their efforts, where successful, excluded unqualified clergy as well as charlatans from practicing medicine. Lay people also gained control of medical education. By the year 1500, for example, only three of the twenty-three members of the faculty of medicine at Paris were clerics.[17]

But despite the efforts of the church and the medical profession to discourage clerics from practicing medicine, the custom persisted. The various medical guilds found it impossible to enforce their monopolies outside metropolitan areas, and necessity forced some priests to minister to their flocks. Many citizens could neither afford a properly credentialed practitioner nor even find one. Consequently, cleric-physicians and other irregular healers flourished in small towns and in rural areas into the eighteenth and even the nineteenth centuries.

Typical of this kind of practice in substance, if not in size, was that of the seventeenth-century Anglican divine Richard Napier, who treated approximately sixty thousand patients during a remarkable forty-year career as rector of Great Linford, Buckinghamshire. A graduate of Oxford, Napier devoted most of his time to seeing the sick, while a curate assumed his preaching duties. Each day patients from surrounding communities flocked to his home, where he offered them an eclectic mixture of classical and astrological medicine, leavened with spiritual counsel and prayer. Rich and poor alike sought his services and paid according to their financial ability.[18]

The Puritan clergy took a special interest in medicine, partly, it seems, as insurance against the prospect of not being allowed to earn a living by preaching. Richard Baxter, a prolific and influential Puritan pastor, began practicing medicine in the mid-seventeenth century, when an outbreak of pleurisy caught his congregation without a physician. For the next five or six years, until he persuaded a doctor to settle nearby, he spent much of his time treating the sick, from whom he took not "one Penny." His reward, he explained, came on Sundays:

> And God made use of my Practice of Physick among them, as a very great advantage to my Ministry; for they that cared not for their Souls did love their Lives, and care for their Bodies: And by this they were made almost as observant, as a Tenant is of his Landlord: Sometimes I could see before me in the Church a very considerable part of the Congregation, whose Lives God had made me a means to save, or to recover their health: And doing it for nothing so obliged them, that they would readily hear me.[19]

In colonial New England, Puritan cleric-physicians provided a significant part of the medical services, especially outside Boston and the larger towns. But clerical medicine in the colonies was by no means confined to New England Puritans. Anglican missionaries, sent out by the Society for the Propagation of the Gospel in Foreign Parts, often treated both Indians and white settlers in the absence of regular doctors. Francis Makemie, one of the founders of Presbyterianism in America, and Heinrich Melchior Mühlenberg, the leading light of American Lutheranism, both undertook healing ministries. "Since doctors are few and far between," wrote Mühlenberg from his Pennsylvania home, "I necessarily had to take a hand myself." Fortunately he had learned a little medicine during his student days in Germany, and he recognized the limits of his knowledge and ability. Although he did not mind treating the sick, he greatly disliked being disturbed for minor complaints, saying that he felt like a "privy to which all those with loose bowels come running from all directions to relieve themselves."[20]

Before departing for America in 1735, the future father of Methodism, John Wesley, spent several months studying medicine in hopes of being "of some service to those who had no regular physician among them." After a disappointing two years in Georgia, Wesley returned to England, where he continued to take a special interest in the problems of the ill. Finding that many were receiving inadequate medical care, Wesley in desperation decided to treat them himself, resolving "not to go out of my depth, but to leave all difficult and complicated cases to such physicians as the patients should choose." Assisted by an apothecary and a surgeon, he opened his own dispensary in 1746. The next year he published a brief medical guide, *Primitive Physick,* designed to provide the lay person with "a plain and easy way of curing most diseases." As an adjunct to pills and potions, it recommended "that old-fashioned medicine—*prayer.*" By the time of Wesley's death in 1791 the book was in its twenty-third edition.[21]

Because patients expected cleric-physicians to be altruistic, many found it difficult to collect fees for their medical services. Nevertheless, some ministers took up the practice of medicine specifically to supplement their clerical incomes. For example, the Reverend Manasseh Cutler of Hamilton, Massachusetts, reported being "driven to the practice of physic" by the financial needs of his family. Most preachers, however, became healers for humanitarian rather than commercial reasons.[22]

In the Catholic countries of continental Europe priests and nuns often filled niches in a medical network that did not adequately provide for the poor or those living in remote areas. Beginning in the seventeenth century, the French government employed rural priests to distribute free medicines from chests of supplies periodically sent out from the capital. Although there was no attempt formally to integrate the rural clergy into a system of health care, the government did expect them to cooperate with authorities in protecting the public health during times of epidemics. In recognition of the important medical role played by the clergy, at least one eighteenth-century physician, S. A. D. Tissot, prepared a manual to assist them in providing intelligent care. As late as the nineteenth century untrained nuns practiced medicine openly but illegally among the peasants, operating unauthorized pharmacies and even making regular rounds in out-of-the-way places. In some respects these sisters aided registered physicians by taking over the least desirable tasks, but in a few cantons they became so active that physicians could not remain in business.[23]

During the Enlightenment, when increased attention focused on the needs of the poor and downtrodden, a number of individuals suggested reviving the old custom of clerical medicine and establishing it on a rational basis. Foremost among the advocates of this plan was Johann Peter Frank, professor of practical medicine at the University of Vienna and an authority on medicine and public policy. Another was the Swedish physician-naturalist Carolus Linnaeus, who during a visit to the hinterland in 1749 met a priest who had made "a considerable reputation for himself as a doctor amongst his parishioners." The encounter apparently inspired Linnaeus to propose giving every theology student an eight-day crash course in the fundamentals of medicine:

> The poor peasant shuns the pharmacy, where life is often sold at a high price, he dreads physicians and surgeons which he does not know how to choose. He puts his greatest trust in his own priest and likes to ask his advice in an emergency. It would be of very great benefit to the state if most rural clergymen would understand how to cure the most common diseases, which destroy so many thousands of country folk every year. Most of them are easily cured like dysentery, scurvy, erysipelas, leg ulcers, acute fevers and intermittent fevers. All this knowledge can be learned by the students while they are still at university within eight days at the most. How fortunate would the peasant be, if their priests could heal these ills with the medical herbs that can be got without cost, as they grow in front of the door of everybody's house. What advantage would that be for the state, what pleasure and honour would this not bring to the priests themselves!

Although Linnaeus's proposal produced no immediate action, the Swedish diet in 1810, over the protests of some clergy, voted to provide fifty scholarships for students at the Universities of Uppsala and Lund who wished to become priest-physicians. But despite this official support, the scheme never lived up to the expectations of its sponsors, and after a couple of decades it was allowed to die.[24]

Early in the nineteenth century, Czar Alexander I of Russia, an admirer of Dr. Frank, issued an imperial edict declaring that "the medical care of patients in rural areas should be entrusted to the rural clergymen, after the latter had been given the opportunity to learn the principles of medicine in addition to their own clerical studies." The Greek Orthodox church opposed the plan, fearing that it would degrade the ministry; and even though some seminaries apparently tried to comply with the czar's wishes, the experiment was soon aborted.[25]

As the unsuccessful Swedish and Russian experiences suggest, the time was fast passing when ministers could participate meaningfully in medical affairs. During the nineteenth century, medicine evolved from an art into a science, and professional barriers became too stout to breach. In the United States the colonial shortage of competent practitioners gave way to a surplus, as Americans fell victim to what one contemporary described as "medical school mania." Physicians competing in an overcrowded profession were scarcely disposed to feel charitable toward ministerial meddling in their affairs.[26] The last quarter of the century saw virtually every state in the union enact some form of medical practice act, making it illegal for the first time in America for clergy without medical training to engage in physical healing.

Occasionally, innovative pastors tried to bridge the gap between the two professions by establishing programs for the psychological treatment of individuals suffering from functional disorders, but generally speaking the separation between ministers and medics was complete. This arrangement seemed to please both parties. Writing in the *Harvard Theological Review* in 1909, the distinguished Boston neurologist James Jackson Putnam suggested that the churches' function was primarily moral. "I should welcome the aid of the clergyman as of real value," he wrote, "but should deprecate the systematic entrance of representatives of the churches into the medical field." About the same time the Reverend Charles Reynold Brown expressed similar views:

> The most friendly relations and the highest form of cooperation between the doctor of medicine and the minister of religion can best be secured where both realize that each one has an entirely distinct function to perform for the service of humanity and where both realize that each can best aid the other by attending strictly to his own specialty.

The once attractive angelical conjunction was thus allowed to dissolve by mutual consent.[27]

HOSPITALS AND NURSES

A similar drift toward secularization can be seen in the history of the hospital, an institution nurtured, if not created, by the church during the Middle Ages. The medieval hospitals were founded by monasteries to provide succor for the needy of every description: the sick, the hungry, the homeless. Although monks and nuns provided the sick with simple herbal remedies and dressed their wounds, they emphasized caring more than curing. The medieval physician had little to do with the hospital. By the late Middle Ages municipalities and other secular organizations were beginning to operate establishments of this kind, but the hospital nevertheless remained closely identified with the church until the sixteenth century.[28]

The Protestant Reformation and its aftermath irreversibly altered the traditional relationship between church and hospital, especially in northern Europe and Great Britain, where the reformers scored their greatest victories. For example, after Henry VIII of England broke with Rome in the 1530s, he confiscated church property, shut down the small monastic hospitals, and delegated the administration of the surviving institutions to secular boards of governors. Similarly, the city fathers of Protestant Geneva, even before the arrival of John Calvin, consolidated all charitable foundations and placed the General Hospital under lay control. Such developments stemmed partly from anti-Catholic prejudice and partly from what seems to have been a peculiar Protestant compulsion to replace indiscriminate charity with a rational, well-ordered system.[29]

In countries that remained loyal to Rome, laicization occurred less abruptly, where it occurred at all. However, the church's inability to continue supporting expensive charities, combined with the ambition of governments to centralize authority, often led to a shift in responsibility even in Catholic lands. In France, for example, Louis XII in 1505 transferred control of the Hôtel-Dieu of Paris from the canons of the Notre Dame Cathedral to secular directors, and a half century later Charles IX placed village hospitals under civil control. Thus by the end of the sixteenth century hospitals in many parts of Europe—both Protestant and Catholic—had drifted from their religious moorings.[30]

But regardless of who owned the hospitals, religious personnel continued for centuries to direct their day-to-day operations and thus to maintain a highly visible Christian presence. In fact, before the rise of professional nurses in the late nineteenth century, few besides members of religious orders were sufficiently motivated to carry out the repetitive and menial tasks that hospital patients required. When the French tried to get along without Catholic sisters during their antireligious revolution in the late eighteenth century, their experiment failed dismally. Among the most prominent of the nursing orders was the Sisters of Charity of St. Vincent de Paul, which, along with numerous other orders, both male and female, came into existence after the Catholic Counter-Reformation successfully restricted the secular activities of the old orders. Although these sisters adhered to hospital regulations in carrying out their nursing duties, their primary allegiance was to the motherhouse. This divided loyalty sometimes created awkward situations, as when nuns refused well into the nineteenth century to nurse in male wards.[31]

As long as the medical profession regarded the hospital as peripheral to its interests, clashes between secular physicians and religious nurses rarely occurred. However, in the eighteenth century, when physicians began to view hospitals as centers for the study of clinical medicine rather than as mere charitable institutions, conflict became almost inevitable, as events at the Hôtel-Dieu of Paris on the eve of the French Revolution testify. At this gargantuan establishment, which housed as many as three thousand patients at a time, Augustinian nurses supervised a large domestic staff and controlled the most important areas of hospital policy. When the First Surgeon of the hospital in 1787 attempted to transform it from a custodial to a medical institution, serving the needs of physicians and medical students as well as patients, the sisters protested loudly:

> Perish the murderous system born in this selfish century, whereby the poor are now only admitted into the hospital to prevent their death, and they should be thrown out just as soon as they cease to be afflicted with sickness. No sooner did this opinion find a single partisan than it is already being practiced in the Hôtel-Dieu of Paris. The religious hasten to rise up against these fatal maxims.

The irate nuns rankled at the sight of hundreds of curious students crowding the hospital and disrupting its religious atmosphere; they wanted to preserve it as a site of solace, care, and charity.[32]

The revolution that soon engulfed France broke the power of the religious orders and gave physicians free rein to utilize the hospital for teaching and research. Under these conditions there arose in Paris in the early nineteenth century a world-famous school of medicine where doctors meticulously observed the natural course of disease in patients and later, if the patients died, correlated their observations with findings at autopsy. Such procedures may have contributed greatly to the advancement of medical science, but they scarcely harmonized with the nuns' view of patients as objects of Christian benevolence.[33]

Unlike the French, who looked to the government to provide medical facilities, the British relied on voluntary organizations, which during the eighteenth and nineteenth centuries populated the island with dispensaries and hospitals. Although the established church did not directly involve itself in this movement, individual clergy often spearheaded local efforts, and Christian piety motivated many of the participants. In arguing for a hospital in Edinburgh in the 1720s, Dr. Alexander Monro noted that "as Men and Christians we have the strongest Inducements, and even obligations to this sort of Charity, as it is warmly recommended and injoyned in the Gospel as one of the greatest Christian Duties." Sermons frequently helped to generate both moral and financial support. In fact, in the mid-nineteenth century many churches instituted Hospital Sunday, an annual event when contributions were collected for hospitals. This device became an important source of funding and soon spread throughout the English-speaking world.[34]

The proliferation of therapeutically active hospitals in the eighteenth and nineteenth centuries created a demand for qualified nurses. Hospitals in Catholic countries could rely on the nursing orders, but Protestants had nothing comparable until the 1830s, when a Lutheran pastor and his wife in Kaiserswerth, Germany, Theodor and Frederike Fliedner, founded a nursing school for pious young women interested in a life of service. These deaconesses, as they were called, lived and worked much like Catholic sisters but retained the right to leave the order when they wished. Beginning with a single room in a small summerhouse, the Fliedners rapidly expanded their operation into a major training center that became a model for deaconess societies in many countries and in several Protestant denominations. In 1851 Florence Nightingale visited Kaiserswerth and returned to England to set up a secular version of the deaconesses.[35]

In the late nineteenth century, as nursing shifted from a domestic to a medical function in response to diagnostic and therapeutic advances, religious nurses began giving way to secular ones, who tended to view nursing more as a career than as a calling. Not only did the secular nurses generally receive superior medical training, but nonreligious physicians often found them to be more flexible. Catholic sisters, for example, disliked catheterizing and bathing patients and in some instances refused to care for persons suffering from venereal diseases. On occasion they were known to place religious duty above medical need, perhaps calling the priest before the physician in cases of emergency or encouraging patients to engage in religious activities, such as fasting and attending religious services, not in their best medical interests. By the early twentieth century nearly half the nurses in countries like Germany were neither Catholic sisters nor Protestant deaconesses, and the trend toward laicization quickened as the century progressed.[36]

In the United States as well as in other countries without established churches, religious groups frequently engaged in operating hospitals. Elsewhere, established churches often felt no need to administer hospitals, preferring instead to shift that responsibility to their governments. The Catholic Daughters of St. Vincent de Paul opened a hospital in St. Louis as early as 1828, but denominational hospitals remained uncommon in America until the 1840s and 1850s, when large numbers of Catholic and Lutheran immigrants began arriving. In response to the needs of these uprooted people, William A. Passavant, a young Lutheran minister who had recently returned from a stay at Kaiserswerth, in 1849 started a small deaconess hospital in Pittsburgh. Shortly after the opening of the hospital, Fliedner himself brought over four German deaconesses to assist Passavant in transplanting the deaconess system to the New World. Inspired by the success of Lutherans and Catholics, all the major Protestant bodies—and not a few minor ones—established their own hospitals, until by the mid-twentieth century church-related hospitals represented one-sixth of all such institutions in the country and cared for over a quarter of all hospitalized patients. Nearly three-fourths of these facilities were Roman Catholic.[37]

Denominational hospitals served a multitude of functions. Many of them, such as the Irish-Catholic hospitals of Boston, bolstered ethnic and religious pride. As Boston's mayor John Fitzgerald declared at the opening of the expanded St. Elizabeth's Hospital in 1914, he was proud that "a new impression will be gained of the strength of the Catholic element of the population by many of those who have been prone to belittle their ability." Church-run institutions also acted as agents for winning converts or, conversely, as barriers against the proselytizing activities of others. Catholics, for example, sometimes feared that Protestant hospitals would pressure them to give up their faith or would deny them last rites. According to one story, a Catholic patient in a particularly insensitive Protestant hospital "had to drag himself off his deathbed and out onto the street, where a priest heard his confession and administered the sacrament in a carriage." Such incidents created considerable alarm and reinforced the efforts of churches to provide for the medical needs of their parishioners in a pluralistic society.[38]

By the second half of the twentieth century, as governments increasingly assumed responsibility for providing health care, church ownership of hospitals was becoming less common than before. In the United States, where the practice continued, it was often difficult to distinguish religious from secular hospitals—except perhaps for their names and, in

Catholic institutions, their distinctive policies relating to reproduction. Overt proselytization had fallen from fashion, nursing orders had lost much of their former attraction, and hospital administrators had come more and more to appoint medical staffs for their competence rather than for their piety. Some church-related hospitals resisted the homogenizing process more than others, but by and large the twentieth-century hospital had become a monument to modern technology rather than a symbol of Christian charity.[39]

INTO ALL THE WORLD

The nineteenth century found Christians throughout Europe and America stirring with conviction to go "into all the world and preach the gospel to the whole creation" (Mark 16:15). These missionaries, like others before them, often employed medicine as an entering wedge in penetrating non-Christian cultures. For centuries Catholics had engaged in foreign medical activities in various parts of the world; in Mexico alone during the sixteenth century they set up over 150 hospitals to care for and convert the Indians. Early Protestant missionaries frequently acquired a little medical knowledge before going abroad. Robert Morrison, for example, briefly attended lectures at St. Bartholomew's Hospital in London prior to becoming the first English missionary to China. Fully trained physicians, however, rarely enlisted as missionaries before the 1830s and 1840s, when the exploits of two Christian doctors, Peter Parker and David Livingstone, touched off a medical-missionary movement that remained vigorous for over a century.[40]

Parker, a Presbyterian physician-minster who reputedly served as the first medical missionary in China, sailed for the Orient a mere three months after graduating from medical school in 1834. Sponsored by the American Board of Commissioners for Foreign Missions, he settled in Canton and opened a hospital. His success in China did not go unnoticed, but it was the work of Livingstone, who went to Africa in 1840, that really fired the popular imagination.[41] By mid-century there were an estimated two or three dozen medical missionaries worldwide, and in the 1870s the number climbed to about one hundred. By this time at least one-third of all American mission stations in China were involved in medical work—and mission dispensaries and hospitals were already far busier than mission churches.[42]

Although medical missionaries sometimes resented being used as bait to lure potential converts, both they and their sponsoring boards clearly recognized that all medical activities were subservient to spreading the gospel. Missionary societies found that physicians were particularly effective in countries "where the Gospel cannot freely be preached by ordinary evangelists" and in regions where "aboriginal and uncivilised peoples [were] likely to be specially impressed by the benevolent influence of medical work." Indeed, the miracles of scientific medicine served as modern-day substitutes for the lost healing powers of New Testament times, allowing missionaries, like the apostles, to gain "authority and influence." To medical missionaries, healing was simply another form of preaching. As one of Parker's friends explained, "in the very act of amputating a limb, in his way, he tells . . . of Him who said, 'I will be their healer.' "[43]

Unfortunately for them, this type of ministry, though it alleviated much human suffering, proved woefully ineffective in winning converts. As early as 1869 a missionary in China observed:

> If we inquire how far these institutions are useful as a means of Christianizing the people, we will be greatly disappointed, if we have been led to expect large results. While we may thankfully observe the few cases of conversion among these [patients], we must admit that [they] bear a very small proportion to the thousands that have been in the hospital wards.

During one twelve-year period the Medical Missionary Society of Canton treated more than 400,000 patients but managed to convert only a dozen of them to Christianity.[44] Missionary doctors discovered that their patients possessed a marvelous ability to explain the success of Western medicine in terms of their own religious beliefs and thus felt little inclination to adopt the religion of the missionaries. To a certain extent the missionaries had only themselves to blame; they had failed to relate their medical therapies convincingly to the spiritual power of Christ, to create a theology of healing that integrated spiritual and medical efforts.[45]

Aware of their poor record as proselytizers, medical missionaries in the late nineteenth century shifted strategies. Instead of trying to reach the unconverted, they increasingly focused their efforts on the needs of the growing Christian community. "If the witch-doctor was to be eliminated, with all that he symbolised of sub-Christian fears and hatreds," explains one African historian, "the missionary doctor must abandon his evangelistic itinerations, stay in his hospital and train African nurses and medical assistants to replace the diviner in village life." Thus, in contrast to the first generation of medical missionaries, who emphasized dispensary and itinerant work that brought them into contact with large numbers of non-Christians, later generations tended to concentrate on hospital-related and educational activities and to stay close to the mission compound.[46]

Although medical missions continued to prosper well into the latter half of the twentieth century, by the 1970s it was becoming clear that the traditional arrangement would not long survive. Lack of qualified personnel had forced the closing of some mission hospitals while others were falling into government hands. In those that remained under church control, nationals were rapidly replacing Western missionaries. Among the medical missions of the Southern Baptist Convention, for instance, the number of national physicians increased more than eightyfold between 1950 and 1974 (from 5 to 424), while the number of national nurses grew from 57 to 705. Some "mission" hospitals no longer included a single foreign missionary on their staffs. The movement inaugurated by Parker and Livingstone seemed to be fast drawing to a close.[47]

THE PERSISTENCE OF FAITH

Thus far our attention has focused largely on the individuals and institutions that have provided medical care during the past five hundred years. We have observed at this level the gradual secularization of medicine, as professionalization, the growth of scientific knowledge, and increased government involvement eroded the once-dominant Christian presence. But we have said little about the beliefs and practices of the anonymous Christians who sat in the pew. Did they too share in the secularizing process? Some may have, but many others—from Jehovah's Witnesses who refused blood transfusions to Catholics who knelt at healing shrines—kept their religious beliefs and medical practices tightly intertwined.[48]

Throughout the entire modern period the Roman Catholic church, the largest Christian communion in the world, actively and officially promoted religious healing, encouraging such practices as praying, lighting candles for particular healing saints, and making pilgrimages to holy shrines. Lourdes, the most popular of these shrines, rests on a site in southwestern France where, according to tradition, the Virgin once appeared. There, since the mid-nineteenth century, the sick have flocked to bathe in the healing waters of a spring that even today attracts about three million pilgrims a year. A visit to such a shrine did not necessarily imply a rejection of secular medicine. As one French medical manual warned, patients often kept "their scapulars, medals, and even the bottle of holy water from Lourdes" right beside the medicine their physicians prescribed.[49]

Leaders of the Protestant Reformation frequently expressed skepticism about the healing miracles claimed by Catholics. Such "miraculous powers and manifest workings," argued John Calvin, died with the apostolic age. The healings of his day, he suspected, were the work of Satan, disguising himself as an angel of light. The Puritan Cotton Mather captured the smug position of many Protestants:

> How ridiculously foolish is the revived Paganism in the Popish Idolatries and Superstitions, applying to such and such particular Saint, for the Cure of these and those Diseases! . . . We are by our happy Instruction in the Protestant Religion emancipated from these Fooleries; and instead thereof, we have so learned Christ as to understand, that we have an admirable Saviour . . . a skillful and faithful Physician will do more for a poor Patient than all the Saints in the Romish Kalender.

Although most Protestants retained at least a theoretical belief in the healing power of prayer, they tended until the late nineteenth century to shun the healing rituals associated with Roman Catholics and the apostles.[50]

The last decades of the nineteenth century witnessed a quickening of interest in spiritual healing among Protestants in both Europe and the United States. Evidence of this can be seen in the faith-cure movement associated with Charles Cullis and Dorothea Trudel, the Holiness Revival among Methodists, and the rise of Christian Science. Late-Victorian evangelical Protestants grew increasingly alarmed by the inroads of higher criticism and modern science, and as part of their effort to defend the faith they sought to prove the truth of James 5:14–15: "Is any among you sick? Let him call for the elders of the church, and let them pray over him, anointing him with oil in the name of the Lord; and the prayer of faith will save the sick man, and the Lord will raise him up; and if he has committed sins, he will be forgiven." As the faith-cure movement grew, participants established special homes and hospitals, and in 1885 one group held a Divine Healing Conference in London that attracted worldwide attention. Although the movement remained relatively small and scarcely survived the century, it helped to draw attention to faith healing in Protestant circles.[51]

The Holiness Revival that swept through American Methodism during the latter part of the nineteenth century spawned numerous Pentecostal sects and independent ministries that kept Protestant faith healing alive during the early twentieth century. Before World War II several Pentecostal evangelists, including the flamboyant Aimee Semple McPherson, won national attention for their healing ministries. But no event before the war compared with the great revival of the late 1940s and early 1950s, when, according to one historian, "the practice of praying for the sick was revived on a scale hitherto unknown." Itinerant evangelists claiming to heal every ailment from arthritis to cancer crisscrossed the country, drawing huge crowds of expectant believers and curious onlookers. The most successful of the new evangelists was a young Pentecostal preacher, Oral Roberts, who launched his career as a healer in 1947 after reportedly curing a crippled polio victim. Wherever he went, the sick flocked to his healing lines, to wait for the touch of his right hand, through which divine power allegedly flowed. By the late 1950s the postwar healing revival had crested. Faith healing, however, remained a vital part of the Pentecostal world, and during the 1960s and 1970s it moved—like Roberts himself, who joined the Methodist church—into the mainline Protestant denominations and even spilled over into Catholic churches.[52]

Although some extreme Pentecostals refused to seek medical care of any kind, many patronized both medical doctors and faith healers. Roberts, who never hesitated to consult a physician, customarily advised those whom he healed to obtain medical confirmation. "I believe that all healing comes from God," he once said, "regardless of whether the instrument is someone like me or a doctor." This philosophy led him in the late 1970s to undertake the building of a large medical center, the City of Faith, on the campus of his university in Tulsa, Oklahoma. God, he said, had told him to use all his healing resources: "Prayer, but more than prayer. Medical science, but more than medical science."[53]

Christian Scientists, who denied the very existence of disease, did not practice faith healing in the manner of the Pentecostals. They traced their roots not to the renewed emphasis on spiritual gifts in the late nineteenth century but to the medical environment of a few decades earlier. In reaction to the bleeding, blistering, and purging of regular physicians, there arose a host of rival medical sects offering alternative therapies: Thomsonians, homeopaths, water curists, mind curists, and many more. As a longtime invalid, Mary Baker Eddy, the founder of Christian Science, acquired firsthand knowledge of several of these

heterodox systems. From homeopathy, which advocated using infini-
tesimally small doses of drugs and which she avidly practiced in the
1850s, she learned that the quantity of medicine made no difference, that
"mind governed the whole question of . . . recovery." From Phineas
Parkhurst Quimby, a mental healer to whom she turned in the 1860s, she
learned that all illness was merely false belief, that curing came from
right thinking. By 1875 she had fashioned from her experiences and from
her reading of the Bible a new system of healing, a description of which
she published in a book called *Science and Health*. A few years later she
formally organized the Church of Christ (Scientist), which by the early
twentieth century counted among its members tens of thousands of
Americans who relied primarily on right thinking to cure their ills.[54]

Two other nineteenth-century American denominations, the Church
of Jesus Christ of Latter-day Saints (Mormons) and the Seventh-Day
Adventists, also displayed a marked affinity for sectarian medicine and
hygienic living. The early Mormons, including both Joseph Smith and
Brigham Young, warmly embraced the botanical system of healing
devised by a New York farmer, Samuel Thomson. As Young explained to
the Saints, herbal medicine nicely complemented religious rituals:

> When you are sick, call for the Elders, who will pray for you, anointing
> with oils and the laying on of hands; and nurse each other with herbs, and
> mild food, and if you do these things, in faith, and quit taking poisons, and
> poisonous medicines, which God never ordained for the use of men, you
> shall be blessed.

In 1834 the Mormon prophet Smith announced that he had been divinely
instructed in a revelation called the "Word of Wisdom" to ban the
consumption of tobacco, alcohol, and "hot drinks," a phrase interpreted
to mean tea and coffee. The church did not strictly enforce these regulations until the last decades of the century, about the same time it
switched its allegiance from botanical to scientific medicine. In part
because they abided by Smith's counsel, twentieth-century Mormons not
only lived longer than the average American, but also suffered considerably less than their non-Mormon neighbors from such maladies as cancer
and heart disease.[55]

The medical history of Seventh-Day Adventists is strikingly similar. In
1863 the spiritual leader of the Adventists, Ellen G. White, claimed that
God had told her in a vision that people should give up eating meat and
other stimulating foods, shun alcohol and tobacco, and avoid drug-

dispensing doctors. When sick, they were to rely solely on nature's remedies: fresh air, sunshine, rest, exercise, proper diet, and—above all—water. Subsequently Mrs. White visited a water-cure institution in upstate New York and returned home to Battle Creek, Michigan, to help establish an Adventist hydropathic institute, the first in a chain of Adventist health institutions that eventually circled the globe. Although Adventists later abandoned much of their emphasis on natural remedies in favor of modern medicines, their abstemious life-styles, often including vegetarianism, helped them, too, to enjoy significantly better health than the general population.[56]

The extent to which religious beliefs influence the health practices of contemporary Christians cannot be determined precisely. We do know, however, that in the United States alone ten million Americans (7 percent of the population), including both Catholics and mainline Protestants, claim to practice faith healing.[57] For these people, as well as for countless others, Christianity and medicine are closely related, no matter how far apart they have drifted at the institutional level. And as long as medicine remains an imperfect science, religion will undoubtedly continue to play an important role in the lives of many Christians during times of sickness and in the quest for health.

NOTES

1. Andrew Dickson White, *A History of the Warfare of Science with Theology in Christendom*, 2 vols. (New York: D. Appleton & Co., 1896), 2:49–63. The quotations about Vesalius come from an early version of this work, *The Warfare of Science* (New York: D. Appleton & Co., 1876), pp. 103–7.

2. Mary Niven Alston, "The Attitude of the Church Towards Dissection Before 1500," *Bulletin of the History of Medicine* 16 (1944): 221–38; C. D. O'Malley, *Andreas Vesalius of Brussels, 1514–1564* (Berkeley: University of California Press, 1964); C. D. O'Malley, "Medical Education During the Renaissance," in *The History of Medical Education*, ed. C. D. O'Malley (Berkeley: University of California Press, 1970), p. 99. See also O. Marcondes Calasans, "Influência do cristianismo na anatomia," *Folia Clinica et Biologica* (São Paulo) 28 (1958/59): 299–319.

3. James J. Walsh, *The Popes and Science: The History of the Papal Relations to Science During the Middle Ages and Down to Our Own Time* (New York: Fordham University Press, 1908), pp. 221–47.

4. John Duffy, *Epidemics in Colonial America* (Baton Rouge: Louisiana State

The Historical Setting

University Press, 1953), pp. 30–32; Otho T. Beall, Jr., and Richard H. Shryock, *Cotton Mather: First Significant Figure in American Medicine* (Baltimore: Johns Hopkins Press, 1954), pp. 104–5. See also Perry Miller, *The New England Mind: From Colony to Province* (Cambridge, Mass.: Harvard University Press, 1953), pp. 345–66.

5. Timothy Tackett, *Priest and Parish in Eighteenth-Century France: A Social and Political Study of the Curés in a Diocese of Dauphiné, 1750–1791* (Princeton: Princeton University Press, 1977), p. 162; Max Bihan, "Mandement de l'Archevêque de Paris en faveur de la vaccination antivariolique," *Histoire des Sciences Médicales* 6 (1972): 169–72.

6. John Duffy, "Anglo-American Reaction to Obstetrical Anesthesia," *Bulletin of the History of Medicine* 38 (1964): 32–44; White, *History of the Warfare*, 2:62–63.

7. Walter Pagel, "Religious Motives in the Medical Biology of the 17th Century," *Bulletin of the Institute of the History of Medicine* 3 (1935): 97–120; Walter Pagel, *Paracelsus: An Introduction to Philosophical Medicine in the Era of the Renaissance* (Basel: S. Karger, 1958); Walter Pagel, *The Religious and Philosophical Aspects of van Helmont's Science and Medicine* (Baltimore: Johns Hopkins Press, 1944); Roland H. Bainton, *Hunted Heretic: The Life and Death of Michael Servetus, 1511–1553* (Boston: Beacon Press, 1953), pp. 101–27, 209; Walter Pagel, *William Harvey's Biological Ideas: Selected Aspects and Historical Background* (Basel: S. Karger, 1967), pp. 136–53.

8. Charles E. and Carroll S. Rosenberg, "Pietism and the Origins of the American Public Health Movement: A Note on John H. Griscom and Robert M. Hartley," *Journal of the History of Medicine and Allied Sciences* 23 (1968): 16–35; Lloyd G. Stevenson, "Science Down the Drain: On the Hostility of Certain Sanitarians to Animal Experimentation, Bacteriology, and Immunology," *Bulletin of the History of Medicine* 29 (1955): 1–26. See also Noël Poynter, *Medicine and Man* (London: C. A. Watts & Co., 1971), pp. 49–52; James C. Whorton, " 'Christian Physiology': William Alcott's Prescription for the Millennium," *Bulletin of the History of Medicine* 49 (1975): 466–81; and John Ettling, *The Germ of Laziness: Rockefeller Philanthropy and Public Health in the New South* (Cambridge, Mass.: Harvard University Press, 1981), which shows the continuing influence of Christianity on public health in the twentieth century.

9. Paul H. Kocher, "The Idea of God in Elizabethan Medicine," *Journal of the History of Ideas* 11 (1950): 29.

10. Ibid., pp. 3–29.

11. Ibid.; Alison Klairmont, "The Problem of the Plague: New Challenges to Healing in Sixteenth-Century France," *Proceedings*, Fifth Annual Meeting of the Western Society for French History, November 10–12, 1977, pp. 119–27; Theodore G. Tappert, ed. and trans., *Luther's Works*, 54, "Table Talk" (Philadelphia: Fortress Press, 1967), p. 53.

12. Carlo M. Cipolla, *Faith, Reason, and the Plague in Seventeenth-Century Tuscany*, trans. Muriel Kittel (Ithaca: Cornell University Press, 1979), pp. 41–74; Kocher, "The Idea of God," p. 7.

13. Charles E. Rosenberg, *The Cholera Years: The United States in 1832, 1849, and 1866* (Chicago: University of Chicago Press, 1962), p. 5. See also Michael N. Shute, "A Little Great Awakening: An Episode in the American Enlightenment," *Journal of the History of Ideas* 37 (1976): 598–602; William Gribben, "Divine Providence or Miasma? The Yellow Fever Epidemic of 1822," *New York History* 53 (1972): 283–98; and R. J. Morris, *Cholera 1832: The Social Response to an Epidemic* (London: Croom Helm, 1976).

14. Rosenberg, *Cholera Years*, pp. 40–54, 121–32.

15. Ibid., pp. 5, 220. On religious views of insanity, see Norman Dain, *Concepts of Insanity in the United States, 1789–1865* (New Brunswick, N.J.: Rutgers University Press, 1964), pp. 183–93.

16. Margaret Humphreys Warner, "Vindicating the Minister's Medical Role: Cotton Mather's Concept of the *Nishmath-Chajim* and the Spiritualization of Medicine," *Journal of the History of Medicine and Allied Sciences* 36 (1981): 278–95; Beall and Shryock, *Cotton Mather;* Wyndham B. Blanton, *Medicine in Virginia in the Seventeenth Century* (Richmond, Va.: William Byrd Press, 1930), pp. 213–14.

17. Darrel W. Amundsen, "Medieval Canon Law on Medical and Surgical Practice by the Clergy," *Bulletin of the History of Medicine* 52 (1978): 22–44; R. S. Roberts, "The Personnel and Practice of Medicine in Tudor and Stuart England," *Medical History* 6 (1962): 363–82 and 8 (1964): 217–34; Paul Delaunay, *La médicine et l'église: Contribution à l'histoire de l'exercice médicale* (Paris: Éditions Hippocrate, 1948), p. 82.

18. Michael MacDonald, *Mystical Bedlam: Madness, Anxiety, and Healing in Seventeenth-Century England* (Cambridge: Cambridge University Press, 1981), pp. 13–71. For a description of clergy-healers in early modern England, see Keith Thomas, *Religion and the Decline of Magic* (New York: Charles Scribner's Sons, 1971), pp. 275–76.

19. Richard Baxter, *Reliquiae Baxterianae*, ed. Matthew Sylvester (London, 1696), pt. 1, pp. 83–84, 89; C. Helen Brock, "The Influence of Europe on Colonial Massachusetts Medicine," in *Medicine in Colonial Massachusetts, 1620–1820*, ed. Philip Cash, Eric H. Christianson, and J. Worth Estes (Boston: Colonial Society of Massachusetts, 1980), p. 104.

20. Brock, "Influence of Europe," p. 104; Blanton, *Medicine in Virginia*, p. 220; Duffy, *Epidemics in Colonial America*, pp. 10–11; Whitfield J. Bell, Jr., "A Portrait of the Colonial Physician," *Bulletin of the History of Medicine* 44 (1970): 504–5. See also Henry M. Parrish, "Contributions of the Clergy to Early American Medicine," *Journal of the Bowman Gray School of Medicine* 14 (1956): 55–64; and James H. Cassedy, "Church Record-Keeping and Public Health in

The Historical Setting

Early New England," in *Medicine in Colonial Massachusetts*, pp. 249–62.

21. Philip W. Ott, "John Wesley on Health: A Word for Sensible Regimen," *Methodist History* 18 (1980): 193–204; Samuel J. Rogal, "Pills for the Poor: John Wesley's *Primitive Physick*," *Yale Journal of Biology and Medicine* 51 (1978): 81–90; Harold Y. Vanderpool, "John Wesley's Medicine for the Masses" (Unpublished paper, 1981).

22. George E. Gifford, Jr., "Botanic Remedies in Colonial Massachusetts, 1620–1820," in *Medicine in Colonial Massachusetts*, p. 280.

23. Robert Heller, "'Priest-Doctors' as a Rural Health Service in the Age of Enlightenment," *Medical History* 20 (1976): 362–64; Jacques Léonard, "Women, Religion, and Medicine," in *Medicine and Society in France*, ed. Robert Forster and Orest Ranum, trans. Elborg Forster and Patricia M. Ranum (Baltimore: Johns Hopkins University Press, 1980), pp. 24–47. See also Tackett, *Priest and Parish*, pp. 161–63.

24. Heller, "Priest-Doctors," pp. 365, 379–82.

25. Ibid., pp. 372–76.

26. James H. Cassedy, "An American Clerical Crisis: Ministers' Sore Throat, 1830–1860," *Bulletin of the History of Medicine* 53 (1979): 26–27.

27. Raymond J. Cunningham, "The Emmanuel Movement: A Variety of American Religious Experience," *American Quarterly* 14 (1962): 61; Charles F. Kemp, *Physicians of the Soul: A History of Pastoral Counseling* (New York: Macmillan Co., 1947), p. 236.

28. George Rosen, "The Hospital: Historical Sociology of a Community Institution," in *From Medical Police to Social Medicine: Essays on the History of Health Care*, ed. George Rosen (New York: Science History Publications, 1974), pp. 274–303; Darrel W. Amundsen, "History of Medical Ethics: Medieval Europe, Fourth to Sixteenth Century," in *The Encyclopedia of Bioethics*, 4 vols., ed. Warren T. Reich (New York: Free Press, 1978), 3:938–40.

29. Richard H. Shryock, *The History of Nursing: An Interpretation of the Social and Medical Factors Involved* (Philadelphia: W. B. Saunders, 1959), pp. 155–61; Robert M. Kingdon, "Social Welfare in Calvin's Geneva," *American Historical Review* 76 (1971): 50–69.

30. Shryock, *History of Nursing*, pp. 162–64; Jean Imbert, "L'Église et l'État face au problème hospitalier au XVI siècle," in *Étude d'histoire du droit canonique*, 2 vols. (Paris: Sirey, 1965), 1:577–92.

31. Shryock, *History of Nursing*, pp. 164–67; Léonard, "Women, Religion, and Medicine," pp. 25–26.

32. Louis S. Greenbaum, "Nurses and Doctors in Conflict: Piety and Medicine in the Paris Hôtel-Dieu on the Eve of the French Revolution," *Clio Medica* 13 (1978): 247–67.

33. Erwin H. Ackerknecht, *Medicine at the Paris Hospital, 1794–1848* (Baltimore: Johns Hopkins Press, 1967).

The Modern World

34. John Woodward, *To Do the Sick No Harm: A Study of the British Voluntary Hospital System to 1875* (London: Routledge & Kegan Paul, 1974), pp. 15–19; Henry C. Burdett, *Hospitals and Asylums of the World*, 3 vols. (London: J. & A. Churchill, 1893), 3:190–94.

35. Shryock, *History of Nursing*, pp. 270–71; Carl J. Scherzer, *The Church and Healing* (Philadelphia: Westminster Press, 1950), pp. 115–21; Cecil Woodham-Smith, *Florence Nightingale, 1820–1910* (New York: McGraw-Hill, 1951), pp. 60–61.

36. William A. Glaser, *Social Settings and Medical Organization: A Cross-National Study of the Hospital* (New York: Atherton Press, 1970), pp. 53–55; Shryock, *History of Nursing*, p. 286; Burdett, *Hospitals and Asylums*, 3:274.

37. James A. Hamilton, *Patterns of Hospital Ownership and Control* (Minneapolis: University of Minnesota Press, 1961), pp. 90, 96, 103; James R. Watson, "William A. Passavant, D.D.," *Surgery, Gynecology, and Obstetrics* 119 (1964): 858–61.

38. Morris J. Vogel, *The Invention of the Modern Hospital: Boston, 1870–1930* (Chicago: University of Chicago Press, 1980), pp. 127–28.

39. Glaser, *Social Settings*, p. 32; Scherzer, *The Church and Healing*, p. 129.

40. Francisco Guerra, "The Role of Religion in Spanish American Medicine," in *Medicine and Culture*, ed. F. N. L. Poynter (London: Wellcome Institute of the History of Medicine, 1969), pp. 179–88; William Malcolm Hailey, *An African Survey*, rev. ed. (London: Oxford University Press, 1957), p. 1064; Theron Kue-Hing Young, "A Conflict of Professions: The Medical Missionary in China, 1835–1890," *Bulletin of the History of Medicine* 47 (1973): 252–53, 270.

41. Young, "Conflict," p. 253; Hailey, *African Survey*, p. 1065; Roland Oliver, *The Missionary Factor in East Africa*, 2d ed. (London: Longmans, 1965), pp. 12–13.

42. Young, "Conflict," p. 253; Hailey, *African Survey*, p. 1065; Peter Buck, *American Science and Modern China, 1876–1936* (Cambridge: Cambridge University Press, 1980), pp. 13, 17.

43. Young, "Conflict," pp. 250–57; Buck, *American Science*, pp. 10–13.

44. Young, "Conflict," pp. 251–59.

45. Terence O. Ranger, "Godly Medicine: The Ambiguities of Medical Mission in Southeast Tanzania, 1900–1945," *Social Science and Medicine* 15B (1981): 261–77.

46. Oliver, *Missionary Factor*, p. 211; Buck, *American Science*, pp. 25–27.

47. Franklin T. Fowler, "The History of Southern Baptist Medical Missions," *Baptist History and Heritage* 10 (1975): 200–201.

48. On the prohibition of blood transfusions, see Timothy White, *A People for His Name: A History of Jehovah's Witnesses and an Evaluation* (New York: Vantage Press, 1968), pp. 391–96.

49. Léonard, "Women, Religion, and Medicine," pp. 29, 32; Kemp, *Physicians*

of the Soul, pp. 158–59. See also Thomas Kselman, Miracles and Prophecies: Popular Religion in the Church in 19th-Century France (New Brunswick, N.J.: Rutgers University Press, 1983).

50. John T. McNeill, ed., Calvin: Institutes of the Christian Religion, trans. Ford Lewis Battles, 2 vols. (Philadelphia: Westminster Press, 1960), 1:1454 and 2:17; Harold Y. Vanderpool, "Dominant Health Concerns in Protestantism," in Encyclopedia of Bioethics, 3:1375; Richard D. Brown, "The Healing Arts in Colonial and Revolutionary Massachusetts: The Context for Scientific Medicine," in Medicine in Colonial Massachusetts, pp. 37–39; Beall and Shryock, Cotton Mather, pp. 232–34.

51. Raymond J. Cunningham, "From Holiness to Healing: The Faith Cure in America, 1872–1892," Church History 43 (1974): 499–513; David Edwin Harrell, Jr., All Things Are Possible: The Healing and Charismatic Revivals in Modern America (Bloomington: Indiana University Press, 1975), pp. 10–11.

52. Harrell, All Things Are Possible.

53. Ibid., p. 101; William J. Broad, "And God Said to Oral: Build a Hospital," Science 208 (April 18, 1980): 267–71. See also E. Mansell Pattison, Nikolajs A. Lapins, and Hans A. Doerr, "Faith Healing: A Study of Personality and Function," Journal of Nervous and Mental Disease 157 (1973): 397–409.

54. Robert Peel, Mary Baker Eddy, 3 vols. (New York: Holt, Rinehart & Winston, 1966–77). See also Walter I. Wardwell, "Christian Science Healing," Journal for the Scientific Study of Religion 4 (1965): 175–81.

55. Robert T. Divett, "Medicine and the Mormons: A Historical Perspective," Dialogue: A Journal of Mormon Thought 12 (1979): 16–25; Linda P. Wilcox, "The Imperfect Science: Brigham Young on Medical Doctors," ibid., pp. 26–36; N. Lee Smith, "Herbal Remedies: God's Medicine?" ibid., pp. 37–60; Joseph L. Lyon and Steven Nelson, "Mormon Health," ibid., pp. 84–96; Leonard J. Arrington and Davis Bitton, The Mormon Experience: A History of the Latter-day Saints (New York: Alfred A. Knopf, 1979), p. 299.

56. Ronald L. Numbers, Prophetess of Health: A Study of Ellen G. White (New York: Harper & Row, 1976).

57. Charlotte Saikowski and Richard M. Harley, "Christian Healing: A Grass-Roots Revival," Christian Science Monitor, March 13, 1979, pp. 12–13. The figure given is based on a 1978 Gallup poll.

PART THREE

A Philosophical Perspective

6

Understanding Faith Traditions in the Context of Health Care: Philosophy as a Guide for the Perplexed

H. Tristram Engelhardt, Jr.

To take a philosophical perspective on the relationship between religion and medicine is to give an account in philosophical terms of both religion and medicine. This results from the fact that philosophy is an enterprise that attempts the most general questions in the most general terms. It explores the nature of knowledge, of evaluations, and of reality. This claim for philosophy's importance in exploring such basic issues requires an explanation, for it may appear that religion, not philosophy, is the more fundamental of the two. However, religion pursues the great questions within particular traditions. Thus there are Protestant, Catholic, Jewish, Islamic, and Hindu understandings of the proper role of medicine. In contrast, philosophy as it has come to be understood is a Western tradition of approaching questions that attempts to be of no particular tradition. In a sense, this commits philosophy to being an enterprise of the least common denominator. It is an attempt to see what is conceptually presumed in the enterprises of humans, including our understandings of the world within which we live. The honest search for such generality will inevitably require abandoning the search for many answers—at least through philosophy. By the time one has framed questions in ways open to their being understood by humans generally, apart from their particular religious and cultural traditions, they may no longer be answerable in great detail, if at all. Philosophical reflection is therefore likely to be humbling, if not disappointing. Where much is sincerely sought, often relatively little is found. Philosophy, for example, is more

A Philosophical Perspective

likely to discover problems with proofs for the existence of God than to be able to conclude that there is a God.

Why, then, seek a philosophical perspective on the relationship of religion and medicine? The answer in part lies in the fact that often neither physicians nor patients share in one religion. Many possess none. One finds a circumstance defined by conflicting viewpoints and competing claims regarding what is right and proper in the practice of medicine. When such conflict and competition define the character of medical practice in a society, one is pressed as a practical measure to find a neutral standpoint. It is as if religion created an embarrassment of riches. By its capacity to deliver numerous relatively concrete and certain answers, it engenders a context of tension in a pluralist society. Though many groups give answers in detail, the detailed answers are at odds. As a consequence, the hope of a neutral albeit sparse standpoint is a natural one. Philosophy is sought as a common vantage point, given a plurality of viewpoints. In a context of conflicting claims about the morality of contraceptives, for example, medicine as a general secular endeavor needs to employ a perspective that does not take one particular religion's side.

Of course, religions also seek a point of consensus. One hopes, after all, to convert others to one's own religious point of view. The feature that distinguishes philosophy vis-à-vis religion, however, is philosophy's commitment to finding a common vantage point without appealing beyond this world and without extramundane grace. In fact, one will need to draw a distinction between philosophy as an enterprise in conceptual analysis and description, and philosophy as it has often been attempted in the past: as a bridge to metaphysical truths. Thus philosophy of the neutral vantage point is not only secular but nonmetaphysical as well, if one includes within metaphysics the objects that Kant enumerates, for example, God, freedom, and immortality. At best it will be able to show that human thought presupposes freedom, rather than being able to prove the existence of freedom, as, for example, the existence of God was proven by Thomas Aquinas.

Philosophy thus appears as a strategy for mapping the grammar of concepts and of values. It is an enterprise in conceptual geography, in critically assessing the competing maps of reality and of values. Even where it does not provide final answers concerning the existence of God or of immortality, it can be used to assess the ways in which such notions play a role in religious value systems and religious understandings of reality. Philosophy, then, is the discipline of conceptual analysis and conceptual description. It is the attempt to become clearer about value presuppositions and the presuppositions involved in particular ways of seeking knowledge and of making claims about the world. When confronted with the plurality of religious understandings in the world, such analysis and description is integral to the conceptual map-making required for the orientation of physicians, patients, and nurses in societies not marked by a uniformity of belief.

On the one hand, philosophy in this sense is to be understood as a set of conceptual disciplines for analysis and description. On the other hand, it is to be understood also as a minimalist account of reality, knowledge, and values. In either case, it makes strong universalist claims. It is the attempt to spell out what individuals can conclude with the aid of reason and without the grace of a particular revelation. In this sense it aspires to be the catholic framework for individuals in their relations to health care.

What roles can and should philosophy play, given the plurality of religious views concerning the proper use of medicine? It can provide intellectual orientation, and this orientation can provide what one might term the logic of a pluralism. That is, philosophy can provide the peaceable matrix within which individuals of varying viewpoints can cooperate in the enterprises of health care. Further, this analytic and conceptually descriptive enterprise can provide the basis for a comparison of the various religious viewpoints regarding proper medical care. Such comparisons are likely to be not only intellectually enlightening but also of use to the health-care professionals treating patients within contexts conditioned by varying religious understandings of the probity of particular medical interventions. Such analytic and comparative regard for religion will also disclose metaphysical prejudices. Religions develop within the embrace of particular cultures and therefore inevitably state their timeless truths in the very timebound idioms of particular cultures with their particular philosophies and metaphysics. A philosophical assessment can provide a final service, namely, a basis for critique. Identifying the outworn metaphysical baggage of a religion may allow it to remain true to its original insights while changing its understandings of the probity of particular medical procedures. For example, a great deal of the theological argument concerning artificial contraception has focused on the extent to which such prohibitions are integral to a particular religious faith commitment, or are instead a function of what was originally a Greek notion of what should count as natural or unnatural acts.[1]

PHILOSOPHY VERSUS PHILOSOPHIES: IN SEARCH OF AN UNDERSTANDING OF RELIGIOUS VIEWS OF PROPER MEDICAL CARE

Just as the history of religion is full of competing sects, so too is the history of philosophy. One finds, for instance, materialists and idealists, rationalists and empiricists. It would seem that philosophy is in no better position than religion to give coherence or direction. However, a similar lament can be added to this if one considers the history of medicine or of science. Though at present there is not the same great division of opinion concerning justifiable scientific or medical theory as there is concerning justifiable philosophical theories or religious viewpoints, over time one nevertheless sees starkly contrasting viewpoints. In this last difficulty a suggestion for a solution can be found. What is most interesting about the endeavor of empirical science is its commitment to the development of intersubjectively examinable and testable generalizations about reality, not simply that particular predictions are borne out or that particular explanations ring true. The latter will surely change over time. Here one finds the clue to understanding the contribution of contemporary philosophy. Philosophy functions as an attempt to frame intersubjectively analyzable and criticizable claims about the nature of values, knowledge, and reality. At this point contemporary philosophy departs not only from religion but also from much of the philosophy of the past. The accent is upon method, as Kant argued in 1781, rather than on an organon of knowledge.[2] Philosophy is closer to science than to religion in this commitment to the goal of intersubjectively substantiable claims.

It should be noted that doing philosophy is not restricted to philosophers. Theologians and physicians, to take two examples, do philosophy when they analyze and assess their claims as arguments, even in terms of particular religious or medical facts or canons. Theologians are, after all, individuals reflecting in an intellectually disciplined manner about the doctrines of a particular religion or of religions generally in order to understand better their value and epistemological commitments. Such reflection does not, in fact, require the theologian to be a believer in order to do well in this enterprise, as common experience will attest.

Philosophy as a Guide for the Perplexed

Also, one should note that medicine, as used here, is secular medicine, an attempt to make intersubjectively testable predictions (e.g., prognoses) about the courses of diseases while giving explanatory accounts of those diseases (e.g., diagnoses) in ways that will in general improve the successful prevention and treatment of diseases and the maintenance of health. However, medicine in any particular time and culture will not only offer historically conditioned explanations, but also treat patients within a medical world view that presupposes a particular ordering of benefits and harms. Still, medicine seeks, as do science and philosophy, to give a culturally undistorted view of reality. So, too, secular humanism is embedded in a particular world view, even when philosophy, which is an element of secular humanism, attempts to step outside the confines of particular cultural presuppositions.

All concrete ways of life presuppose particular hierarchies of values and harms. They instruct regarding which goods are more important than others and what harms are to be avoided at what price. However, any such ordering presupposes a particular moral sense. Thus, for example, philosophical theories that appeal to impartial observers or rational contractors must, in order to determine such an ordering, project a particular moral sense onto such observers or contractors. John Rawls's *A Theory of Justice* can be seen as a rational construction of the moral sentiments of a liberal member of the Cambridge, Massachusetts, community.[3] Even though his work does not provide a reconstruction of a concrete universal morality (to do that, one would need to decide which moral sense was normative, and how could one do that except by appealing to some particular moral sense, which would beg the question), it makes an important intellectual contribution. It offers a conceptual map of the consequences of a particular moral point of view. Alan Donagan makes a similar contribution by attempting in *The Theory of Morality* to give a rational reconstruction of Hebrew Christian morality.[4]

Such philosophical endeavors of limited scope fall within the more general undertaking of sketching the lineaments of morality itself, that to which one has committed oneself in deciding to ask ethical questions (e.g., to resolve disputes about the probity of alternate lines of conduct on the basis of reason, not force). The more general ethical endeavor is likely to deliver only very abstract statements that depend on the nature of the project of ethics itself (e.g., the peaceable resolution of moral controversies on the basis of reason). The reconstruction of particular ethical viewpoints will bear the same relation to the endeavor of sketching the foundations of ethics, as attempts to reconstruct particular scientific endeavors (e.g., Immanuel Kant's reconstruction of Newton's physics in *Metaphysical Foundations of Natural Science* [1786]—Kant would not gladly accept this more restricted interpretation of the significance of this work) do to accounting for empirical science generally.

Western religion, however, usually holds that there is indeed a unique and impartial observer whose viewpoint one could in principle appeal to in order to resolve ethical and epistemological disputes. The deity offers an authority who stands outside time and culture. Moreover, the deity's authority can in principle answer epistemological and ethical questions concretely and in detail. Since there are many competing views of the deity's concrete answers, philosophy is useful in offering an endeavor for finding common conceptual and ethical ground, or at least conceptually placing the competing accounts. It seeks a common vantage point as a regulative ideal even when that goal is beyond reach as a concrete viewpoint.

Religions also seek to surmount the cacophony of competing claims. They make this attempt through an appeal to a particular revelation or special grace, at least in the case of revealed religions. The particularity of the revelation may be divisive in a pluralist society. And in the case of natural theology, skepticism concerning the capacity to sustain particular metaphysical propositions leads to a similar bar to general agreement. In order to move with certainty to a conclusion, one will have needed first to accept premises that will not be open to general substantiation. Thus, in talking about philosophy's role in understanding religion's relations to medicine, one will need to specify a particular sense of philosophy. The sense of philosophy that will serve best in a context of religious pluralism is that of a disciplined endeavor of analysis and conceptual description. One will want to discern how one can talk across religious boundaries and how one can weigh the reasonableness of the claims made by the various religions one encounters. Here philosophy functions through its regulative ideal of seeking to criticize claims concerning values and knowledge through generally defensible, rational criteria. Even where philosophy fails to produce final answers, it will always be attempting, as does science, to resolve a conflict of conclusions through a common commitment to the fragile capacities of mundane human reason.

This view of philosophy is surely uninspiring; it is plodding and tedious. It lacks the bold proposals and detailed ontological vistas provided by revealed religions and metaphysics. However, in recurring always to the general capacities of finite human reason, it offers a way back from the diversity of religious and metaphysical opinions to a common task of outlining the possibilities for true knowledge and justifiable evaluation. It is, after all, precisely this endeavor that is called for when faced with the plurality of beliefs concerning the proper ways to intervene through medicine in human life and death.

This is not to imply that philosophy ought not to take an interest in religious or metaphysical questions. Though philosophy may not be able to answer such questions, it can provide suggestions concerning the conceptual grammar one would have to employ in answers if they are forthcoming and if they are to be put in rational terms. After all, religions that speak simply in the quick embrace of mystical grace need not give justifications to anyone. Those that feel the spirit know where it lists and follow. However, insofar as inspiration must be put into rational form, the confines of reasonable discourse constrain. It is here that philosophy can do more than offer a sense of what would fit, where and when, given a particular syntax of values and of concepts of reality. It can also provide a conceptual map by interrelating competing viewpoints. For example, religious claims framed in the language of natural law draw upon a language of nature and of norms that is indebted, at least in the West, to Stoic, Aristotelian, Platonic, and other Greco-Roman sources. In analyzing them one can show their conceptual origins and display what premises lead to what conclusions.

Consider a traditional Roman Catholic proscription of contraception:

> What is said of feminine contraceptives is true *a fortiori* of the use of a condom, as well as of the onanistic practice of withdrawal with ejaculation outside the vagina. In both these cases, not only are the natural effects of *coitus* impeded, but the *coitus* itself is rendered unnatural, because the minimum essential of natural *coitus* is ejaculation within the vagina.[5]

To understand the account offered of the immorality of the act, one will need to understand the author's interpretation of "natural" and "unnatural" and terms such as "unnatural sexual acts" and "natural coitus." One will need to know as well what is held to be an "onanistic practice" and wherein its evil lies. Moreover, one will need to know why unnatural acts should also be considered immoral acts. For someone outside the Catholic tradition, a secular philosophical assessment of these viewpoints will place such views within general intellectual concerns to explore concepts of the natural and to understand their bearing on the morality of particular medical interventions. They can be given a place in the geography of human concerns.

It is helpful to see how the Catholic position contrasts with traditions that have not articulated their viewpoints on contraception in such metaphysical language. A good position for comparison is the Jewish view, which is relatively innocent of such Greek or Roman understanding of the natural or unnatural. The Jewish viewpoint relies instead upon a tradition in which divine injunctions are not amenable to the rational accounts sought by the Greeks. Thus the Jewish understanding of contraception is framed in terms of the commandment to "be fruitful and multiply." "The Jewish rulings on contraception, therefore, derive their form and authority neither from the whims of the human conscience nor from the laws of nature, but simply from the positive divinely-ordained obligation to propagate the race."[6] What one discovers within the Jewish argument is an interpretation of an injunction in Gen. 1:27–28 to increase and multiply as well as similar statements such as Deut. 7:13. As a consequence, the interpretation of onanism has a different valence. The act of Onan was immoral not because it was unnatural but because he failed in the fulfillment of an obligation to reproduce, in this case disobeying his father by not providing his brother's widow with a child. One has as a result a quite different view of how the morality of contraception is to be developed.

Health-care professionals interested in understanding the religious bioethical issues raised by contraception will thus need to place these issues not only within particular religious traditions but also within particular metaphysical idioms—and this within the terrain of philosophical questions. For individuals accustomed to contemporary understandings of evolution, such conceptual orientation will be necessary in order for them to comprehend what concerns are at stake in the moral views of those opposed to the use of contraception. In evolutionary terms it becomes difficult to talk of *a* human nature (i.e., one would presume that there would be variations within populations with respect to traits adapted to particular environments). As a deliverance of blind forces of natural selection, "the natural" would not bear moral force because it was "natural." One finds, for example, William Clifford, a follower of Charles Darwin and Herbert Spencer, arguing in 1875: "And we may then say that, since the process of natural selection has been understood, *purpose* has ceased to suggest design to instructed people, except in cases where the agency of man is independently probable."[7] In contrast to many traditional views, the contemporary ontology of human nature loses the conjunction between the unnatural and the immoral. Indeed, the epistemology of current scientific studies of the evolution of human sexuality is free of Stoic or Aristotelian notions of the natural or the unnatural on which such conjunctions were based. Further, if one were disposed to draw a general conclusion from the empirical data, one would suggest that other than immediate reproductive consequences of sexual activities played a central role in the evolution of human sexuality. Theodosius Dobzhansky stressed the social role of sexual intercourse in the evolution of Homo sapiens. "Continuous sexual receptivity of the female made monogamous family life possible and thus freed the male from the constant necessity of warding off interlopers."[8]

As a consequence, in order to orient physicians, nurses, and others to what is at stake in moral claims about the propriety or impropriety of the use of contraception according to particular religions, one will need to place such claims within a conceptual geography. That geography will need to identify how particular views of the authority of historical divine injunctions, views of concepts of the natural and the unnatural and their relations to moral structures, and views concerning the extent to which human biological function may be properly harnessed to individually chosen goals can be related to the assessment of the morality of contraception.

A similar analysis can be offered for religious bioethical views on abortion, the definition of death, euthanasia, or other issues on which particular religions have developed characteristic accounts. Such analyses can serve the role of placing conceptually the relationship of particular religions to particular medical practices. Such conceptual orientation is necessary to aid physicians and nurses who are not members of such religions to understand opinions on the part of their patients that would otherwise appear strange, if not bizarre. Philosophical bioethics should, after all, increase the capacity of health-care professionals to treat their patients as persons by indicating the assumptions that make particular proscriptions and ways of acting appear to be reasonable to their patients. Good patient care requires an adequate appreciation of the opinions and felt needs of the patients being treated. Since medicine bears dramatically upon the conditions of reproduction, illness, and death, and since these circumstances are freighted by humans with strongly held values, a knowledge of the geography of such values can increase the capacity of health-care givers to deliver care that patients will find acceptable. In providing a conceptual matrix for orientation, philosophy discharges one of the major social obligations of a secular humanism. It provides a cynosure in circumstances that would otherwise be intellectually disorienting.

Even where philosophy does not succeed in providing a single, generally acknowledged account of bioethics' goals and obligations, it offers the sole mode for peaceable, cognitive resolution of disputes and for dealing with conflicting bioethical views regarding the provision of health care in a pluralist, secular society. That mode is critical assessment and analysis of claims. How else could one understand which claims to credit and how to appreciate the claims one does not credit but respects as the cherished beliefs of a particular patient or colleague? Here philosophy becomes catholic even when it is itself beset by sectarian divisions. It embraces the rational hope for the intersubjective weighing of conflicting claims in a community of peaceable reasoners who may not share the same religious traditions.

RELIGIOUS STORIES AND THE STORY OF STORIES: SECULAR HUMANISM AS THE CYNOSURE

Since health care is delivered in communities marked by divisions of religious beliefs, philosophy is sought as a neutral rational fabric. As indicated, though it springs from the traditions of a particular culture and is marked by its history, it is unique in its attempts to step beyond those particularities. It seeks to weigh its claims and the claims of others regarding values, knowledge, and reality in terms of criteria of reasonableness that would be open to all. Philosophy thus aspires to be the general human story. It attempts to be true to its tradition of attempting always to step critically outside its own particular traditions. As such it provides a general, abstract framework in terms of which one can identify the reasonable, clarify ideas, and test claims. Philosophy thus seeks to provide the grammar of grammars, to offer canons for the syntax of any particular story. However, it does not offer a concrete way of life.

Ways of life are to be found in particular traditions, particular stories.[9] There is thus a dialectical relation between philosophy on the one hand and ways of life on the other. Because religions are second only to such major ideologies as Marxism in providing a general metaphysics and *Weltanschauung*, they will inevitably be tightly bound to philosophical reflections. To live a concrete life, one must fashion it within understandings of what is meaningful, beautiful, good, and true. Such understandings must be drawn with a completeness that falls beyond the capacities of general philosophical arguments. Philosophical arguments can rule ways of life in or out as reasonable accounts, or as fulfilling general rational criteria of morality. However, very little can be said about what the concrete lives of individuals ought to be like. Thus philosophy is likely to be able to give an account of promise-keeping. But in most of the interesting areas of life it will do little to suggest what promises one ought to make. For example, ought one to contract for polygamous, monogamous, or polyandrous marriage? Secular philosophy is likely to have little of use to say on such matters. Guidance will be found instead in the traditions that provide accounts of heroes, saints, and patriarchs. Through their stories one is able to learn how the particular virtues of a particular way of life can be assembled into a living whole. One comes to know through such instruction what it is to flourish in a particular ethical mode.

Religions are among the primary tutors with regard to the virtues of particular ways of life. Through them one learns in detail why it is virtuous to bear up under sufferings of a certain kind, how one is to understand the significance of pain, disability, and disease, and when it can be redeemed within a transcendent understanding of the purpose and meaning of human life. Such metaphysical accounts fall beyond the ken of secular philosophy. In fact, the accent upon transcendent realities and meanings in giving accounts of the significance of copulation, birth, illness, disability, dying, and death distinguishes religious stories from secular ones. Examples of the latter can be found in the accounts of what it is to live and die as a Southern gentleman or a good old Texas boy. (Marxism, due to its peculiar metaphysical claims, probably falls as a *tertium quid* between such secular stories and those of religious traditions.)

Philosophy is thus always stepping back to gain a perspective on the particular traditions within which we all actually live our lives. It is a merely abstract endeavor apart from those traditions (here read the religious faith traditions) in which it lives and to which it directs its attention. Philosophy solves the conceptual problems that particular traditions engender for themselves and for those outside those traditions who are puzzled about their meaning. Through such solutions philosophy has concrete purpose and application. Through philosophy the particular traditions gain rationality and a place in the general intellectual endeavor of the community of reasoners. Philosophy is thus not a luxury but an intellectual necessity. It is a practical necessity for the coherent, peaceable practice of medicine in a pluralistic secular society. Medicine needs a general story through which to integrate the various stories of the particular traditions that fashion the lives of its members and of its patients. Philosophy as the core of the secular humanistic endeavor provides the grammar of this general story: the endeavor of critically and analytically regarding and relating the various claims of particular traditions, chief among them the religious faith traditions.

CHART-MAKING

The argument of this chapter has been that in order to understand the relations of the various religions to medicine, one will need a vantage point outside any of them. The vantage point offered is that of critically analyzing and describing the conceptual claims of religions bearing on medicine. A philosophical approach to the relation of religion and medicine will thus lead to exploring both the epistemological dimensions and value-theoretical dimensions of this relationship.

Concepts of Disease

Different religions have at different times had radically varying views with regard to the significance of diseases. The Hippocratic corpus, for example, contains a treatise *(On the Sacred Disease)* in which the author argues that epilepsy should not, any more than any other disease, be considered to have a special divine origin.

> It is not, in my opinion, any more divine or more sacred than other diseases, but has a natural cause, and its supposed divine origin is due to men's inexperience, and to their wonder at its peculiar character. Now while men continue to believe in its divine origin because they are at a loss to understand it, they really disprove its divinity by the facile method of healing which they adopt, consisting as it does of purifications and incantations.[10]

One finds captured in this passage a step in the process of the separation of religion and medicine. The history of medicine and religion has been marked by a separation of prerogatives regarding not only the healing of diseases but also their explanation.

Disease language is complex.[11] It identifies certain states of affairs as worthy of treatment because they are associated with pains, dysfunctions, deformities, and losses of physical or psychological grace that are held to be beyond the natural or tolerable course of things. It includes explanations through which these phenomena are accounted for in order to predict outcomes and to guide treatment. Further, disease language is performative; it creates social reality (consider, for example, what happens when a sheriff says, "You are deputized"; an army physician says, "You are 50 percent disabled"; or a bishop says, "You are excommunicated"—social reality is being made, not just described). Disease language thus possesses descriptive, evaluative, explanatory, and performative dimensions. Religions and medicine are likely to have disagreements regarding each of these four dimensions.

Particular religions may differ with medicine regarding what circumstances ought to be described as diseases or objects of medical intervention. Differences may lie, for example, in evaluations regarding what ought to be borne patiently or treated by medicine. Here one will find disputes about the extent to which it is permissible to use anesthesia to blunt pain, especially that of childbirth, or to use medicine to terminate unwanted pregnancies or to control unwanted fertility. Here too will be disputes regarding whether teenage masturbation is a sin or a wholesome part of developing sexual awareness (and, in the case of women, orgasmic capacity).

In addition to disputes with respect to what ought to be acknowledged as bona fide states of pathology to be treated, or of health to be supported, medicine as a science is likely to speak somewhat differently regarding the proper ways in which one should explain the contradiction of diseases or the processes of healing. There is a long history of contention with regard to the role of divine and malevolent spirits in the production of disease and illness.[12]

Finally, because of the differences in evaluating circumstances as proper goals of medical care or as open to medical or religious interventions, religion and medicine will variously cast individuals into sick roles or penitent ones (as well as supplicant roles, and the like). Consider, for example, a homosexual coming for treatment of sexual dysfunction in order to perform better as a homosexual. Here there are likely to be disagreements regarding whether an individual should be cast into a therapy role or into a role of a penitent. Some religious groups would see such a use of a therapy role to be immoral, while some physicians are likely to see casting a patient into a penitent role in such circumstances as injurious to the patient's health. In other circumstances, the roles offered by medicine and religion are likely to be mutually supportive.

Since religions vary in their views regarding the propriety of different medical interventions, it will often not be clear to physicians or nurses when they are likely to find the ministers of a particular religion as their colleagues in treatment or their adversaries. On the other hand, a conceptual understanding of the views of religion in these circumstances can support cooperation. That is, a better understanding of each other's positions may avoid conflict in many circumstances. One might think, for example, of how a better understanding of the approaches of medicine and of the views of Jehovah's Witnesses can allow compromises to be fashioned in many circumstances, given the availability of plasma expanders and other blood surrogates. Without such an understanding, there may be actual conflict about the propriety of casting a patient into a particular therapy role. The extent to which accommodations can be usefully achieved will depend in part upon the general commitment to a peaceable society. It should be noted that these disagreements have been wide-ranging and have included incidents regarding when pain and disability should be suffered in patience as punishments for sin rather than seen as unfortunate states of affairs to be prevented or treated as far as possible through medical science. An example here would be the opposition to variolation on the grounds that it involved an attempt to thwart the will of God.[13]

It should be stressed that what is at stake in conflicts over what should count as diseases or as medical problems precedes moral conflicts. The physician is seeing a circumstance to be undesirable or improper through a nonmoral evaluation. When a physician decides a state of affairs is pathological, the judgment involves values (this is not proper), but not moral values. Compare, for example, "this is a beautiful woman" versus "this is a just women"; or "this is an ugly man" versus "this is a bad man." Compare, as well, "he is diseased" or "he is a pervert" with "he is a sinner." The moral judgments in the second element of the contrasts involve views regarding worthiness for happiness. Medical judgments concern appropriateness for treatment. In the case of the homosexual seeking treatment to enhance his function as a homosexual, one may have a conflict between medical and religious judgments, between a judgment on the one hand, "he ought to be treated" versus "he ought to repent of his sins." Of course, such judgments can also be compatible.

Consider: "he should be treated for his alcoholism," and "he should repent of his sin of drunkenness."

Whether there is compatibility or tension is dependent upon the coincidence of somewhat independent views of the significance of reality: one view informed by a secular scientific technology, the other informed by a particular religious tradition. As the above suggests, there will be areas of both overlap and disagreement between the two genres of systems of concepts and values. The areas of disagreement or tension spring from the fact that the two languages serve quite different purposes. The language of medicine is framed in terms of concepts of health and disease, illness and disability, and focuses upon distinguishing between the therapeutic and nontherapeutic. The language of Western religion, in contrast, maps the same world in terms of concepts of grace and sin, of the damning and of the redeeming. The result is two quite different understandings of what humans ought to be, one focusing on salvation and on justification before God, and the other focusing on health and the control of disease.

As indicated, these languages need not be in tension. However, they need not be in harmony either. Compare two questions: "Does it advance public health to give contraceptives to the poor who could otherwise not afford them?" And "Is it a mitzvah or an act of Christian charity to give contraceptives to the poor who could otherwise not afford them?" Though the questions concern the same behavior, they involve somewhat different actions because the intentions of the actors are different. In one case health is being sought, in the other case individuals are attempting an act of lovingkindness that is seen to be praiseworthy by the Deity. Whether the questions produce answers that can be co-ordinated will depend upon the viewpoint of the particular religion with regard to contraception. Philosophy can make a major contribution by analyzing, within a secular language that can speak across religious boundaries, the conceptual and value presuppositions of medical practice. In this fashion not only will areas of disagreement be better understood, but areas of cooperation will be secured as well.

Rights, Duties, Goods, and Virtues

The major proportion of the areas of religious concern with medicine, which are clearly distinguishable from secular concerns, involve the issues of sex, euthanasia, and dying, as well as special areas of difference

A Philosophical Perspective

such as that regarding blood transfusions for Jehovah's Witnesses and medical treatment for Christian Scientists. The bulk of contemporary analysis of the concepts of justice, of rights to health care, and of rights to consent to treatment spring from secular interests or are for the most part at least articulated in secular terms. Unlike the arguments regarding contraception, abortion, or euthanasia, these latter areas appear to engender no special points of tension. However, even where religious and secular medical concerns appear to be in concert, the ways in which goals are understood differ. To understand claims regarding rights and duties, one must first be clear regarding their foundations. A right to consent to treatment based on the conditions for the possibility of a moral community is a different right from that claimed on the basis of a calculus of the on-balance beneficial consequences that would derive from such a practice. Both these rights are different from claims to rights to consent based upon what is held to be the will of God. They differ in their force and foundations. In the first case, to violate such a right would be to set oneself outside any moral community. In the second case, to violate such a right would be to act in ways that have long-run adverse consequences. In the third case, it would be to offend the deity and divine interests. One needs to specify the grounding of a right (or of an obligation) in order to see what it would mean to violate it, and thus to know how serious a right or an obligation is at stake.

The same is the case in comparing the goals of religious and medical concerns with illness, disease, and disability. One will need in each case to know what hierarchy of goods or goals is presupposed. For instance, a physician faced with a dying patient who wishes to refuse further treatment may see the circumstances quite differently from a minister who wishes the patient to repent and be saved before dying. The minister has a moral observer to whose viewpoint an appeal for an authoritative ranking of goals can be made. The physician practicing medicine in a secular context may despair of such an authoritative viewpoint. In fact, it is the general absence of such an authoritative viewpoint that makes the appeal to the consent of individuals such a central element of secular society. Where one cannot discover what individuals ought to do, one will establish procedures to allow them to invent or choose their own destinies. In a secular society the right to consent, as a consequence, plays a practical role beyond any arguments for the right of individuals to self-determination. Even where physicians hold that they can indeed discover a proper ordering of goods, the ordering of secular medicine will be focused on health, not on salvation. One might think of the Middle Ages in which would-be patients were required to show a certificate of confession prior to receiving medical treatment.[14] Secular medicine, in having mundane goals, will not possess the concerns of religion, which tend to transcendent destinies. As a result, pain, suffering, disability, and death will be appreciated differently in the view of secular medicine from that of religion. A satisfactory understanding of secular medicine's relations with religions will require a critical comparison of their axiologies.

Such axiologies reveal the terrains for ideas and values that fashion the concrete world in which particular virtues flourish and others are excluded. In choosing one set of virtues, any particular tradition excludes others. Consequently the sense of a just or virtuous person will vary from tradition to tradition. Such differences often exist even within what is termed one faith tradition. One might consider the differences in virtue exemplified by Saint Francis of Assisi (1182–1226), who tended to all with kindness, and Saint Olaf Haraldsson (995–1030), who led Christians into battle at Stiklestad. The virtues that Saint Francis embraced excluded the virtues of bravery and courage that Olaf embodied, and the reverse. So too one will find different senses of what will count as virtue in suffering illness, disability, and death, given the stories told within particular religious traditions. One might think of the differences between the Jewish tradition, which fairly uniformly valued medicine and care by physicians, and the Christian tradition, which has shown greater ambivalence, the extreme example being Christian Scientists. Further, religious traditions, which hold that there is an afterlife and a transcendent economy in which suffering can gain merit, will endow the patient endurance of pain with special meaning and will not rank as highly the goal of increasing the pleasures of this life as will a secular account. Within secular medicine it will make sense, all else being equal, not only to seek to diminish pain, but also to increase the pleasures of this life (consider, for example, sex therapy). The importance of such satisfaction is greater in hierarchies of values that do not include transcendent rewards and punishments. And insofar as the language of rights and obligations is reducible to interests in goods or values, or differences in their deontological foundations, there will be a discordance between religion and secular medical understandings of rights and obligations.

Rights, duties, goals, and virtues must be seen within moral systems. Understanding the relation of religion to medicine will require analyzing these systems in order to disclose what is in fact at stake. One will need to determine what kinds of claims are being made and how they can be brought into harmony in order to aid health-care professionals in seeing what particular sufferings and disabilities mean to their patients. Thus a religious patient's rejection of euthanasia may not exclude an interest in exercising a right to reject "extraordinary" means of treatment, though in some classifications of euthanasia the latter would be a species of it. Senses of "extraordinary" can only be parsed within the confines of a tradition. A study of what it is to relate the goals of religious patients and ministers with those of secular medicine will, then, require one to study the ambiguity of the good and the multiple senses it carries in divergent circumstances. This is a philosophical task.

THE TASK OF A PLURALIST SOCIETY

A peaceable society which embraces individuals with divergent religious viewpoints (including atheists) will need to fashion a common standpoint within which to pose and answer important questions it cannot avoid in providing health care. When may individuals refuse lifesaving treatment? What are the rights to health care? Should these include rights to contraception and abortion on request? What are the goals to be sought through health care? To what extent should the happiness of patients be pursued through cosmetic surgery? These and other similar issues can be discussed and assayed only through a common language and perspective.

Philosophy as the core of a secular humanism offers this lingua franca. In being a part of no particular tradition, it will not be fully satisfactory to any and will be the focus of suspicion on the part of all. However, despite its shortcomings, it provides a conceptual perspective that is otherwise not available. It is, after all, nothing more or less than the commitment to the critical assessment and analysis of claims, and the rational description of the conceptual presuppositions and values that frame our lives. Such analysis and description is a major cultural endeavor in self-understanding.

Philosophy as a Guide for the Perplexed

NOTES

1. John T. Noonan, Jr., *Contraception* (Cambridge, Mass.: Harvard University Press, 1965); Charles Curran, "Natural Law and Moral Theology," in *Contraception*, ed. C. Curran (New York: Herder & Herder, 1969).

2. Immanuel Kant, *Critique of Pure Reason*, A12–B25.

3. John Rawls, *A Theory of Justice* (Cambridge, Mass.: Harvard University Press, 1971).

4. Alan Donagan, *The Theory of Morality* (Chicago: University of Chicago Press, 1977).

5. Gerald Kelley, S.J., *Medico-Moral Problems* (St. Louis: Catholic Hospital Association, 1958), p. 160.

6. Immanuel Jakobovitz, "Population Explosion: The Jewish Attitude to Birth Control" (Lecture delivered October 28, 1968, edited and annotated transcript of the Jewish Marriage Education Council Annual Lecture, London, England, 1969), pp. 5–6. A similar view is expressed by Dr. Rosner: "The Jewish attitude toward contraception by any method is a nonpermissive one if no medical or psychiatric threat to the mother or child exists. The duty of procreation, which is primarily a commandment on man, coupled with the wife's conjugal rights in Jewish law, mitigates against the use of condom, coitus interruptus or abstinence under any circumstances." See Fred Rosner, "Contraception in Jewish Law," in *Jewish Bioethics*, ed. Fred Rosner and J. D. Bleich (New York: Sanhedrin Press, 1979), p. 95.

7. William Clifford, "On the Scientific Basis of Morals," *Contemporary Review*, September 1875, p. 295.

8. Theodosius Dobzhansky, *Mankind Evolving* (New Haven: Yale University Press, 1962), p. 199.

9. I am indebted here to the ways in which Stanley Hauerwas has developed the notion of the moral narrative of a particular community through which one comes to understand its moral viewpoint. Though Hauerwas may not be in agreement with me, his account shows a very Hegelian viewpoint. The concrete moral life is to be understood in particular societies. For a development of Stanley Hauerwas's viewpoints, see *A Community of Character* (Notre Dame, Ind.: University of Notre Dame Press, 1981).

10. W. H. S. Jones, trans., *Hippocrates*, Loeb Classical Library (New York: Putnam's & Sons, 1923), 2:139.

11. H. Tristram Engelhardt, Jr., "Clinical Judgment," *Metamedicine* 2 (October 1981): 301–18.

12. Lester King, "Some Basic Explanations of Disease: An Historian's Viewpoint," *Evaluation and Explanation in the Biomedical Sciences*, ed. H. Tristram Engelhardt, Jr., and S. F. Spicker (Dordrecht, Holland: D. Reidel & Co., 1974),

pp. 11–28; "Values in Medicine," in H. T. Engelhardt, Jr., and D. Callahan, *Science, Ethics, and Medicine* (Hastings-on-Hudson, N.Y.: Hastings Center Press, 1976), pp. 225–41.

13. See, e.g., G. Miller, "Reaction and Controversy: 1722–1729," in *Adoption of Inoculation for Smallpox in England and France* (Philadelphia: University of Pennsylvania Press, 1957); J. Blake, "The Inoculation Controversy in Boston: 1721–22," *New England Quarterly* 15 (1952): 499–506.

14. This can be traced at least to the twenty-second constitution of the Fourth Lateran Council. See *Conciliorum Oecumenicorum Decreta*, ed. Centro di Documentazione Istituto per le Scienze Religiose Bologna (Basileae: Herder, 1962). For a canon based on this constitution, see H. Denzinger, *Enchirdion Symbolorum Definitionum et Declarationum de Rebus Fidei et Morum* (Rome: Herder, 1964), p. 265.

PART FOUR

Theological Perspectives

7

Topics at the Interface
of Medicine and
Theology

KENNETH L. VAUX

If popular tastes in reading gauge a society's interests, then our generation is fascinated, if not obsessed, with health. In August 1981, for example, one-third of the fifteen nonfiction best sellers on the *New York Times* list dealt with some aspect of health. Judy Mazel's *The Beverly Hills Diet* topped the list, followed closely by Richard Simmons's and Miss Piggy's guides to better nutrition, better life-style, better mind-set. In this volume, Ernst Wynder promises longevity as the reward for a life free from tobacco, alcohol, and fat consumption. A recent *New York Times Magazine* article alerted readers to the hidden harm in excessive (and unfeminine) slimness. Health, it seems, whether won through thinness or plumpness, jogging, or meditation, is the prize to seek.

The pursuit of good health engages us with varying degrees of playfulness, fascination, or fanaticism. If we successfully hold disaster at bay, squeezing a few more years out of a body all too fragile, then life seems merry indeed. Yet, as fervently as we seek our own good health we are fascinated by ill health: stories of patients' struggles with disease or their pilgrimages toward death from cancer. Their fight becomes our fight, their distress or their victory the prototype of that debility and death which comes to all. Whether our interest springs from compassion or fear cannot always be determined easily; what we can acknowledge is that the struggle of others with disease and death involves us closely. Concern with our own health and our own bodies may in fact kindle an interest in the fate of others, for often when we scrutinize our life-style and its attendant health practices, we are forced to examine the values which led to such a life-style—for ourselves and our society.

Both health and disease touch us at our core. Widely publicized medical dilemmas (such as Karen Quinlan's predicament or the birth of the Danville, Illinois, Siamese twins) have engaged great numbers of people in what must be called values debates. We strive to gain control over our own bodies through salutary health practices, yes, but what shall we do with situations over which we have no control? The Danville parents had sought a good birth by taking Lamaze classes, nourishing the young mother properly, and seeking the best prenatal care. They could not have foreseen or prevented the conception of conjoined children who could neither thrive nor die. What forces have we unleashed on nature to cause that tragedy or the series of other Siamese births this year? We read of such cases and recognize the signs of our time—pesticides, pollutants, nuclear sources, a host of factors new in our century, even our lifetime—and weep for the sorrow of parents or children destroyed by these forces.

But then there have always been mutagenic or teratogenic births even before we despoiled the good earth. Are we perhaps railing against the inscrutable purposes of the Creator? Are we in futile and furious pursuit to "relieve our estate"?

We sympathize too with the pain of parents removing their children from "orthodox" cancer treatments, searching desperately for a miracle. Technology both aids healing and causes pain—that too we recognize from our lives as we read of injurious spinal taps or life-support systems prolonging nonresponsive life. Once we have questioned technology's role in our own lives, or have cried over a physician's (and a patient's) agonizing case, or have asked a friend, "What would you do in this situation?" we have acknowledged our kinship with all sufferers and our own commitment to ask questions about ultimate beliefs and values.

Who are the healers in such cases as these? Who copes with the parents' sorrow, the child's agony, the law's strictures? Who is forced to reconcile the power of medical technology with economic necessity or individual volition (what if the patient cannot pay, or wants to die naturally)? Nurses, physicians, and other health-care professionals deal daily with cases no profession should have to face alone. Their power to aid has undeniably been enhanced through the biomedical advances of past decades. But along with these advances, medical costs, numbers of patients, patient expectations, and chronic disease have also risen. Who then can help, and heal, the healers?

Through Project Ten those persons and resources which can assist medical practitioners will be identified. Once medicine and religion walked side by side and indeed were often bound up in the same person (as in the medicine man, the shaman, or the Puritan divine). Scientific advancement has forced a separation of the two disciplines; still, in both disease and health and in all degrees of malaise which hover between the two states, religion and medicine fulfill common, complementary roles. Both disciplines grew from a common desire to heal the sick and wounded and to promote good physical, psychic, bodily health in other persons. Practitioners in both fields concern themselves with others from the time of birth to death's last gasp. The end, care for "our fellow travelers on this pilgrimage to the grave," merits a full-hearted sharing of burdens and opportunities common to both.

How can such mutuality be fostered? Project Ten treads the path between the two disciplines, seeking to contribute in a lasting way to philosophical and ethical knowledge about medicine. It seeks to involve health-care professionals who must live out their faith and ethics daily, and pastors, teachers, and lay people who guide our minds into belief and our hearts into service of other human beings. Project Ten isolates ten themes common to the work of medicine and religion and explores them in the light of ten faith traditions. The project will spread out over several years, engaging the world's leading scholars in health and religion.

THE RATIONALE FOR THE SELECTION
OF THE THEMES

The ten themes selected for exploration during this project follow a logic created by life itself: well-being sets the norm, followed by the spectrum of human experience from birth to death.

1. Well-being	6. Madness
2. Sexuality	7. Healing
3. Passages	8. Caring
4. Morality	9. Suffering
5. Dignity	10. Dying

Theological Perspectives

As we outline the story of our lives, we can identify certain powers, certain moments, certain passages which are both basic and transcending. The union of conjugal love, the inception of new life, the flourishing of vitality, the exhilaration of thought, the mystery of suffering, the sublime drama of dying—all are life events which emerge in the biophysical stratum of our bodies and are dealt with throughout life in cooperation with the human services of medicine, yet lift us beyond. They take us to the gates of heaven or hell, as in crisis they bear ultimate meaning. The ten chosen themes represent the human lifeline, punctuated at spike points of high significance. Theology and medicine alike interpret and intervene at each critical point.

Our care, then, envelops the human creature in health and disease, life and death. Pastor and physician follow the model "Persoun of a Toun" who in Chaucer's *Canterbury Tales* ministered to a parish "Wyd" and "fer asonder":

> . . . He ne lefe not, for reyn ne thonder,
> In siknesse nor in meschief to visite
> The ferreste in his parisshe, muche and lite,
> Upon his feet, and in his hand a staf.
> (General Prologue)

But both medicine and religion are systems not only of actions but also of ideas. A similar theoretical architecture undergirds the healing enterprise in both disciplines.

The logic and grammar of medicine moves from the inception of life to its conclusion within the ongoing dialectic of well-being and disease. The logic of theology moves from creation to eschatology, from conception of a world in time and space to its consummation within the ongoing dialectic of redemption and fall.

Textbooks of classical systematic theology and the philosophy of medicine resemble one another in plan, with an underlying assumption of a norm, an ideal state to be gained: physical well-being ("health") in the one and integration ("wholeness")—reconciliation of God and humankind—in the other. The principles governing the disciplines—their agendas, the healing of the human person—are the same. Theology deals with God's relationship with the human community. It speaks of unity and integrity (potential and fulfillment) as well as disintegration and alienation; it embraces both the giving and the ending of life and provides covenants for these. All religions speak of creation, of a loyalty or a resistance of the creature to God. Religious language speaks in images of sexuality, parent and child, madness and violence, sanity and peace. The natural world, historical events, and life spans of individuals exist within, are constituted and sustained by, and are given purpose through the divine will. Wolfhart Pannenberg has written that prior to our creation we possess minds and wills because God is mind and will, that the divine being and activity forms structures and capacities within the human being. Sigmund Freud argued conversely that we project human characteristics onto the world beyond, making God into our image. These conflicting perspectives need not be reconciled; it remains true that human experience corresponds in pattern with that of divine revelation.

The ten themes we have chosen are fraught with meaning because divine revelations sanctify them. Each of ten world religious traditions will confront these ten themes, probing the interface of theology and medicine.

1. Judaism
2. Eastern Religions
3. Roman Catholicism
4. Eastern Christianity
5. Islam
6. Lutheran Christianity
7. The Mainline Reformation Traditions
8. The Evangelical Communions
9. Nineteenth-Century Religions
10. The Native Traditions

Do certain aspects of our living take us to depths that require theological understanding? Do certain stipulates of our belief and constraints of our conscience force us to see biological existence in a different way? How does medicine require religion? How does religion shape medicine?

Project Ten is designed to draw from the various religious heritages that constitute our common human experience those underlying beliefs and values by which we live and choose. This background volume sets forth the rationale for an enterprise of such magnitude and scope. Further volumes will create a treasury of history, insight, and memory which health-care professionals and all other healers may consult as they seek guidance. Both the programs and the publications will carry scholarship in theology, medicine, and medical ethics beyond the superficial casuistry, econometrics, or facile cost-benefit analysis popular in the literature a few years back—toward profound questions concerning issues of life and death.

Theological Perspectives

Recent inquiry has moved in this direction and indeed has set the stage for the appearance of Project Ten. Questions of human rights and analytic motifs such as equity, autonomy, and distributive justice have arisen. When the surface of problematic cases (known to many now through mass media) is probed deeply, currents of freedom, beneficence, justice, and mercy—the stuff of theology—are stirred. The distinguished reference work compiled by the Kennedy Institute, *The Encyclopedia of Bioethics*, dealt with many practical issues and inquired into fundamental topics.[1] Further advances in scholarship have been made by The Hastings Institute's inquiry into the foundations of medical ethics and the Engelhardt and Spicker series in philosophy and medicine.[2] It is on these beginnings that Project Ten builds.

THE THEMES: ISSUES AND INTERPRETATIONS

1. Well-being

ISSUES

The Good Life, Disease, Health, Sin, Sickness, Illness, Wellness, Health Habits, Prevention of Illness

ANALYSIS

How did we as thinking, acting creatures conceive the concept of health as a desirable (and disease as a regrettable) state? In older societies surely disease in its many forms—and certainly child and young adult deaths—afflicted the majority of the population. Visions too, and unusual powers, often came to the ill or maimed. Those who were hale, hunted; those who were not, prophesied or saw visions. Women gave birth in pain, and such suffering ensured the continuity of the human race. How did we first begin to shape the notion of health as some optimal condition toward which we must strive?

This idea can be found in most religions: that the creator wills health or wholeness for that which has been created. The striving itself springs from hope and from confidence in divine providence, particularly in religions such as Judaism and Christianity, which share a linear conception of history—that God and humanity are moving together through history toward some end point, the eschaton. Health itself—wholeness or integrity—might be defined as that physical, psychic, or spiritual state in which the creature becomes most nearly "himself" or "herself"—that is, what the creator intended him or her to be.

Primitive religions discerned some necessary connection between health/disease and the greater powers. They often concluded that affliction was the punishment of the gods, a disruption of the primary alliance between Creator and creature through either a cosmic "fall" or personal disobedience. Job searched his heart in vain for some memory of a duty or prayer not performed and found none, but his friends believed nonetheless that personal sin caused his disease.

If sin brought about sickness, then righteousness assured blessing and prosperity. This belief, common in Old Testament writings, anchored in Judeo-Christianity the confidence that a wholesome and just personal life would bring health. "Stewardship of the body" issues from the positive side of this belief; health as a sign of salvation and disease as a mark of sin or divine disfavor issues from its perversion. Recent fads in nutrition and body-building may represent vestiges of this primitive desire to invoke, or manifest, divine blessing.

The notion of health as an optimal state, then, arises from the idea of a creator, and a creature to be wooed toward wholeness. Yet "health" in this religious sense embraces more than vitalism (vigor, absence of all disease, and longevity). The worship of vitality alone can become an idolatry—the idolatry of vitalism. Religious definitions of health, well-being, or "the good life" usually include more factors than physical perfection and functional power. All religions accent human finitude. Spiritual health or wholeness can flourish alongside physical disease, weakness, or deformity: serving one's neighbor, sacrificing one's life, or mortifying the flesh—all motifs of faith—contrast vividly with any definition of health as physical strength alone.

If by these widened interpretations of physical well-being we may mean not only strength but also weakness, what of psychic health? Do we define this only as inner confidence, comfort, and contentment, happiness, complacency? Here too the paradox of strength in weakness punctures our sure composure. Humility is perceived to be as crucial to being "whole" as are confidence and control. Anger at injustice and anguish over others' sufferings mark the unquiet, not the satisfied, mind. The desire to change oneself or the world fuels the process. Further, those persons most often called saints possessed no common minds; they trafficked between the realms of nature and supernature and might have been called schizoid. Phrases such as the "wounded healer" or the "broken victor" capture the paradoxical nature of religious definitions of psychic "health."

What then becomes of the imperative to heal the sick, if "health" is conceived so multidimensionally? Here enters the need for dialogue. With powers to extend life, replace or modify limbs, bend minds, or alter genetic material, some goal—some working concept of health and disease—must guide us. After four decades we still shudder at the memory of Nazi Germany, where medical skill served warped ideas about human (racial) health. What qualities do we seek to perpetuate in the human race? What traits do we sanction and reinforce? Do we breed for perfection or allow some deformity? Do we urge the power of biomedical advance toward achieving longer and longer life? Each underlying definition of health and disease affects health-care policy, genetics policy, research priorities, and allocation of available money across a spectrum of needs. It determines the decisions we make as individuals, families, institutions, societies.

Medicine and theology must grope together toward such insight. Medical knowledge can supply parameters for interventions. For example, whether there is a natural limit to the life span is a question for which scientific inquiry can at least approximate an answer. Sophisticated feedback insight will be able to project the consequences of interventions. Will genetic programs, life-style modification, surgery, or transplants be the best solution for heart disease? Science and technology can help us with value questions. Theology, with its great doctrines of the impartiality and judgment of God, the human soul, and immortality, will not only enable us to generate prophetic critique against the inhuman misuse of medicine but also offer positive visions of the directions biomedicine ought to take.

2. Sexuality

ISSUES

Procreation, Genetics, Abortion, Contraception, Fertilization

ANALYSIS

The cluster of issues surrounding the joining of two persons involves love and the transmission of life, engages theology, and provokes some of the most perplexing questions in medical ethics. Judaism conceived of God as the lover who remained faithful even when that love was unrequited (Hosea). When the great Hebrew writers wished to describe the closeness and the steadfastness of their Savior God, they used terms of intimacy, intercourse, and love's devotion. God's love, they wrote, is like that of a wife for her husband, a father for his son, a mother for her child. The old radical in the Hebrew language that translates into the Greek word *charis*, or grace, is the word used to imitate the sound of a mother camel searching in the desert for her lost son. From our treasury of human experience, these are the closest images we have to describe the constancy and searching quality of God's love.

In the New Testament as in the Old, human sin or departure from healing relatedness to God is cast in images of sexuality. *Porneia*, pollution, adultery, and apostasy are prevalent concepts. The focus of Augustine and other early church fathers on celibacy, sexual sins, and the desires of the body was not an aberration; it was a central theme in the Hebrew and Christian Scriptures. Religion concerns relationships within the setting of the divine-human relationship. The logic of faith requires that human sexuality be taken with utmost seriousness. That most religions accent these issues is grounded in the fact that God is not apathetic; rather, God is love.

The knowledge and art of medicine also require the examination of normative issues of human sexuality. Medicine is asked through surgical, medical, and psychiatric intervention to determine sex when physical, hormonal, or psychic ambiguity is present. Diagnostic manuals must gauge whether variant forms of sexual expression are pathological. This requires that fundamental values about health and normalcy, disruption and deviancy be considered.

Biomedicine and its cognate fields are called upon to make decisions and intervene at the inception of life. This involves safeguarding the normal processes of conception, gestation, and birth. It includes developing new ways of making babies, finding problems before babies are born, and doing something about these problems. Conception control and interruption, fertilization and fetal diagnosis, indeed, all the techniques used in the transmission of life, involve both basic religious and moral values and biomedical interventions. The dialogue is unavoidable and imperative.

3. Passages

ISSUES

Birth, Adolescence, Aging, Extending the Life Span, Beginnings and Endings

Theological Perspectives

ANALYSIS

In Jewish faith God is the giver and guardian of life's passages:

> Naked I came from my mother's womb, and naked shall I return; the Lord gave, and the Lord has taken away; blessed be the name of the Lord (Job 1:21).
> The Lord will keep you from all evil; he will keep your life. The Lord will keep your going out and your coming in from this time forth and for evermore (Ps. 121:7–8).

Similarly, the vestigial primitive faiths (e.g., Hopi, Navaho) and the Eastern religions (Hinduism, Buddhism) imbue life's transitions with sacral significance. Coming of age, becoming a man or a woman, becoming an elder and assuming functions of wisdom and guidance, these are all events where divine blessing and benediction is present. Buddhism, in fact, extrapolates from the transitions of life a total view of reality wherein transiency of life is stressed to the point that life's spiritual secret is found in the escape from the transitory.

God ordains life's passages, constituting biological life so that growth, maturation, and reproduction mark the life cycle. The transaction of these moments of transition are crises. They open life to new possibility. They render life spirited rather than static. As Erik Erikson has shown, movement along the life cycle involves movements of venture and consolidation, of risk and retreat. Passages are the mechanism by which the deity who is eternal transforms lives that are bound by space and time.

Initiation and graduation are features of most religions; certain risks and rituals mark the passage from observer to participant, from follower to leader. In the divine logic, preparation is necessary to receive insight and take on responsibility. Christian faith, claims the apostle Paul, is given to the human race in "the fulness of the time" (Gal. 4:4, KJV). When the time was ready, when the ancient religions and Judaism had prepared the collective soul, when the Roman peace had unified the world, when the Greek tongue had given a new power and universality to language, in the *kairos*, this potent moment, the passage into a new age was accomplished.

The divine Being, it can be said, is leading the cosmos through the epochs of evolution, is guiding the human race through passages where greater knowledge and power are bequeathed to make possible responsibility. God watches over, indeed precipitates, the transitions in the lives of each one of us. They are the instruments of divine providence.

Not a sparrow falls to the ground without God's knowledge, claimed

Jesus of Nazareth. Every vicissitude of adaptation and natural selection is ordered in the divine activation of nature. Every passage, every rise and fall of the species, every generation and blowout of a solar system is ordained in the divine drama. This theology of nature requires that any inquiry into religion and medicine ponder deeply the passages of life.

Biomedicine also concerns life's passages. Medicine has laid claim to and has been given power over some of these natural transitions. Ivan Illich has warned of the danger of "medicalizing" such life events as adolescence and the passage to death.[3] While the usurpation of life events by the medical establishment is a violence to be challenged, it remains true that some aspects of life's passages have of necessity become concerns of medicine. Pregnancy and birth can be overseen and monitored, insuring appropriate prenatal care. Proper maternal diet can be recommended, toxic influence from cigarette smoking or overwhelming depression can be treated so that the noxious influence does not cross the placental barrier to the fetus. Traumas of birth— prematurity, hyaline membrane disease, wrapped cord, and the like— can be anticipated and corrected.

Another passage of life, adolescence, also has an essential endocrinal and psychological dimension. The life sciences (biological and psychological) afford us knowledge of that transition. Aging, menopause, and the other modes of our passage toward senescence and death are processes increasingly comprehended and by implication safeguarded by medical knowledge and techniques.

Another way that consideration of life's passages is crucial to the goals and activities of medicine is found in research that concerns life events, the prevention of disease and the onset of illness. A growing body of knowledge is developing which shows that people stay well or become ill in terms of the way in which they respond to life's changes. The data show that people tend to get sick when they are unable to process the passages of life in a salutary fashion. Thomas Holmes and his colleagues at the University of Washington compiled a list of life events, ordering them in terms of the disruption they bring.[4] Points were designated for each life event, and the patient was asked how many of these events had transpired in his or her recent experience. The accumulation of points was then correlated with the intervening variable of coping ability. Causal associations were then drawn in retrospect, or prospective predictions were made. When these life crises and celebrations cluster, buffeting the organism with inordinant change, resistance and immunity is compromised, physical and psychic compensation occurs, and disease very likely begins. Not only the psychosomatic and stress-related disorders, but also infectious, parasitic, neoplastic, cardiovascular, musculoskeletal, even traumatic disorders crescendo in these moments of vulnerability.

TABLE 1

LIFE EVENTS SCALED IN DESCENDING ORDER OF SIGNIFICANCE

1. Death of spouse
2. Detention in jail
3. Divorce
4. Death of close family member
5. Major personal injury or illness
6. Marriage
7. Marital separation
8. Being fired from work
9. Major change in health of family member
10. Sex difficulties
11. Retirement from work
12. Major business readjustment
13. Pregnancy
14. Change to different line of work
15. Marital reconciliation
16. Death of close friend
17. Mortgage loan foreclosure
18. Son or daughter leaving home
19. Mortgage loan of $10,000 or more
20. In-law troubles
21. Major change in financial state
22. Major change in responsibility at work
23. New member in family
24. Outstanding personal achievement
25. Wife starting or ceasing work
26. Major change in living conditions
27. Troubles with boss
28. Minor violations of law
29. Revision of personal habits
30. Mortgage loan of less than $10,000
31. Major change in work hours or conditions
32. Beginning or end of formal schooling
33. Major change in arguments with spouse
34. Change to new school
35. Major change in sleeping habits
36. Major change in eating habits
37. Change in residence
38. Major change in recreation
39. Major change in social activities
40. Major change in family get-togethers
41. Vacation
42. Major change in church activities
43. Christmas

SOURCE: Kenneth L. Vaux, *This Mortal Coil: The Meaning of Health and Disease* (New York: Harper & Row, 1978).

Topics at the Interface of Medicine and Theology

This area of medical epidemiology and prognosis is just one frontier where clinical interests touch on classic theological themes. Mention can also be made of the interest within adolescent medicine of the new knowledge emerging in endocrinology of how hormones and peptides bathe the brain and create not only mood and disposition alteration, but also stimulate basic growth and development. The study of human growth hormones and of the basic biochemistry of aging are research frontiers that will be fraught with ethical significance. We will be forced to declare our normative values about these momentous passages of life so that we can decide in personal, professional, and policy situations what we must do with these new capacities.

Finally, the frontiers of genetic engineering and cloning raise fundamental moral considerations that our theological traditions must help us evaluate. Do we wish to modulate and modify life's passages and crises? Do we wish to ameliorate the human situation when these painful, often morbid and even mortal transitions set in? Will we seek to modify the estral cycle? Should we seek alterations in female menopause and the male change of life? Will we be tempted to avoid the basic transmutability of life by replicating the genetic substance of individuals and recreating them by cloning, or immortalizing individuals after death by freezing them in liquid nitrogen in hope of a cryogenic resurrection? The dialogue between medicine, where potential modifications and treatments for life's passages are developing, and theology, where the meaning of these passages is explored, is now imperative.

4. Morality

ISSUES

Sanctions, Warrants, Sources of Moral Insight, Authority, Inspiration

ANALYSIS

What has theology in general and our religious faith in particular to do with moral action and the moral life, especially as it is contoured by the challenges of health and disease, life and death? While we would expect an answer that religion has much to do with these two features of human experience, we are surprised to find very little written or spoken about this interface. As Stephen Toulmin relates in the Hastings Center Report, we have tended to analyze ethical dilemmas of medicine with the philosophical categories of Rawlsian, utilitarian, or Kantian thought. The themes of justice, benefit-risk, and autonomy have been invoked to resolve clinical and policy quandries. Only recently have we turned to the case wisdom of Jewish Halacha, Catholic *casus conscientiae,* and Protestant case ethics.[5]

This inability at the level of formal discussion to position ethical dilemmas of health care in the context of theological ethics is striking in light of the fact that at the personal level those who struggle at the great borderline horizons of life and death inevitably perceive crises in terms of their deepest beliefs and values. When the chips are down, not only the imperatives for specific action but also the broad motifs of meaning and the impulses to pursue virtue and avoid evil are most often theologically mediated. Similarly, public moral deliberation is shaped by spiritual commitments and the derivative moral values. In recent years theologians have attempted more carefully to correlate basic theological beliefs with concrete actions. Good examples of this endeavor are Helmut Thielicke's *Theological Ethics*[6] and James Gustafson's new study.[7]

Specific guidelines for action are found in more detail in religious traditions that stress casuistry. In Orthodox Judaism, for example, one can find an elaborate system of rules for actions as specific as sterilization or using electric doors on the Sabbath. Protestantism and the liberal traditions stress freedom of conscience, fundamental values, and intermediate-level guidelines, as opposed to highly specified rules.

Religious convictions can be seen shaping the ethics of medicine and health care in several ways. In any society the moral atmosphere is created, at least in part, by those fundamental visions, values, and senses of meaning that constitute the religious culture. Three of the many ways that religion can and does affect human ethics are (1) forming the system of justification, sanctions, warrants, and reprieves; (2) providing the stimulus for character formation by nurturing virtue and proscribing vice; and (3) providing moral guidance in ethical promulgation, teaching, and counsel.

Initially religion provides salience and structure for morality by insisting that our life comes from God, before whom we stand responsible. Our existence is telic; that is, it is purposive. Whether, as in the classic view, we are thought to pursue goodness in obedience to God and in self-realization of potential or, as in the modern view, we are found to be free and undetermined and thus able to create value, we are nevertheless responsive and responsible beings. Religion contends that life is not absurd and that God orders the world with moral expectation, empowers moral action, and renders moral judgment. From this fundamental theological structuring of human existence flow the sanctions, warrants, goals, and guides of life.

All religions lay a claim of personal accountability on us in terms of our relationship to God, to our fellow beings, and to the natural world. The fundamental axis of responsibility is that of person to person, which includes the self-relation. In Judeo-Christianity we are to care for our neighbors as ourselves since we are loved by God. This interaction of the horizontal and vertical moral relationship is often accompanied by the sanctions of benefits and punishments.

In doctrines of creation and fall, grace and sin, forgiveness and judgment, the context of moral responsibility is framed, the imperative to right action founded, the sanctions of misdirection made known, and the availability of forgiveness assured. In some theological systems natural law subsumes the moral law, giving both knowledge of what is good and the price of transgression within nature herself. Nature and revelation concur with reference to the wholesome manner of sexual expression, contend Roman Catholic and Calvinist natural law. If this manner of expression is violated, the very fabric of personal and familial existence will be torn. Other religious systems find the moral life shaped by free human reason or by the active will of God mediated to a person's conscience through faith, hope, and love.

Most religions place emphasis not so much on moral rules or action but on moral being. One is righteous. The person develops character. The young person builds a moral life; one becomes virtuous. Religion's great contribution to medical ethics is not rules or guidelines, not even noble principles and values, but the formation of people who are just and caring. A moral tenor is introduced into medicine when it is practiced by health-care professionals who are fair, honest, just, trustworthy, and sympathetic. These are the qualities of being that undergird specific values and moral life. Unfortunately religion has often been used to justify immoral action and has contributed to the formation of moral pathology in individuals. For this reason it is essential that the great themes of theology—providence, responsibility, grace, and forgiveness— always be called on to critique and inspire the moral life. Prayer to the living God alone can save us from the malevolence that ensues when devotion ends with the penultimate deities we construct.

Finally, religion has introduced great systems of ethical wisdom to the activities of medicine. From the prudential stipulates of the Hebrew

Theological Perspectives

Proverbs or the Wisdom of Sirach, to the Prayer of Maimonides, from "The Hippocratic Oath as a Christian May Confess It" (third century) to the directives for physicians in John Wesley's *Primitive Remedies,* we find a treasury of specific teachings that bear on health care. Jewish rabbinic teaching has pondered many of the moral dilemmas of life and death in the Halacha and has proffered this perennial wisdom. Pope Pius XII often spoke to medical associations and delivered insightful directives on many concerns sustaining the magnificent strength of the Roman Catholic promulgations of medico-moral thought.

The churches have come to grips with many of the moral questions of health and disease and have offered helpful guidance. Part of the purpose of Project Ten is to assemble this wealth of material generated through the ages by individuals and religious communions and make it accessible to us today as we face decisions so profound that only these deep texts can help.

5. *Dignity*

ISSUES

Soul, Sanctity of Life, Freedom, Autonomy, Respect for Life

ANALYSIS

Paul Ramsey, in his landmark work in the theological ethics of medicine,[8] has forcefully articulated the sine qua non value of medicine. Care for a person because of his or her inestimable inherent worth is the moral foundation of medical care. In identifying this central quality which condemns any view of human value based on utility, Ramsey moves to the quick of religious conviction. Religion—with its understanding of the human being as a divine creation imbued with an immortal soul, possessed of inalienable dignity, and given to a destiny beyond the boundaries of space and time—alone can anchor the pivotal conviction of medicine. This doctrine we call the inviolability of human life.

In this brief analysis of the concept of human dignity, we can discover both an affirmation of the notion and a threatening tendency in the logic of medicine and religion. With the deciphering of the DNA code and genetic knowledge in general, science has corroborated the ancient religious claim about the distinctive uniqueness of each person. While there is correspondence at the elementary level with all nature (the ingredients of DNA) and a biological continuity with parents and descendants, each life is a unique, unrepeatable occurrence.

This individuation of unique human beings even at the naturalistic level is often invoked in medicine to establish a moral position. In abortion cases the argument that the fetus is only a tissue of the mother's body is weakened now that we know the exquisite lottery of genes that congeal in conception. In potential questions of cloning, the argument against replicating individuals rests not only on the scientific argument that diversity enriches and enhances the species, but also on the moral argument that human beings ought to remain unrepeated instances of life, since meaning is found in that unique story and destiny.

While science can suggest and corroborate sanctity of life, it cannot establish or verify it. We find ourselves in the strange situation where the virtue without which medicine cannot exist cannot be established with the tools of that discipline. Theology therefore becomes a necessary companion to medicine. We understand why the two disciplines emerged simultaneously. With its own powers, science has sought to establish the existence of the soul or some other basis for human dignity. Some have sought to prove the physical reality of the spirit of a person by weighing the body before and after death. On the serious side, science has conceded that human beings are of infinite value because of the highly developed frontal cortex of the brain.

John Lilly, a neuroscientist, has called a halt to his work with dolphins because he has perceived with a sense of awe and wonder that they are intelligent creatures. Neurological criteria have become the basis for saying "this is a human person." This judgment pertains both to questions surrounding abortion and the question "When does life begin?" and questions of the cessation of life and the definition of death.

Respecting the presence of reason in another is now imperative. The liberties of manipulation, experimentation, and killing—liberties we take with nonrational animals—are prohibited in those beings who possess reason.

Theology also has a great stake in asserting the underlying dignity of personal life as this evokes our respect and restrains our violence on human beings. Humans are created *imago Dei*, proclaim the biblical writers. We share reason, responsivity, responsibility, power, freedom, and will with the Creator. This is the ground of our dignity. This is what is meant when we say that people have inviolable and immortal souls. While all religions revere the natural world and its living creatures, it is humankind, capable of faith, hope, and love, that bears the divine imprint. Harming a person, then, is nothing short of blasphemy.

Establishing and delineating the contours of human dignity is central to the purposes of medicine and theology. The yield of Project Ten on this theme will help reestablish the moral foundations of medicine. It will help found new guidelines for the protection of human subjects in medical research. It will reinvigorate the striving to develop new knowledge about life and health for the benefit of humankind. It will reemphasize the bases of respect for all people, especially the sick, the handicapped, the poor, and the young—those who in expediency we despise but whom in transcending concern we value.

6. Madness

ISSUES

Guilt, Shame, Anxiety, Depression, the Daemonic, Evil, Psychic, Emotional Health, the Life of the Mind, Exorcism, Loss of Reason

ANALYSIS

When we ponder the nature and working of the human mind, we find ourselves at the crossroads of medicine and religion. The mind and the soul are closely associated, if not identical, phenomena. Mental therapy and soul-healing (*Seelsorge*) are cognate, indeed interpenetrating, functions. Belief and faith generate peace of mind. It can be argued that the greatest force in our world for serenity, sanity, and the altruism that rescues us from narcissism is the ecstasy of religious experience wherein we are released from self-obsession and the fear of death and in the divine love given over to care for one another.

Religious elements are also often found in diseases of the mind. With the exception of the organic brain syndromes and some of the personality disorders, almost all the neuroses, obsessions, and fantasies can be seen as belief gone haywire. Idolatry or sin, in theological nomenclature, is misdirected devotion and penultimate obsession. Delusion or illusion is the failure to understand oneself over against others within the reality of God. Debilitative anxiety is the verve of life loculated, choking its creative expression; neurotic guilt is blindness to the mercy of God and nonacceptance of our human fraility. Alternately, religion offers release from the self-condemnation and judgment of others that so greatly contributes to mental sickness.

Topics at the Interface of Medicine and Theology

What in the logic of medicine requires examination of theological insight as it deals with the life of the mind? Psychiatry tore itself away from religion in the nineteenth century as the theory of the divine or daemonic etiology of madness waned and neurological, endocrinal, and psychological explanation was found to be more helpful and humane. Witch-burnings still occurred, albeit rarely, in places within Judeo-Christian civilization. Yet even that society, steeped in the vision of life offered in that scripture and tradition, still punished the demon-possessed and the visionary in asylums and other inhuman hovels reminiscent of the caves where Jesus met the Gerasene demoniac (see Luke 8:26–39).

In bringing the human brain within experimental reach, thus allowing causes and cures for mental illnesses to be explored, a great liberation of humankind was achieved. This required that our ideas about insanity be demythologized. Lithium deficiency, not the cursing of gods, sometimes caused brooding depression. While some felt this development repudiated religion, as in one sense it did, in a larger sense it continued the work of the Hebrew creation theologians and of the rabbi Jesus Christ in salvation-history as each began to strip the daemonic of its power over our lives.

Psychiatry and psychological counseling can now profitably examine the knowledge emerging from the theological disciplines both to refine theory and strengthen practice. Likewise, theology needs to look to the behavioral and biomedical sciences of the mind both to rid itself of outmoded concepts and to support its pastoral ministry. It remains a most important medical fact that the front line of preventive and interventive mental health care in our society is the church, the clergy, and the religious community.

7. Healing

ISSUES

Concepts, Practices, Practitioners, Institutions, Pricing, Professionalism

ANALYSIS

Soteria, salve, salvation, heal, whole, hale, pain, purification, punishment—all the words with which we describe the processes of disintegration and restoration of the human being come from the common source of medicine and theology, that is, that primal consciousness which seeks to understand the how and why of this breaking and healing. These experiences have always been imbued with transcending significance. The diabolic forces that tear our lives apart, epitomized in disease and death, and the symbolic energy that mends and integrates our being are supernatural in origin. The experiences of illness and healing take on meaning against that divine backdrop.

Medicine has known from time immemorial that healing is both natural and divine. Hippocrates, who captured the wisdom of ancient civilization about healing in his phrase *via mediatrix naturae*, constantly affirmed nature's own power of health and healing. In the discussion of epilepsy as the "holy disease," he stressed not only that this ailment must be understood in terms of natural forces, but also that all diseases, and by inference all healings, are divine in origin. There is nothing especially sacred about epilepsy. All disease and all wholeness are based in the divine ground of the universe.

Healers have always known the secrets that the body heals itself, that most diseases are self-limiting, and that gracious or uncanny, even unjust, forces from beyond usually determine health outcomes. Yet they have offered their services to the ailing and injured. From the dawn of human life there have been five major types of healers: the bone-setter, the surgeon, the midwife, the herbalist, and the shaman or soul-healer.

In the modern world, people in need have turned to trained specialists. At the same time, the medical profession has laid claim to all these ancient offices and has slowly repudiated the folk healers and excoriated them with the label "quack." This expropriation of healing has been both salutary and dangerous. On the positive side, modern medicine has retained some of the deep wisdom of traditional knowledge and skill. It has corrected harmful errors of theory and practice (e.g., demon possession and bloodletting) and added new knowledge and technique. On the negative side, it has delimited the great art of medicine by granting hegemony to scientific positivism as the basis of theory and empirically verifiable technique as the basis of practice. This has dangerously constricted the theory and practice of medicine, since so much truth about life is not objectifiable or verifiable.

As an example, since the Renaissance the psychosomatic and certainly the spiritual dimensions of sickness have largely been repudiated and neglected. Healing has become a technological manipulation by means of the arts of pharmacology and surgery. Antimicrobial therapy is introduced to challenge infectious process. Insulin is injected to bolster that flaw in metabolism. The occluded vessels supplying the heart muscle with blood are replaced. Healing is ridding oneself of some noxious, toxic, or malignant invasion. Perhaps more accurate, medicine is the attempt to offset the body's own destructive resistance to these assaults.

Modern science is coming to understand the pathogens that start disease. It is learning about the genetic bases for vulnerability to disease and the triggers of disease onset. It is developing a multitude of therapies that safeguard the patient with as much function as is possible in the face of these assaults.

But when we think comprehensively, we realize that at one level healing is cutting and mending, resecting a lesion; the body then heals the wound. At another level, healing is resisting an infection, going through the long hot nights, struggling with what the prayer book calls "the fever of life." At another level it is adapting to or living through a psychotic episode with the possible aid of drugs and psychotherapy. At another level it is saying "I'm sorry" and repairing a relationship that was broken. At another level it is coming home to peace with God after sojourn in some far country. Each of these instances is an experience of healing, of restoration, of wholeness.

This spectrum of instances of healing illustrates the need for a medico-theological understanding. Even rudimentary healing at the tissue level is a psychosomatic event. People who through mental concentration can self-inflict stigmata or hemorrhagic lesions on their bodies supply evidence for the interplay between mental and physical process. Most healing in human experience is in the realm of relationships, the self or intrapsychic relation, the relationships between people. The divine-human relations all bear the possibility of yielding discord and disease, or wholeness and wellness.

Many possibilities for creative research into the phenomenon of healing exist at the interface of medicine and religion. For example, the amenability of immunologic response to belief forces such as peace, immortality, faith, and community (*koinonia*) would be fascinating to explore. Why is cancer incidence roughly one-half the expected rate among the Seventh-Day Adventists? Why do blood-pressure values vary predictably with the adherence to and declension away from orthodoxy among the Amish? Why is there scarcely any alcoholism among Jews? Why was there no psychotic disease and insanity in the concentration camps? All these questions point to the conjunction between medical disease and symptomology on the one hand and religious belief and behavior on the other.

Inquiring into the topic of healing is thus pivotal to collaborative exploration by medicine and theology. The logic of each discipline is incomplete without this consideration. Unilateral exploration would yield only partial insight. The work must proceed together.

8. Caring

ISSUES

Medical Missions, Ministries of Health, Pastoral Care

ANALYSIS

Theologically conceived, morality involves first and foremost the act of caring for and not harming oneself or another. In medicine this primal value means respecting the person through care and not bringing injury. The primary positive imperative of medicine has been stated in various ways: respect life; do your duty; preserve health; save, heal, rescue the wounded and sick; prevent disease; cure disease; serve the human project; develop medical knowledge; care for the person; prolong life.

For Hippocrates this basic commitment involved trying to understand better the imbalances that caused sickness and getting the sick person back in the salutary flow of airs, waters, places, and humors. For Paracelsus this basic commitment meant trying to understand chemical responses in the body and concocting elixirs to expel noxious substances and restore health to the vital body fluids. For Benjamin Rush, it meant standing by the bedside, struggling pragmatically with what would help the victim of yellow fever. Was it more bleeding, purging, or just standing there doing nothing? Like the great physicians before and after him, Rush discovered the therapeutic wisdom of this latter course.

For Salk and Sabin, caring meant testing the polio vaccine in people after long trials in the lab and in animal studies. For Ken Rosen, George Jackson, Bill McGuire, or Stan Schade (University of Illinois chiefs of medicine) or any other academic clinician or the village doctor today, response to the first commandment of medicine means coming to the aid of sick people with the knowledge and technique at hand. It also means seeking one small increment of new insight through investigation or observation. It might be a new electrophysiological parameter for understanding cardiac function, or another angle on viral replication, or a new cytotoxic cocktail that does a little better with a little less side effect. From the community physician, it might be the suggestion of how one patient might cope better with stress while on Cimedidine for treatment of a peptic ulcer.

"I suggest the word 'care,' " writes Paul Ramsey, "as the source of particular moral obligations and our court of final appeal for deciding the features of actions and practices that make what we do right or wrong." The distinguished Princeton ethicist, the first to be named to the National Academy of Medicine, goes on to say:

> Care has the advantage of locating medical ethics within the ethics of a wider human community. It also locates our model for decision-making alongside other models: Jewish ethics, whose ultimate norm is based on steadfast fidelity to the covenant of life with life; and Christian ethics, whose final appeal and criteria of judgment is Christian love and compassion.

We might add that in ethics, caring also resonates not only with the moral sense of Islam, Eastern religion, secular humanism, and the other great philosophies of life, but also with the universal dictum to treat others as one would wish to be treated.

Ramsey continues by saying that in specific cases, after carefully gathering the facts, the options, and the consequences as precisely as these can be projected, we should ask, "What specific action takes most care of human life—present lives and (in the case of research) future lives?"

> What singular deed or design of ours is most likely to embody or convey care or respect for human life? We ask, will this or that procedure care for the patient more? Or we ask will this or that research design be productive of the more significant benefit for the ongoing community of medical care?[9]

Medicine today is being forced to declare what care requires in a wide variety of cases. Does care require the notification of others at risk in the situation of genetic or infectious disease? Does care in the confidential and trust relationship with one's patient prompt one not to inform? What does care dictate in a situation where a woman is pregnant with a Down's syndrome baby which has been detected by amniocentesis? What do you do when care for the unborn and the present family seems to present contradictory imperatives? What of the situation where the good of other people and future people requires some suffering or even sacrifice from the person at hand? Patients are sometimes invited to undergo a procedure or treatment that will not benefit them but may help others, even though it will entail some suffering.

In theology the theme of caring is taken to greater depths. Not only is the requirement to be concerned given in religion, but the power and inspiration to be helpful to others is also conveyed. Sacrificial love is most possible in the context of religious faith. It defies rationalization in any egoistic or even utilitarian system of ethics. In Christian faith the central paradigm of the life of sacrificial love is the Crucified One. Here is found not only the example for the caring life but the ability to do it. "Greater love hath no man than this," wrote John, "that a man lay down his life for his friends" (John 15:13, KJV).

In Charles Dickens's majestic *Tale of Two Cities,* two men are identical in appearance. Out of love for the woman, the one man who has lived a dissolute life stands in at the gallows for his look-alike who has been wrongly accused. When asked why, he says: "It is a far, far better thing that I do, than I have ever done; it is a far, far better rest that I go to, than I have ever known." Caring is a residue of religious faith that lives on in a secular culture and is a cornerstone of medical practice. The continuing search for concrete implications of medical *care* is an urgent agenda priority for medicine and theology.

9. *Suffering*

ISSUES

Pain, Interpretations, Responses to Suffering

ANALYSIS

As we move to the deeper reaches of the logic of both medicine and theology, we confront the theme of suffering. Medicine is in the ultimate reaches of its raison d'être committed to the alleviation of suffering. But this is an impossible and unreasonable objective. Medical measures to relieve pain, from the great prescription "Take two aspirin and call me in the morning" to the sophisticated neurological blocks in advanced cancer treatment, are commendable and merciful. But suffering itself cannot and probably should not be seen as a problem to be solved. The pain of life that we call suffering, whether it be anxiety, anguish in the face of disease and dying, or grief itself, may be a message to us of our humanity, finitude, and contingency. In its more profound ministries, medicine concerns the relief of pain and the creative endurance of suffering. Most religions embrace the theme of suffering near the heart of their belief system. Buddhism speaks of the travail of human experience and counsels contemplative disregard. In Judaism a suffering messianic people becomes the secret of redemptive history. In Christianity the clue to the meaning of the universe is the Suffering Servant: Jesus, called Christ.

Suffering is a problem because of theology. If there were no account that a God existed and that this world is a divine handiwork, suffering, and indeed the entire problem of evil, would be merely a brute fact. It would simply "be there" without value or disvalue. But as Dostoevski wrote, the death of a child is an affront to our sensibility precisely because there supposedly is a creator who is caring and just. Theology therefore brings a particular explanation and intensification to the question of suffering. The crucifixion of Jesus, the Righteous One, helps me understand and accept the cancer death of a young woman in the prime of life. It is unfair and unjust, but it is somehow embraced in the cosmic event at the center of history.

Theology assists in explaining or rationalizing suffering. At the same time, theology intensifies the problem of suffering. If suffering is "just there," it demands no explanation and gives rise to no efforts of amelioration. Theology both demands an answer and prompts a response to the problem of suffering. In one sense the whole enterprise of biomedicine is a theological response to the enigma of suffering. The physician seeks to cure. In these activities of therapeutics and investigation, the physician is seeking to ameliorate suffering. Medicine and theology go hand in glove as vehicles by which the human race comes to grips with the problem of suffering. Project Ten will study this collaborative consideration.

10. Dying

ISSUES

Death, Immortality, Care of the Dying

ANALYSIS

Life in the midst of death is the final word in both medicine and religion. Modern biomedicine has recognized the filaments of life called

DNA. These basic structures, similar in composition to all created matter and life forms, replicate and die, forming a tape that binds life today back to the dawn of life when the first complex molecules formed. That tape will wind out toward the future if we have the sense to avert the catastrophe now possible because of our splitting of the atom and our unraveling of the genetic code. Life begets life, then collapses toward death. Even the disintegration into the inanimate is a form of continuity. The physicists remind us that nothing is lost. Matter is transformed into energy; the inanimate penetrates the animate.

In humans death intermingles with life. Conception is a spark of life amid an ocean of death as germ cells die. The female child has millions of oocytes in the ovaries. The store rapidly diminishes, leaving few at age forty-five. Most sperm and ova never fertilize, most embryos never implant, most implanted embryos do not have the perfection to go to term and create a new life. In early adulthood we begin to lose brain cells. All our days are numbered; we are dying slowly from the moment of conception.

Animals die around us all the time. The microbiotic world is a teeming mass of death and regeneration. The small creatures, birds and squirrels, go away to hidden places to die. The elephants also haul away their deceased to hidden crevices. The whales swarm in ritual around beached colleagues as if to foster the ongoing illusion that life, not death, reigns supreme.

In biology and medicine, vitality and finality are constant pressures. Diseases as prefigurations of death are the object of the medical challenge. To understand and explain the etiology and natural history of disease and to develop preventive and interventive strategies is the sustaining activity of medical practice. One might argue that medicine is our human warfare with death. It is at least the effort to name, control, and eventually overcome the vectors of death. All this is the magnificent energy one writer called the "raging thirst for life."

Yet death inevitably comes. All medicine concerns itself with the pilgrimage toward death. Sensitive medical care always involves euthanasia—accompanying persons to a good death. Often it involves treatment decisions that guide persons toward "better" deaths than might otherwise transpire. While positive gestures to cause death are proscribed in most medical ethics, the powers at hand can often be selectively employed so that one death meets us before another. The person with a head-neck carcinoma may die from exsanguinating after the tumor erodes the carotid artery, or after metastatic pressure on a vital structure in the brain, or after obstruction from a lung metastasis. Medical care can sometimes guide the falling life-trajectory toward one of these options.

In treatment of terminal disease, pain-killing medication is sometimes used at levels that not only alleviate pain but also hasten death. Great controversy now gathers around the question as to whether suicide is licit when one is affected with intractable, incurable, and excruciating disease. Should measures less violent than staged auto crashes, a gun to the head, or a leap from a bridge be proffered? Should medical counsel participate in any way in that deliberation?

In summary, medicine is inspired by the pursuit of life: saving life, preventing disease, rescuing the injured, resuscitating the arrested, prolonging life, extending the life span. Its grand vocation is found in sustaining vital power in us while we are being bombarded by morbid and mortal forces. Yet medicine lives surrounded by death. Eventually every patient slides into rest and death. The lifesaving efforts always fail, and death has the last word. Medicine endures in an ongoing atmosphere of life and death. It must nurture the *ars vivendi* and the *ars moriendi*.

Theology also lives in the service of life and concerns itself with death in the midst of life. Vivification and mortification are two of the prime functions of religion. Jesus claimed to have come to give the human race life, and life abundant. The life of the Spirit brings new birth and vitality in the midst of decadence, and eternal life within and beyond our space- and time-bound life.

Theological teaching in all religions, with the exceptions of those who believe that existence is an illusion, contend that sustenance of life and breath itself is a divine gift. In Hebrew the *ruach Elohim*—the wind of God—breathes life into the person. When one inspires, it is the sustaining energy of the divine Spirit. When one expires, God has withdrawn life.

Theology seeks to imbue existence with a sense of verve by instilling meaning and value to experience. Most faiths believe that one can live a living death unless life is activated with this quality. To be "truly alive," the spirit must be animated. The moral qualities of reciprocity, kindness, and justice are, in the religions of the world, not only desirable virtues, but also preconditions of happiness, fulfillment, and life itself.

Theological Perspectives

It is not life but vital anguish that gives rise to religion. In health and wholeness we feel self-sufficient, and the sense of radical dependence wanes. It is sickness and the premonition of death that prepare the human soul for spiritual awareness. Salvation is being saved to life from death.

One finds in religion a great ambivalence about death. On the one hand, death is the enemy, and faith is a challenge to death. On the other hand, death is a welcome friend. In the conflict with death, the structure and style of the spiritual life is formed. Life in the Spirit, new life, eternal life, is juxtaposed to the old life, life that is death-bound. Yet many faiths think of spiritual vitality and growth as mortification. To be truly alive to God is to die slowly to oneself, slowly to disengage oneself from this world and to make ready for, indeed to celebrate, death. "Welcome Sister Death," sang Francis of Assisi. Said Dietrich Bonhoeffer as he was led to the Flossenberg gallows, "For you it is my end; for me it is the beginning."

Many problems of mutual intrigue lie in the subject of death at the interface of medicine and theology. The questions of "natural death," the artificial extension of life, suicide, and definition of death need to be explored collaboratively by medicine and theology. Joint exploration of the practical and pastoral issues is also needed. How do we care for the dying? How do we move away from the disregard that kills, the negligence that makes life a living death?

We have considered a number of themes selected from myriad possibilities of mutual concern to medicine and theology. An attempt has been made to move across the internal logic, the development, the momentum of these two great activities of the human mind. If we held before our eyes two transparent sheets—one with the progression of philosophical themes in medicine across the life cycle from birth to death, the other with the outline of systematic theology from creation to anthropology to eschatology—the inner architecture of each discipline would show striking coincidental concentrations at the thematic points we have raised.

Project Ten will seek to examine the theology and ethics of medicine in an unprecedented way. It will take the great faith traditions of our world and examine from within these categories, within these logics of faith, the deep questions of medicine.

This chapter is a small road map for the journey soon to begin.

Topics at the Interface of Medicine and Theology

NOTES

1. Warren T. Reich, ed., *Encyclopedia of Bioethics*, 4 vols. (New York: Free Press, 1978).

2. H. Tristram Engelhardt, Jr., and Stuart F. Spicker, eds., Philosophy and Medicine Series, multiple volumes (Hingham, Mass.: Kluwer Boston, 1975).

3. Ivan Illich, *Medical Nemesis: The Expropriation of Health* (New York: Bantam Books, 1977).

4. Kenneth L. Vaux, *This Mortal Coil: The Meaning of Health and Disease* (New York: Harper & Row, 1978).

5. Stephen Toulmin, "Marriage Morality and Sex-Change Surgery: Four Traditions in Case Ethics," *The Hastings Center Report*, August 1981, p. 8.

6. Helmut Thielicke, *Theological Ethics*, 3 vols. (Grand Rapids: Eerdmans, 1978).

7. See the forthcoming work on James Gustafson's systematic ethics from the University of Chicago Press.

8. See esp. *The Patient as Person: Exploration in Medical Ethics* (New Haven: Yale University Press, 1970); and *Ethics at the Edges of Life* (New Haven: Yale University Press, 1978).

9. See "The Nature of Medical Ethics," in *Ethics in Medicine: Historical Perspectives and Contemporary Concerns*, ed. Arthur J. Dyck and Stanley Reiser (Cambridge: M.I.T. Press, 1977), pp. 123–28.

8

Theological Foundations
of Medical Ethics

KENNETH L. VAUX

No words can better set the stage for these reflections than those of James Gustafson. In a 1979 issue of *The Journal of Medicine and Philosophy,* he writes:

> Many of the persons who have published widely in medical ethics were trained in theology. Indeed, until the recent discovery of moral philosophers that practical moral questions were philosophically interesting and of deep concern to students and members of the professions, most of the literature in medical ethics was written by persons with theological training and religious affiliations. The last twelve years have seen an increase in the contribution of moral philosophers, physicians and others to the field. As medical ethics became a growth industry in the academic world, and as the traditional religious and theological bases for the word apparently lost significance, many of the theologically trained speakers and writers repressed, denied or became indifferent to theology as a field.[1]

Gustafson's indictment rings true. Nevertheless, we are not witnessing a permanent theological amnesia. What may be occurring is a temporary acknowledgment by many of the pluralism and radical secularity of our time and a willingness, much in the spirit of the apostle, to be all things to all people and to introduce oneself initially on the Athens agora as familiar with one's own poets and idols. But Gustafson is right to contend that today both secular analysis and technological imperatives are calling medical theologians, now in secular disguise, back to their confessions.

Theological Perspectives

It must be acknowledged that it is not an easy time to formulate one's witness. In the Western world the times are luxuriant and lazy, and our confessions do not possess the precision and power of those formulated in moments of suffering and challenge. Theological language is confused; moral prophecy is muted. Systematic work has deteriorated into topical work and from there into pop theology. Only in recent years has biblical, hermeneutical, and apologetic science focused to the point where it can respond meaningfully to the profound questions being raised so rapidly in the human sciences. Until now the theological ethicist laboring in the biomedical sphere could offer only vapid clichés and shallow moralisms. We can hope that fundamental theological work has at last come to the point where it can ground a witness that is fresh and convincing.

Such a witness is desperately needed. The great philosopher Alasdair MacIntyre has pleaded for a vibrant theological witness in the arena of biomedical ethics. Today, he argues, the idolatry is so pervasive, the divine image in people so disregarded, and the imperatives of social justice so violated that a new *religio medici* is urgently required.

Certainly the obsessions of contemporary medicine, obsessions of both consumer and provider, verge on the idolatrous. In the consumer sector, our manias for health, beauty, and youth are unashamedly religious. They are put forward with the full fervor of belief and devotion. "This is our theology," the ads seem to say (see Figure 1). "Yes, we believe," reply the buyers.

Adulation of health and body is also found among the providers. Basic scientists and clinicians are so caught up in efforts to intervene, to modify functions, to manipulate vital powers, and to alter human nature itself that they fail to sense the dimensions of suffering, feelings, historic continuity, and hope in those they supposedly serve. They see human substance as immediate, infinitely malleable, and plastic.

The idolatry of contemporary biomedicine is most acutely expressed in its underlying anthropology. The body-machine image of Descartes and Francis Bacon has become the operative paradigm. Indeed, we have reached the absurd point where ideas like wholism and the hospice are seen as dangerous new precedents, and healing faith is perceived as an unnecessary appendage to real healing.

The desanctification of the person and systemic injustice, points one and two of MacIntyre's critique, are self-evident. When added to the

---

Come to our Country Growth Center at Oz
In Port Arena, California

Join the Oz Staff for a lovely country vacation

Here are the Saving Experiences you can have:

- **Zen running on the beach . . .**
- **Yoga—hot tubs—sauna—massage . . .**
- **Nature and art walks . . .**
- **Delectable organic meals . . .**
- **Sights and smells in the country renewing your appetite for life . . .**
- **Body archology . . . Urban development through isolation tank and human body workshop with pingpong . . .**

This 5-day program will include 10 sessions on human body as archetype. A systematic approach to natural coordination and release of vital body fluids—to remove excessive tension—shallow breathing, and toxic relationships in an otherwise exologically unbalanced world.

FIGURE 1.

FROM A BROCHURE ADVERTISING A HEALTH AND
HUMAN RELATIONS CENTER IN CALIFORNIA

threat of idolatry, they adequately justify a new *apologia pro vita sua*. MacIntyre states his expectation of theologians in the area of medical ethics:

> First—and without this everything else is uninteresting—we ought to expect a clear statement of what difference it makes to be a Jew or a Christian or a Moslem, rather than a secular thinker, in morality generally. Second, and correlatively, we need to hear a theological critique of secular morality and culture. Third, we want to be told what bearing what has been said under the first two headings has on the specific problems which arise for modern medicine.[2]

This essay responds to the declension noted by Gustafson and the challenge issued by MacIntyre. Five motifs of theology—hypotheses of faith—will be correlated with hypotheses of meaning and value in medicine. The affinity of the theological concept to the biomedical gives instructive moral insight to guide that medical quest.

Theological Perspectives

The five theological ideas move from the general and universal to the distinctively Christian. While the author addresses these issues from his own standpoint, which is Judaic and Christian, the reader is invited to think about these normative questions of medicine within the context of other secular and religious faiths. The themes, with their counterparts from biomedicine, are these:

Theology	Medicine
1. Creation/Redemption	Archaic Law
2. Sin/Fall/Judgment	Responsibility for Health
3. Providence	Disease Endurance
4. Soteriology/Wholeness	Healing
5. Eschatology	The Goals of Medicine

1. CREATION/REDEMPTION: ARCHAIC LAW

The doctrine of creation and redemption signals the energy of God in time and history and in space and nature.

> When I look at your heavens, the work of your fingers, the moon and the stars which you have set in place,
> What is man that you think of him, and the son of man that you come to him.
> Yet you have made him nearly a God and crowned him with glory and honor and given him to rule over your handiwork putting all things under his dominion (Ps. 8:3–6).[3]

The One who activates time and space and who creates history in nature is moral to human beings, who are the epitome of the creation. From these beings the One elicits response to and cooperation with the tasks being undertaken. The doctrine of creation is therefore about moral management of the natural world and moral living in reciprocity and mutual realization within the human community. Martin Heidegger and Paul Tillich, following the Psalmist, spoke of a structural ontic and moral relation that humans have within nature, using the words *Zuhandensein,* *Verhandensein,* and *Miteinandersein.* People are the mediation of God into the world, the instrumentality with which God's task in the history of nature is being pursued. In the light of this analysis, we see that not only the knowledge and technology of medicine but also the moral imperatives relative to that sphere are derived from divine creation.

As medical practice has sought to guide its activity ethically, it has searched for a universal moral substance, a generic, basic norm. What might be called archaic or primal law, natural law, Noachian law, is sought by medicine. Science has quested not for high and holy calling but for a rudimentary law found in the structure of the life world. This is the law Thomas called *lex naturalis* and *lex aeterna*, as opposed to *lex divina*. This is what the Nuremberg judges called the "laws of humanity." Rooted in the moral sense that emerged in prehistoric and primitive people, expressed in the customs and jurisprudence of the first civilizations that formed around the world as the last ice age withdrew, this law is biological and social; it antedates the preception of a singular deity who is a moral being. This is the cosmic moral sense that Paul acknowledged in the first chapter of Romans.

The aspects of this primal law, recognized in Judaism as Noachian law, included proscriptions of anarchy, blasphemy, idolatry, murder, sexual promiscuity, theft, and brutality to animals. In most cultures in the Orient, Near Orient, and Africa the same ingredients (violation of the given relationship to fellow human and beast, to the community, to the deity) were recognized in the law of nature.

As the Holy Roman Empire and the classic Christian era waned, as homogeneous and pervasive conscience broke down, society looked again for this primal, rational law. Kant and the rationalists sought stipulates of reason that could govern human affairs. Today medicine too looks for values, guidelines, and policy norms, not from theology but from these primal, prereligious moral perceptions.

Take, for example, the ethical corpus that proceeded from Nuremberg and the trial of the German physicians in 1945. Accusation was grounded on the so-called "laws of humanity." Nuremberg asked how we protect people from the violations of medicine committed to experimentation, intellectual intrigue, torture, iatric death, ktenology, or medical murder. At Nuremberg we did not and could not invoke the radical Hebrew cry that spilling human blood is blasphemy, for it was on the body of Jewish humanity that the atrocity was inflicted. That divine law had long been forsaken. Instead we invoked general moral wisdom: the doctrine of autonomy; the right to refuse or withdraw from what is being offered; the requirement to test innovative techniques *in vitro* and on animals before they are tested on people.

The attempt at Nuremberg to define "laws of humanity" reflects the search of medicine for a universal moral culture. Today, as Oriental Buddhists, Indian Hindus, and Near Eastern Muslims practice medicine in towns and villages across America along with Jews, Catholics, and Protestants, the clarification of basic moral guidelines for medical practice is imperative. The universities and research centers where the training of these doctors and nurses takes place are usually steeped in scientific rationalism, secular humanism, and a disposition of sympathy to a syncretistic moral atmosphere called by one physician "the golden rule in medicine."[4]

Medicine and theology therefore have much to offer each other in understanding creation and the moral architecture of life. It would be enlightening to see what correspondence exists among sociobiological instincts, cross-cultural values, and primal theological virtues. Medicine will call forth what is fundamental and universal out of the rich body of morality that includes much that is time-bound, culture-bound, and supererogative. In the moral teaching of the faiths of our culture, the treasury of directives on procreation, sexuality, and living and dying offer much to be appropriated and much to be discarded.

Conversely, by introducing concepts of transcendence and universality, theology can rescue contemporary medicine from the sterile morality of secular humanism and cultural syncretism. General morality most often deteriorates into utilitarianism, expediency, econometrics rights theory, and eventually adversarial or Machiavellian power play. The absurd vacillation of the courts on the scandal of life prolongation cases from Quinlan and Saikewicz to Spring and Brother Fox illustrates this moral confusion: affirming one time that it is licit to terminate treatment, then later that it is not. Clarity in case law, public policy, and the more common decision-making requires more substantive moral insight. Theology may be able to offer this.

2. SIN/FALL/JUDGMENT: RESPONSIBILITY FOR HEALTH

Ideas of primal and continuing transgression of divine law are thought to affect health in two important ways. First, there is the belief that a fall from primeval innocence introduced disease and death into the cosmos. Most religions remember either a historic or a mythic moment which was free from disease. There is also the implied belief that such a lost paradise must be restored. Second, there is in all times and places the pervasive association of getting sick with doing something wrong. This inferred connection between morality and morbidity prompts us to clarify with some care the Judeo-Christian beliefs about sin, fall, and judgment.

> Because you listen to the enactments (*mishpatīm*) and do them, Yahweh, your God, will keep his covenant of mercy with you. He will love you, bless and prosper you. He will bless your offspring and bring the earth to fruition; the grain, the wine, the fresh oil, the cattle and flocks on the land sworn to your ancestors. Above all people you will be blessed and neither your wives or your cattle will be barren. And Yahweh will take from you all sicknesses; and none of the diseases that you knew in Egypt will afflict you (Deut. 7:12–15).

As we consider the first point of primal fall, there is great interest today in biomedical philosophy as to whether disease and death are natural and necessary to the world or whether they can be alleviated and therefore are problems to be solved. An important new book, *Life Span*, edited by Robert Veatch, has recently been published.[5]

A fascinating literature has emerged in recent years asking whether there is a "natural" age to die, whether the life span is biologically determined and specific, whether aging is a disease, and whether cancer or senility is the last disease. In a recent issue of the *New England Journal of Medicine*, Dr. James Fries of Stanford argues yes and no. Yes, there seems to be a natural boundary to life; the capacities of vital organs diminish on the arc of the life cycle even in the absence of pathology. No, acute and chronic diseases are not necessary. They can be cured and are being cured. White women in the Western world will soon reach this ceiling, and many will die natural deaths—unless, that is, sociological counterforces set in. Fries feels that natural death at age seventy-seven to ninety-three, free from disease, will become more commonplace. Unfortunately the other morbid and mortal vectors—pathogens, genetic determinants, environmental toxins, and socioeconomic factors—will continue to cause premature deaths.[6] Dr. Ernst Wynder, president of the American Health Foundation, argues that corrections in life style habits and diet will move us closer to a day when most of us will "die young of old age."

Theological implications of this idea are obvious. Are diseases demonic intrusions into the created order? If so, what measures of science and experimentation are justified in explaining and counteracting these forces? What coercions, societal and personal, are allowed—genetic screening, proscribed procreation and sterilization, fetal diagnosis, infanticide?

Theological Perspectives

If disease and unnatural deaths fall within the sphere of human control, in what sense are we responsible for their resolution? As the environmental etiology in disease becomes clear—as in mesothelioma or some forms of leukemia—what is our societal duty in preventing disease and in bearing the cost of treatment? What of the economic and industrial tradeoffs? How long can we live with the fact that black men in our country have a one-third greater incidence of cancer deaths than white men? When we suddenly realize that it is a small group of people who are sick most of the time and that most of these are poor, unemployed, or stressed to the breaking point by the exhaustion of surviving, will we have the resolve to do something about this?

The theodicy question collapses into an anthropodicy question at many points. Why do we willfully inflict disease and shortened life opportunity upon other people? The question of human sin and what the early church fathers called its antidote comes into focus. The sacrament of life that binds the community in life and death to the eternal sacrifice must become the moral paradigm of our life-style.

There is also a personal dimension to the theologico-medical theme of sin and responsibility. If personal habits and behaviors are deleterious to health, is one individual to be held to account in any way? The dramatic health status indices of the Seventh-Day Adventists, for example, point to the salutary effect of beliefs, practices, and habits that are born in the theological covenants. Are people with alcoholic liver disease or smoking-induced cancer or high anxiety secondary to discontent and compulsion sick because of their sin? Do we overlook, forgive, or take care of such people? Recently several cases of PCP (an addictive street drug) overdose have occurred. In such cases the patients are rushed to the emergency unit, physically, psychologically, and neurologically in great danger. They are then pumped out, lavaged, chemically neutralized, and detoxified—only to come back, confident that medical technology can again rescue them from the pit. Sometimes a patient will even say, "I'm not scared to take the stuff; I know you'll take care of me." I have little doubt that we are entering a new age where inferences between misbehavior and the onset of illness will be drawn. We will be thrown back to previous ages where sin and sickness were associated. Our moral response will be posited on the basis of the theology underlying the culture. If we become neo-Puritan we will respond to people who are both physically and mentally ill in one way. If we become laissez-faire liberal we will respond in another way. Whatever paths we take, the theology of the culture will be the principal force in shaping our health policy ethics.

3. PROVIDENCE: DISEASE ENDURANCE

The theme of providence takes us to another theological level and another bioethical application. If archaic law is the offering of Noachian theology, and responsibility for health the offering of deuteronomic covenant, the moral understanding of providence is the offering of apocalyptic Judaism and messianic Christianity. This passionate theology of suffering arises among a very specific people under unique conditions and therefore entails a deeper and more intense moral calling. The theology of the Exile and the Second Temple acknowledges that even the righteous suffer and die. In Deutero-Isaiah, the exilic Psalms, and Job, the conventional identification of righteousness with health, and sin with sickness, was shattered.

In late Judaism, eschatological and messianic consciousness came to influence piety and literature, and sickness and suffering slowly came to bear redemptive significance. A theological transformation occurred at this point. The revision of the idea of God then altered the meaning of morality and also revised any evaluation of health, disease, and death.

In theology and worship, Yahweh now came to be known not so much as the Akkadian sovereign or the aloof Egyptian sky-force but a pursuing, beneficent spirit. Although sovereign and immutable, God was a being who was known as a loving, caring, yearning, pain-bearing savior. God, in this mode of Hebrew scripture, is a pathetic being who feels for and with humanity. God reaches out to people in need and suffers with them. God heals; God saves. Two passages from the period of the Exile stand out. The Royal Servant is seen in grotesque leprous visage:

> He has not form or grandeur that we should look at him and no loveliness that we should desire Him. He was despised and abandoned by men, a man of sorrows, who knew sickness and pain. Shunning him we could not bear to look at him. Yet he has borne our pain and diseases. With his wounds we are healed (Isa. 53:1–5).

The doctrine of providence undergirds the blended virtue of courage and patience which one might label endurance. If the basic doctrine of creation elicits moral *reaction* to disease and the doctrine of fall elicits a sense of *responsibility* about disease, then the doctrine of providence elicits the virtue of *resignation* within disease. In this view, human frailty and finitude is not a problem to be solved but an enigma to be borne with equanimity. Beyond this, messianic theology contends that suffering and dying are not absurdities but rather provide clues to the deeper meaning of life. They initiate one into the deeper structure of reality—the reality of God.

The virtue of patience and courage, along with caring and serving in the face of disease and death, was expressed by the last days of one of our colleagues, a theology professor. Note the way that the suffering Messiah paradigm controlled his moral response:

> Bubba died of malignant melanoma in one of our university hospitals. He was a young man, in the flowering of his vocation, splendidly trained, a minister and theological professor, when a mole appeared on the back of his leg. A careless oversight, a bungled diagnosis, finally a belated excision and a positive biopsy ensued. Bubba was preaching a mission when the truth hit. He felt something radiating up from the mole into a lymph node. He knew he was dead. Although dread swept over him, he also related a deep pervasive sense of calm. Then followed months of intermittent, then fulltime, hospitalization, finally that admission from which there would be no return. He carefully chose his physician. The energy of hope and the yearning to live prompted him to come to an advanced medical center and work with a distinguished physician who was advancing frontiers of treatment. He also selected his surgeon-oncologist on the basis of his writings, which showed heightened and somewhat exceptional sensitivity to the psychodynamic dimensions of catastrophic illness. He forced his physician to be just that: one who would move with him as a partner into those profound transactions of hope and fear, radical treatment and restraint— one who would help him maximally relish the life that remained and courageously go to meet death. He would not allow his doctor to withdraw. He asked all who accompanied him on this last adventure to remain open and honest—retaining, as he did, that earthy sense of humor that Dostoevsky found to be the essence of humanness and humility. He taught all who knew him the gracious sense of mingled terror, mystery, and comfort that is in the profound biblical sense of the meaning of disease.
>
> Memorial services were held in cities around the country—his home town, his schools, towns where he had served as pastor. As he had wished, the text for meditation was John 13. Jesus, on the eve of his death, surrounded by the threat of violence, the foreboding of the unknown, amid a rush of events absurdly senseless, took the basin and the towel, knelt and washed the feet of his friends.
>
> For Bubba, this Last Supper act became the paradigm of a human response to disease and death, the only way that the Christian could imbue

this trauma with meaning. There is no easy rhyme or reason to our being and destiny in this world. Life is cruciform; and the important thing is that our being is faithful as it is embodied in life together. In this precipitous night, like that night of nights, we can only kneel and serve one another. In suffering and in death, Bubba witnessed to the truth of life's deepest paradox: "In dying we live."

As Jesus died on the cross, he cried in dereliction: "Why hast thou forsaken me?" He is recalling the ancient servant cry in Psalm 22. The question is, as theologian Jürgen Moltmann argues, the root question of all theology. It is also the question of the atheistic rebellion against God. It is surely the fundamental question of any theological treatment of the meaning of health and disease. The deepest meaning we can derive is that, in some profound sense, God bears and shares our pain and disease. In some mysterious sense, suffering draws us to the heart of the meaning of reality.[7]

4. SOTERIOLOGY/WHOLENESS: HEALING

Now let us look at the doctrine of salvation and wholeness as it correlates with the medical concept of healing. This is a day of great interest in wholistic health care. Nowhere can theology and medicine contribute more to each other than in the phenomena we call healing and salvation. Indeed, one might argue that only in understanding physico-mental healing can we save our doctrine of salvation from spiritualized subjectivism. Conversely, only a discerning soteriology can rescue medicine from the materialism and technomania which lead ultimately to the destruction of the human.

> Proclaim as you go, saying, "the kingdom of heaven is at hand"; heal the sick, cleanse the lepers, raise the dead, throw out demons. Freely you have received, freely give (Matt. 10:7–8).

> Having called together his twelve disciples, he gave them power and authority over all demons and to heal diseases. And he sent them out to announce the kingdom of God and to cure those sick in their very being (Luke 9:1–2).

The preaching, teaching, and pastoral care of the primitive Christian community sustained Jesus' estimate of the human condition as fractured and wounded, needing mending and healing.

Human disease, as Tillich reminded us, is the disintegration of life. "Many diseases," he wrote, "especially the infectious ones, can be understood as an organism's inability to return to self-identity. It cannot eject the strange elements which it has not assimilated." We might add that sometimes this throwing-off requires a healer, a savior.

> But disease can also be the consequence of a self-destruction of the centered whole, a tendency to maintain self-identity by avoiding the dangers of going out to self-alteration. In order to be safe, the organism tries to rest in itself, but since this contradicts the life function of self-integration, it leads to disease and disintegration.[8]

Healing in the physiological and psychiatric sphere is found in that delicate equipoise between saving oneself and surrendering oneself. Many diseases—metabolic, infectious, neoplastic, and psychoneurotic—penetrate one's being as one either centers too intensely in self-control and self-obsession or loses oneself in self-negation and self-depreciation. That Levitical and Christian wisdom of altruism evoked by self-esteem, "loving the neighbor as oneself," seems to be the secret of health and healing.

The Bible commands this mingled regard and disregard for oneself and one's health in the Old Testament by depicting flesh as the grass that withers and blows away (Isa. 40:6). In the New Testament we are counseled not to be anxious about life and the body (Matt. 6:25). *Christus Soter*, the healer, saves us from ourselves to be ourselves.

What moral implications of this doctrine bear on biomedical issues? Salvation in biblical context has two dimensions. The first is related to salvation as movement beyond the world. We are saved from this world, the flesh, and the devil; we are rescued from life's terror. This is the Persian and Hellenistic contribution to biblical thought. The other notion of salvation is wholeness in life, being made well in and through the salutary gifts of this world: medicine, rest, friendship. As a result two moral imperatives appear to be rooted in Christian soteriology. The first is a prophetic critique of the excesses of vitalism. Great thinkers in all traditions of medical theology have contended that there are values higher than life itself. The positive norm, though, prompts a concern for social justice and secular commitments that will safeguard and ensure health in the community.

The medical enterprise today desperately needs moral authorization for releasing life when such is called for. The agonies of case litigation and policy formulation in cases like Quinlan, Spring, Saikewicz, and Fox, and in policies like "natural death statutes" and "do not resuscitate" orders, witness to the perplexing value conflicts in this area. Because we do possess awesome powers to prolong life even at vegetative levels, we need to determine when such tools should be used and when they should be neglected. Legal verdicts have been rendered for and against medical heroism. We have torts for wrongful termination of life and for wrongful prolongation of life. Only a theological vision wherein our personal existence is being saved within space and time, within the body, and *beyond* this world—only that kind of profoundly paradoxical theology can guide humane medical decisions at the conclusion of life.

A salvation-grounded ethic is committed to health care for all as part of a social justice that guards the poor from injury and exploitation and seeks life-enhancing opportunities for all people. Some of the great moral impulses are generated by this belief: those to find the cause of diseases, to learn new therapeutics, and to make this knowledge and technique universally available.

5. ESCHATOLOGY: THE GOALS OF MEDICINE

Finally, the doctrine of eschatology is morally informative for health care. Since morality is most often motivated by self-justification, we need a moral message that has bearing both within and beyond this existence. The religious doctrine of the future, of consummation and judgment, elicits here and now both hope and condemnation, moral encouragement and critique.

> I reason that the agonies of the present time are not worth comparing to the forthcoming glory that will be revealed in us. For the creation eagerly expects the revelation of the sons of God. For the creation was subjected to futility not of his own will but by the will of Him Who subjected it in hope (Rom. 8:18–20).

The doctrine of eschatology is complex and profound in its bearing on the present. Through images of hope of things to come, of end-time events, of eternal life, of the final transfiguration of reality, resistance is generated to what is when viewed against what ought to be or what will be. Positive images of what a future could be or ought to be are also fashioned in eschatology. The implications of this doctrine for bio-medicine are many.

Do we seek to build upon our present control of the bacterial plagues and assault the world of the virus and seek a world free from microbial disease?

Do we build on the discoveries of psycho-pharmacology and seek pain-free life?

Do we build upon the transplant age to achieve a world where all human parts are replaceable and physical immortality comes within reach?

These questions and many other challenges of the biomedical agenda will require the theological task of cleansing our hope of illusion, seeking rather the human future that is rooted in the divine promise.

A final note: All our penultimate moral acts seem to express those basic beliefs and senses of destiny which undergird our culture. For four thousand years biblical religions have seen the control of nature and the suppression of malign and morbid forces as the work of humanity. We hunt the horsemen of the apocalypse, all the while fashioning our own warhorses, famines, and diseases. Now we need to clarify that sense of purpose and recover our awareness of boundaries and a vision of reciprocity with our surroundings. Above all, we need to learn to live with that consideration of others that the apostle called *agape*. Then and only then can faith and hope transmute into that greatest gift.

NOTES

1. James Gustafson, "Editorial," *Journal of Medicine and Philosophy* 4 (1979): 345.

2. Alasdair MacIntyre, "Theology, Ethics, and the Ethics of Medicine and Health Care . . ." *Journal of Medicine and Philosophy* 4 (1979): 435.

3. Unless otherwise specified, all translations in this chapter are by the author from the original Hebrew and Greek.

4. Michael E. DeBakey, "Medical Research and the Golden Rule," *Journal of the American Medical Association* 203 (February 19, 1968): 574–76.

5. Robert Veatch, ed., *Life Span: Values and Life-Expectancy Technologies* (New York: Harper & Row, 1980).

6. "Doctor Says 85 'Natural' Age to Die," *Chicago Tribune*, October 26, 1980, p.6.

7. Kenneth L. Vaux, *This Mortal Coil: The Meaning of Health and Disease* (New York: Harper & Row, 1978), pp. 30–31.

8. Paul Tillich, *Systematic Theology* (Chicago: University of Chicago Press, 1963), 3:35.

PART FIVE

Medical Perspectives

9

Preventive Medicine and Religion: Opportunities and Obstacles

ERNST WYNDER
and
MARY-CARROLL SULLIVAN

Such diseases as smallpox, typhoid, and cholera presented almost insurmountable obstacles to physicians of yesteryear. Heart attacks, strokes, and cancer present equally imposing challenges to the physicians of today. The latter diseases cause some 60 percent of all deaths among modern American adults. The data from the U.S. National Center for Health Statistics are disheartening. Examination of a recent survey of the ten leading causes of death shows that at least six of these directly reflect the state of disrepair, physiological or emotional, into which our society has fallen. Ranking first is heart disease, followed by cancer, then cerebrovascular disease. Fourth is accidents, seventh cirrhosis of the liver, and suicide is ninth.[1] If we are to reach the ultimate goal of medical care, that is, to allow people to live long and healthy lives, these are the diseases that must be conquered. These diseases—particularly when we add to them chronic pulmonary diseases and conditions related to alcoholism—account for a substantial part of the health-care dollars spent in this country. It is therefore a matter not only of medical and social importance but also of economic importance to overcome these successfully.

An observation that must be made immediately is that our society is experiencing an epidemiological shift. The morbidity and mortality of our society is no longer a condition of "acute onset." Rather, chronic ill health is too frequently a common and accepted way of life. The question to be answered is whether, given the knowledge we hold concerning causes of these diseases, we can bring about a significant reduction of the incidence of these killers, thereby not only gaining years of productive life but also reducing the cost of our health-care system. Why cannot such knowledge properly be applied to man-made diseases?

Cancer and heart disease, the leading killers in our society, do not arise inevitably from aging but, like most of our diseases today, are man-made. Clearly, then, these diseases should also be man-preventable. To say that a disease is man-made is to say that its etiology can be directly related to the life-style humans have created for themselves. A cursory reading of the lay press—for example, the *Chicago Tribune* and the *New York Times*—reveals an ongoing roster of what could be termed the carcinogens of the week: DDT and DES, saccharin and cyclamates, nuclear energy and water pollution. The general reaction of the reading public is unanimous: "Isn't it terrible that the environment in which we live causes all these diseases?" True, the presence of pollutants in our environment does indeed cause disease, and we the public ought not to tolerate those that are not absolutely necessary for life. However, it is our deliberately chosen and cultivated Western life-style—what we eat, drink, and smoke—that causes most illness.

Nature meant that human beings should die from old age, not from disease. Few subjects have caused people as much apprehension, fear, and fascination as death. Throughout history, humans have tended to delude themselves into believing that their being on earth was just a finite part of an eternal, tranquil existence in the beyond. The closer they came to death, the more readily could they be persuaded to believe in the hereafter. Even as people increased their knowledge of the biological and astronomical phenomena of the universe, they could not cope with death in scientific and realistic terms or verify an existence after death. It is a basic human reaction to deny those events that one does not understand or finds unpleasant. To deny death, therefore, may be regarded as a natural reaction to its reality.

Such denial clearly has its virtues, particularly to those facing imminent death due to a fatal disease or the hazards of combat. A belief in the hereafter also may be helpful to those severely or chronically depressed, as well as to those eking out a miserable existence on earth. However, to deny death and have an illusion of an eternal existence is often detrimental to health. When people are unwilling to face their mortality, they may indulge in health practices that are likely to invite illness and hasten premature death. Such interplay between medicine and religious belief can be illustrated dramatically by analyzing some notions of mortality and immortality as these affect health practices.

Preventive Medicine and Religion

OBSTACLES TO PREVENTIVE MEDICINE

Louis Pasteur has said that successful scientists must not only discover but also apply the knowledge they have discovered. But the discovery is often a good deal easier than the application. Examples from the field of epidemiology abound to testify to the rarity of seeing newly discovered knowledge utilized. A notable example is the seeming disregard for the knowledge gained by the investigators who first related the smoking habit to lung cancer. Possession of knowledge cannot cure where the will to change life-style is absent. Furthermore, our attitudes toward health practices are conditioned by training and/or economics.

A visit to most medical schools today, a look at departmental budgets, or a walk through the wards of today's hospitals makes it obvious that the power of our hospitals and associated medical schools lies in the hands of the "treating physician"—in therapy rather than prevention. The basic attitudes toward medical care and medical practice carried by physicians throughout their lives are deeply influenced by their experiences as medical students. The power of a physician clearly lies in the academics if not the economics of therapy, or at least so it seems to the young student. Most students regard the physician's role as that of a healer rather than a preventer. When selecting an internship and subsequently a residency, it again becomes apparent that most of these training periods are geared toward treating rather than preventing illness. Moreover, when young doctors open their first office, they find that reimbursement schedules from the insurance carriers by and large pay only for therapeutic services, not for preventive services.

In a capitalistic society financial reimbursement holds the greatest incentive for most people. Thus several other factors inhibit the advancement of disease prevention. It is not to be expected that the tobacco industry will give up producing products that a large segment of the public continues to desire, that the alcohol industry would take the lead in prohibiting the sale of liquor even to the alcoholic, or that the food industry would take major steps to reduce the high fat and cholesterol content of the Western diet. Therefore proponents of preventive medicine often feel like Don Quixote dreaming an impossible dream. Although one often gets verbal or written support when discussing these problems with medical or lay audiences, verbal support cannot be equated with the economic incentives being given to therapeutic or crisis-oriented medicine.

Medical Perspectives

There are no pressure groups in Congress in support of preventive medicine, as there are for catastrophic illness. Twenty victims with kidney disease, in their demand for dialysis, can generate more letters to their representatives than all the millions of Americans who theoretically believe in the advantages of preventive medicine. Heart transplants made television headlines for years, but the health and economic benefits resulting from polio vaccination are rarely referred to in the daily press. Crisis medicine is news; preventive medicine is like a war that never happened.

As stated, the majority of the diseases in the Western world today are related to factors we ourselves could control, and herein lies another dilemma. We can no longer put the blame on outside forces, but rather have to assume responsibility ourselves. More than merely receiving our immunization shots, we must modify our life-styles and develop a new sense of discipline—a price that many of us are unwilling to pay, because of yet another problem which faces the proponents of preventive medicine: our "illusion of immortality." There is a fundamental need for people from a variety of disciplines to examine the reasons human beings continue to indulge in a life-style that seems to defy their mortality. In conducting this examination, people must consider whether or not this belief is fundamental to their being able to live through the day-by-day hardships of life and whether a constant reminder of their mortality would hinder their ability to conduct properly the affairs of life.

RELIGION AND MEDICINE

The metaphysical nature of the questions we are asking, and the very physical ramifications of the conclusions we come to, place the forum for this discussion comfortably within the realms of both religion and medicine. Conversation between these fields is not new. However, the thrust of the dialogue we shall commence here is one that has not been seen in the past as either desirable or necessary, since historically medicine and religion have been partners in the healing enterprise.

In primitive society, the role of the medicine man was seen in various guises, many of them more related to magic or faith healing than to the practice of any scientific method. Documented cases of cures from the administrations of the shaman or the exercise of voodoo or black magic, when all attempts at herbal healing or bleeding or trepanation have failed, abound in the annals of medical anthropology.[2]

Preventive Medicine and Religion

The combination of priest-physician (*iatros*) who appeared in the Hellenic literature was succeeded in the Judeo-Christian scriptural literature by the rabbi/teacher who healed. The historical link between religion and medicine became more evident as both the church and health care took more visible institutional forms from the days of the Roman Empire through medieval times. It was a function of religious societies within the church to establish dispensaries, clinics, and the first hospitals, which were staffed by monks and religious brothers and sisters.

The relationship between religion and medicine in modern times is of a decidedly different texture. As medicine became a more highly developed science, it became clear that full-time practitioners of the art/science would shape and determine its future. It also became clear that the work of the church was not *primarily* technological.

So as medicine in the last two and one-half centuries set out on a course of incredible technological development, it lost "official" contact with an institution whose major input into that development would have been more philosophical than scientific, more "otherworldly" than the technical concerns of the "here and now."

We have reached a point where the very technology that we have expended so much human effort, time, and talent in developing has become our nemesis. If the statistics are to be believed, the changing patterns of health and disease referred to earlier are directly attributable to our technology. These technological advancements have created a two-headed monster that seriously threatens the health of our global society.

First, we have let loose upon our environment a myriad of pollutants, many of which are yet to be identified. Ironically, this identification often comes about by virtue of diagnosing a new disease syndrome. Only in analyzing the condition do we come to discover its etiology.

Second, our technological "advancements" have invested us with a sense of superiority that is in itself life-threatening. We view our accomplishments as the outward manifestation of our obedience to the God-given mandate to "fill the earth and conquer it" (Gen. 1:28). We are the masters of the universe. It is this latter result of our scientific growth that accounts for our "illusion of immortality." The consequences of such an illusion can be seen in the indisputable findings of some of our studies.

For example, while a significant proportion of the more educated white males in this country have stopped smoking, the antismoking propaganda has had relatively little impact on the public at large. The smoking habits of young boys are similar to those ten years ago, and cigarette smoking among girls has doubled—all this in spite of the fact that a Gallup poll has shown that about three-quarters of all Americans believe smoking is a major reason for lung cancer. When it comes to disease or infirmity, those of us who inhabit a society which can catapult people to the moon and engineer genetic structure suffer from a serious case of "it can't happen to me." The direct result of the unmerited self-assurance is an unwillingness to abide by the admonitions of those who would like to guarantee that "it" doesn't "happen."

This false sense of security is almost ludicrously widespread. This country has some twelve million alcoholics; half of all highway fatalities are known to be related to alcoholism. Obesity is a national disease; attempts to reduce it relate not so much to fear of disease as to the ungainly appearance of the condition. Only a small fraction of all drivers wear seat belts, though most know that wearing them reduces traffic fatalities. In one study, it was shown that only about 17 percent of the drivers of older cars (that is, those without buzzer warning signals) wore seat belts. The same study showed that the number of drivers of the newer cars (that is, those with warning signals) wearing seat belts was about the same! People would rather overcome such technological warnings than protect themselves from possible injury.

It would seem that in our quest for a technological utopia we have at least reached a point of diminishing return. Perhaps we have passed that point and have created a paradoxical situation. The theory that Western technology and access to it must be critical factors in the incidence of disease occurrence has been borne out by many studies. One investigation into the demographic distribution of cancer in the American Northeast concludes: "The nation is moving toward a common pattern of cancer mortality, a pattern consistent with the many studies that have shown that second and later generation immigrants manifest cancer mortality patterns of the new nation rather than that of their parents."[3] That technology, upon which we pinned our hopes for a panacea for all evil, has become instead a wellspring of further problems.

Rather than eradicating illness, we have become victims of an unhealthy life-style. That those ills from which we suffer are within the boundaries of our control and yet we continue to suffer them indicates a more radical shift in the societal schemata. We submit gladly, recklessly, to those ills we have willed ourselves.

OPPORTUNITIES FOR PREVENTIVE MEDICINE
AND RELIGION

We have, then, the picture of a changing value system as well as a change in life-style. What we must concern ourselves with now is what we are going to do about what we have done. We have so entwined ourselves in a slick and efficient life-style, one which gratifies desires without reference to need, that we have neglected to question the values that lay at the base of our new life-style.

At this juncture we must resurrect the dialogue between religion and medicine. The true test of the value of a new insight or a new theory or policy lies in its ability to stand up to scrutiny and analysis. Religion is the realm into which value-testing falls. Values deal with the intangibles, those attitudes and beliefs which transcend the mundane. They are observable and verifiable characteristics of scientific data. However, they are neither quantifiable nor necessarily reobtainable, even when conditions that originally produced them are unchanged. Therefore they are not the "stuff" of science and must be tested in a nonscientific, or at least not exclusively scientific, arena.

There are other reasons for channeling this discussion along the tracks of both religion and medicine. The many contiguous points along the paths of both disciplines could provide the common ground necessary to get beyond the impasse we call the "illusion of immortality."

The notion of immortality is very definitely religious. It refers to the concept of a life after the one in this world. In many cultures and faith traditions, the presumption in such a notion is that the life hereafter is one of greater importance,[4] that the life we have here on earth is one we endure or the means by which the nature of our life hereafter is determined. Because of this underlying belief in a life hereafter, it is extremely important that those institutions and resources whose business it is to deal with religious belief and its effects on the behavior of its members become involved with the medical phenomenon which results from this "illusion of immortality." The World Health Organization (WHO) defines health as "a state of complete physical, mental and social well-being and not merely the absence of disease or infirmity."[5] This professional goal of the practice of medicine as defined in a charter document of the only universal body of health-care practitioners is important in several respects. First, it defines health clinically in two ways: negatively as the absence or privation of illness, but positively and primarily as the presence of well-being in all aspects of human existence.

This elucidation by the WHO establishes the first of the contiguous points between medicine and religion that are relevant to our discussion. Obviously, one of the underpinnings common to both religion and medicine, historically as well as sociologically, is that both are seen as caring or healing ministries. However, there are ramifications of the religious concept of health that exceed the notion of curing or healing. These religious ramifications are more in line with the concept of disease prevention and health maintenance. They derive from the Old Testament repetition of the word *shalom*, which is the Hebrew word expressing the fullness and well-being of life.[6] *Shalom* is a blessing one seeks for oneself and wishes for others, "in every sphere of life whether physical, mental and spiritual, or individual, social and national."[7]

In the New Testament the notion of well-being becomes a moral responsibility. The body is viewed as a temple of the Holy Spirit. "It is life with the quality of eternity where God himself dwells. It is the life of God himself."[8] Again, a scriptural mandate to health maintenance: "May God himself, the God of peace, make you holy in every part, and keep you sound in spirit, soul and body, without fault when our Lord Jesus Christ comes."

We can see that there is a historical connection between health and religion in the literature. However, one must ask whether there is any evidence of a connection between religion and health in praxis.

- Mormons in Utah have a 30 percent lower incidence of most cancers.
- Seventh-Day Adventists have from 10 to 40 percent fewer hospital admissions for epidermoid and nonepidermoid malignancies.
- Regular church-attenders in Washington County, Maryland, have 40 percent less risk from arteriosclerotic heart disease.
- Jews living in Brooklyn have twice the expected incidence of leukemia.
- Jewish men in New York City have decidely lower rates of lung cancer than Protestant or Catholic men.

  Research on the correlation of religious faith and health attitudes and behaviors will be difficult because of the subtlety and elusiveness of these beliefs. Beliefs prompt moral behaviors; these in turn affect health.[9]

One cannot say with certainty that the adherence to a religious belief will have a beneficial effect on one's health. Nor can one say that rejection of religious belief is detrimental to one's well-being. However, we can make the empirical observation that sometimes religious beliefs result in a pattern of behavior which includes good health habits and excludes bad ones.

Having pointed out the common viewpoint of medicine and religion that the state of health or well-being is seen as a good or desirable trait, we can point to other areas of common ground. In many instances the fields of health and religion share the same language and symbols. The words "life," "healing," "caring," "purging"; the concepts of "birth," "death," "purification," "breath"; the symbols "water," "fire," "air"; and rituals "anointing with oil," "exorcism," "laying-on of hands"—all these and more are shared by the two disciplines.

Perhaps the attribute most pertinent to our topic, one shared by both religion and medicine, is the common intentionality of these disciplines. That is, neither religion nor medicine exists in a vacuum. Each carries with it a societal responsibility. There is a responsibility on the part of physicians to exercise their knowledge and skills in the service of others. Religious believers similarly are obliged to do good for others. We have illustrated above some of the scriptural basis for that moral dictate in the Abrahamic faiths, and facsimiles of the golden rule can be found in the writings of Confucius, the Rig-Veda, and other sacred books of the East. It is on the point of commonality that the only possible solution to the dilemma under discussion can be reached. On the issue of commonly understood societal responsibility, religion and medicine can move from an area of conversation to an area of collaboration.

In a recent editorial review, epidemiologist W. E. Waters remarked on the need for medicine to recognize the demand for its active participation in active interdisciplinary collaboration, and to recognize that solitary efforts on the part of medicine will be ineffective in coping with today's health problems and issues:

> In both affluent and developing countries many health problems can be tackled either through health services or by interventions in other aspects of social policy, such as public health measures involving clean air and water as well as accident prevention, nutrition and taxation policies and health education. Epidemiology has an important role in providing a perspective of the *relative* importance of medicine as *just one* of a large number of determinants of health care.[10]

However, one can postulate government-sponsored programs forever, and to no avail. First, as already noted, the ability to engage government bureaucracies to the point of their appropriating funds is not one that has been easily demonstrated. Second, the efficacy of an externally imposed standard is always questionable. There are two concepts, both prominent themes in applied theology, which are very important to the discussion at hand: a notion of accountability and a sense of autonomy.

Accountability can best be described as an awareness and acceptance of responsibility by an individual for an ongoing project or idea. Surely the concern of one's own health ought to carry with it this element of accountability. The individual is charged with responsibility to himself or herself to maintain and preserve (or in some cases reestablish) to whatever extent possible his or her own bodily integrity. This charge is also a duty which is "owed" society as well, since that is the group upon whom the burden of care falls when one's bodily integrity is not maintained.

The second concept, that of autonomy, is understood as the inherent freedom of the individual to act. People are agents in their own behalf. There are also occasions when people's actions result in changes for the community around them. The motivation and reasons for a person's actions vary, but they are ultimately the result of some kind of value-ranking. That which motivates a person to act, whether the outcome is a desired goal in his or her own behalf or on behalf of others, is adherence to or adoption of a fundamental value.

Autonomy, however, is not license. Freedom is tempered by its position within a value system which is ranked by "weight." Certain values or qualities take preeminence over others. Clearly, while freedom or autonomy has a high ranking, the freedom of all people can be safeguarded only by recognition of other rights and values. These safeguards are guaranteed by observance of the golden rule—"Do unto others as you would have them do unto you"—which is a part of all religious traditions.

It is the acknowledgment and application of this series of religious themes (accountability and autonomy in the light of the golden rule), then, which points out most clearly the common concern of religious tradition and medicine. This combination of religious belief in a principle which has elements of beneficence (doing good for others) and nonmaleficence (avoiding harmful acts) bestows a sort of moral mandate for prophylactic health care. In order to avoid harm and do well, one must enact measures to prevent disease. Given the present lack of receptivity to such measures in Western society, a praxis of prophylaxis calls for a change in life-style.

Preventive Medicine and Religion

Sociologists and theologians agree that changing life-styles depends almost exclusively on the acceptance of the values or beliefs that provide the foundation for the new life-style. Acceptance of values depends entirely on the degree to which they are understood. The explication and subsequent comprehensibility of these values are functions of education. This, then, is the area of collaboration between medicine and the resources of religion that is so desperately needed: clarification and adoption of value systems.

If one were to ask today what it is that we can really do about preventive medicine that will have the greatest impact, one would have to say, "Let's concentrate on our children." Several years ago the American Health Foundation conducted a study called the "Know Your Body" (KYB) program. The findings showed that many thirteen-year-old boys already had a high cholesterol level, smoked, drank, were overweight, had elevated blood pressures, and had a poor recovery index of the heart. We have not even listed here the drugs and other abuses which harm our children's health.

We must begin an effective health education program like KYB when the children first enter school. The key to this program is a "health passport" that records the children's health data. Someone wisely has said that our children need to become involved in the learning process, that they cannot only be taught didactically. One puts one's hand on a child and says, "Look, I care for your health. I want to do an examination of you." The child is much impressed by such personal attention and is likely to say to you, "If you care for me, let me see what I can do to care for myself."

The KYB program has been introduced to thousands of children in the New York area across socioeconomic lines. Other KYB programs are now being conducted in various parts of the country. Whether it is this program or any other meaningful cost-effective program does not really matter. What is important is that, by doing nothing we are condemning our children to death from our diseases because they have not learned to take responsibility for themselves. We are one of the few countries that has no centralized system of health education. Such education is left up to each of the states—which means it is left up to seventeen thousand different school boards.

We often think that all we *must* teach are the three Rs. When asked, "What do you think health is?" the response is that it is something that needs to be self-taught. Health education is relegated to the parents and the community. If the children continue to do what we do as adults and what we do as a community, it is no wonder that early in their lives they will have developed the same risk factors for diseases that we have.

The American Health Foundation is an interdisciplinary institution for epidemiology and disease prevention. It interrelates chemists and biologists in their efforts to develop experimental models to show mechanisms by which certain diseases occur and what preventive measures will help. It works in health education and in health maintenance studies and industry product modification (e.g., lowering the tar and nicotine content of cigarettes and changing the fat content of American food). It works for legislation, where indicated, and for occupational health. This is the kind of institution that should be developing throughout the world.

How can all the accumulating scientific data be applied? Imagine a benevolent dictator in the health area: First, health education might be made obligatory in every school system. After all, there is not a church or a dictator in this world who has not recognized that the time to educate people is early in their lives. There is no question that if one takes six-year-olds and begins to teach them good health education continuously for at least eight years by having them learn to appreciate their own bodies the children are more likely to have good health practices. Occasionally someone asks, "Is this an attempt to indoctrinate and brainwash our children?" The answer must be, "Yes, that is exactly what we are trying to do." If we do not, we are neglecting our children. One should add a fourth "R" to the three Rs that we classically call the three basics—the "R" of responsibility. In the areas of disease prevention and health, we as parents, as a school, as a church, or as a hospital must educate our children in responsibility.

Ours is not a time of great economic prosperity and stability, but a time for economic belt-tightening and budget-trimming. A key issue concerning health educators, then, should be whether it is possible to educate significant numbers of the population to modify their life-styles or to have some form of physical checkup.

Perhaps this is the place for the intersection of religion and medicine to recur. The tradition of education is one that is intrinsic to religion: instruction, proselytization, evangelization. All are part and parcel of the religious heritage.

This historical function, together with the clear need for educators in an area that would clearly be an addendum on the list of budget priorities, if indeed it has any place in these days of human-services cutbacks, provides the churches with a service that will remain unfilled if they do not assume the position. If health education can reach only a limited segment of our population, then we ought to concentrate on that segment. If we come to recognize that broad-based health education is not successful because of the inability of most people to recognize their own mortality, then we must seek alternative measures. However, it is essential that we have presented the problem to those affected by it in the proper context. Given the religious implications of the question, it is not only appropriate but also necessary that we expend all the religious resources available to us to couch the question, to explain it, and to provide any further information on related subjects that those being faced with the problem might require. In other words, we in the field of medicine can only benefit from close collaboration with those who can share with us the wisdom of the faith traditions. To those who would object to the assumption of health education by religious bodies, we would offer the reminder that health maintenance is a religious concern of the individual and of society.

If we conclude that people cannot or should not be confronted with educational efforts to remind them of their mortality, this fact should be recognized by our physicians and health educators alike and alternative steps advanced. There is a Greek saying which has been adopted as a motto for the American Health Foundation: "It should be the function of medicine to help people die young as late in life as possible." How else can we achieve that goal except through preventive medicine? We will need all the assistance we can get in working toward that achievement.

NOTES

1. These statistics and others are cited in *CA* 8 (January–February 1980): 23–28.

2. For an excellent exposition of the relationship between faith and healing, see Unit V ("Divination and Diagnosis") and Unit VI ("Sorcery and Witchcraft in Sickness and in Health") in David Landy, ed., *Culture, Disease, and Healing* (New York: Macmillan Co., 1977).

3. Michael Greenberg, Frank McKay, and Paul White, "Cancer Mortality Patterns in New Jersey–New York–Pennsylvania," *American Journal of Epidemiology* 2 (February 1980): 166–74.

4. This belief is present not only in the Judeo-Christian religious heritage but also in the concept of Nirvana in Eastern religions.

5. World Health Organization, *Basic Documents* (Geneva: World Health Organization, 1948), p. 1.

6. John Wilkinson, *Health and Healing: Studies in New Testament Principles and Practice* (Edinburgh: Handsel Press, 1980), p. 4.

7. Ibid., p. 5.

8. Ibid., p. 14.

9. Kenneth L. Vaux, "Religion and Health," *Preventive Medicine* 5 (1976): 523.

10. W. E. Waters, *International Journal of Epidemiology* 8 (September 1979): 199–200. Emphasis added.

10

Religion and Medicine: The Physician's Perspective

DANIEL W. FOSTER, M.D.

The marrow of the tragedy is concentrated in the hospitals
. . . . Much of a race depends on what it thinks of death and
how it stands personal anguish and sickness.

—Walt Whitman
Memoranda During the War

The religious dimension may be considered universally present in serious illness provided the word "religious" is allowed to function unrestrictedly to indicate thoughts and actions concerned with primal matters, particularly the ultimate issue (for most people) of life and death. Religious questions may be overtly expressed or deeply hidden. They arise, invited or uninvited, whenever there is suffering or whenever the potential for an end to being is perceived. They may also appear in the context of trivial illness, provided symptoms are interpreted as threatening by the patient.

The historical intertwining of religion and medicine has been dealt with elsewhere in this volume. Here I wish to consider them together at the operational level—in the interaction between the physician and a single sick human being. The great corporate and social issues that join religion and medicine (e.g., defining life and death; preparing rules for human research and informed consent; weighing risk-benefits of promising scientific breakthrough such as recombinant DNA techniques; coming to grips with the economics of medical care; solving worldwide problems of hunger, malnutrition, hygiene, and population control) will not be addressed.

To my mind there are at least four reasons that the physician must deal with religion in the routine care of patients: (1) Religion influences the feelings and actions of a significant number of people. (2) Patients often place the physician in the role of secular priest. (3) Illness induces serious (religious) questions. (4) Physicians' own belief systems impinge on and influence patient care.

THE INFLUENCE OF RELIGION ON PATIENT BEHAVIOR

All people live out their lives against a background of some kind of belief structure. That belief structure may be minimal, even to the point of nonbelief, or highly organized. In this section the impact of formal religious belief on the care of the patient who holds it will be considered. The simple point to be made is that such religious beliefs are often intensely held and that they may exert powerful influences on inter-actions between physician and patient. If unrecognized or not taken seriously by the medical team, the results can be disastrous. This is particularly true if physicians and hospital personnel consider the beliefs of the patient to be irrational or a barrier to the delivery of proper care. An excellent example is the case reported by Redlener and Scott.

> A nine-month-old child was admitted to a teaching hospital of the University of Miami with a history of lethargy and convulsions of two days duration. Bacterial meningitis was suspected and subsequently confirmed. Because there was evidence of extensive central nervous system injury, an arteriogram was requested by the physicians to rule out the presence of pressure-producing accumulations of fluid beneath the covering membranes of the brain. The family refused on religious grounds, initiating a conflict with the hospital and its personnel that lasted for more than three months. The child's medical care was compromised and he ended up grossly disabled. In addition, destructive elements were introduced into the family structure at the conclusion of hospitalization when the baby was placed, under court order, in an institution for the neurologically damaged with visitation by the mother severely restricted.[1]

Problems in the clinical management of this patient arose because the mother was a devout member of the Holiness Church; she believed that her baby was ill because he was possessed by an evil spirit or demon. She brought the baby to the hospital only because the father insisted.

Religion and Medicine: The Physician's Perspective

She herself believed that it was a sin to bring the baby since healing could come only in response to prayer. Moreover, because she and the father were not wed (and nonmarried sex was condemned by the church), the specter of illness sent by God as punishment for sin also hovered in the background. Her lack of trust in the orthodox health-care system (as opposed to belief in the Divine Healer) was confirmed when the child did not get better with treatment and she tried to take him home.

The hospital then appealed to the judicial system of the state of Florida on the grounds that the child's life was being endangered by the religious beliefs of the family. The medical record described family members as "fanatic in their religious beliefs," invoking frequent "ritualistic" prayers around the crib. The formal description of the mother by the social worker captured the picture well:

> Affect is animated when she speaks of the boy. She becomes very verbal during conversations, often injecting phrases such as "Praise Jesus," "Hallelujah" and continually refers to her belief that her son will be returned to her. Mrs. ——— has strong maternal bonds to [her child]. He is the object of great investment for her. She continues to visit but has greatly impaired ability to do reality-testing or make proper judgements on his behalf.

Following this and other testimony, the petition of the hospital was granted and emergency protective custody was awarded to the state. Unfortunately, the neurological damage was irreversible despite additional hospitalization, and eventually custodial care was required. Throughout, the mother denied that the baby had medical problems.

In this case the clinician-scientists prevailed in court, but in reality no one won. There is little question that the interpretation by physicians and hospital personnel that the baby had been irreparably damaged by the religious beliefs of the family was correct. It is also clear that in retrospect the doctors felt that they had not handled the situation well because of failure to respond seriously and sympathetically to a religious ideology foreign to their experience and in conflict with the scientific demands of modern medicine. As a result there was a strong desire to help others avoid a similar trap. Their forthright presentation of the problem in the published analysis is a model of honesty and insight. The authors recognized that the "disparate value systems of the hospital staff on one hand and the family on the other resulted in the breakdown of effective communication and led to feelings of bitterness and anger on both sides." They concluded that maximum benefit for patient, family, and health-care team would have been secured by compromise and reciprocity. For example, the medical staff might have allowed religious ritual (including prayers and chants) to have been carried out at the bedside without restraint in exchange for allowing the baby to remain in the hospital. Doubtless it would have been helpful to ask the family minister's "help in healing the child" (without condescension or manipulation). In short, every attempt should have been made not to overcome or destroy the religious beliefs, but to work around or even through them. In essence the doctors would be saying to the religious family and their advisers, "You approach God directly for healing, and at the same time we can be used by God to help with the medicine God has allowed us to learn." Such an approach is not cynical or hypocritical even if the physicians find a particular religious belief naive or abhorrent, since the aim is to help a sick and otherwise helpless patient. Obviously attempts at cooperation may be rejected, but at least the effort would have been made. The conclusion that religious beliefs should be taken seriously and only as a last resort overturned by legal means has also been recently expressed in the case of blood transfusions for children of Jehovah's Witnesses.[2]

While religious faith only rarely interjects itself so dramatically into clinical care, disrupting diagnosis and treatment, it is not unusual for patients to express beliefs considered primitive or unrealistic by medical personnel and thus cause problems in relationships. Sometimes a patient will accept medical care as prescribed but maintain that he or she will be divinely healed through prayer or some direct action of God. More often a person of strong religious faith does not expect healing or special treatment by the Divine, but simply faces difficulty with calm and courage because of that faith. Surprisingly, even such a mind-set, which ought to be considered a strong positive attribute, may also cause discord between patient and physician. A prototypic case known to me serves to illustrate:

> A sixty-five-year-old Presbyterian woman developed a cancer of the colon, which on discovery was already metastatic to the liver and thus beyond surgical resection. Since this particular lesion is not susceptible to chemotherapy, the physician informed her of the grave prognosis. She did not respond with either fear or depression, and the absence of these emotions was considered worrisome by the doctor, who felt that she was practicing a form of denial that was unhealthy. She explained that her "faith was

in Christ" and calmly quoted Scripture: "I know whom I have believed, and am persuaded that he is able to keep that which I have committed unto him against that day" (2 Tim. 1:12). After several days of similar conversations the physician shouted, "Woman, don't you realize you are dying!" Her response was to break into tears for the first time. In relating the story to a friend she said poignantly, "Why couldn't he just let me believe?"

It seems clear that in this case the physician, not having experienced the supportive effect of religious faith, felt it necessary to attempt to alter his patient's affect because he thought her response to terminal illness was unrealistic. In so doing he came close to rupturing their personal-professional relationship at a time when the patient was extremely vulnerable, and risked conversion of a peaceful final period into one of anxiety and turmoil.

These two cases illustrate the powerful influence religious faith can have on medicine and the delivery of medical care. There are a thousand variations on the theme; even when religious feelings are not expressed they often exert major pressure on feelings and behavior. The problem is very real in the United States, where a majority of the population specifically believe in God and a significant proportion actively participate in formal religious practice. Piety may actually be increasing. For example, in "Middletown, U.S.A.," a midwestern community whose religious beliefs were studied in depth at two intervals half a century apart, the following was found. In 1924 only one-quarter of married couples regularly attended church, while in 1978 the figure had increased to one-half. In the 1920s over one-half the population never formally worshiped, but by the 1970s, only one-sixth reported that they never attended services. In 1924 only one of one hundred families tithed (gave at least one-tenth of their income "to the Lord"), while in 1978 almost one-third of active church members did so. While these findings apply specifically only to one community, other surveys indicate similar trends in the broader society.[3] My personal experience is limited to medical care in the United States, so I am unable to say whether religion has a similar influence on clinical affairs in other countries. Based on a variety of studies, one can reasonably conclude however that religious beliefs influence perceptions of illness and approaches to therapy in multiple cultures.

All this suggests that it is not possible to divorce religion from medicine. If the physician chooses to ignore a patient's beliefs because he or she is uncomfortable with religious expressions, the ability to deliver optimal care may be impaired and the patient may be damaged. Doctors are not required themselves to believe, but they need to know that others believe, sometimes intensely.

THE PHYSICIAN AS SECULAR PRIEST

According to myth, the genealogy of physicians traces back to Aesculapius (Greek, Asclepius), son of the great god Apollo. For centuries the capacity for healing was considered vested in those with divine power; priest and physician were one and the same. The religious and medical roles have long since been separated professionally, but even now it is not unusual to find references to the "priestly function" of physicians in secular medical literature. That phrase refers to the third component of the classic expression of a physician's duty in the fight against illness: to cure disease and prevent premature death (when that is possible), to relieve suffering (when cure is not possible), and to comfort (always). The preservation of a term like "priestly function" in common discussions of medicine implies that patients want more from their physician than simple medical care, no matter how expert or technically sophisticated that care might be. It is easy to understand that a seriously ill patient wants communication with and support from the physician who guides therapy. What may not be as widely appreciated is the frequency with which people come to the doctor with trivial symptoms (or occasionally no symptoms at all) for reassurance, guidance, or even confession. This has led some to distinguish between *disease,* defined as disordered function of some organ or system of the body, and *illness,* the perception that one is sick or that something is wrong with the life.[4] The former is considered to be biologic in origin, while the latter may arise in response to disease or be independent of it. It has been pointed out that well over two-thirds of patients reporting to a physician's office have no serious physical disorder and that the most common single diagnosis made in general practice in nondisease.[5] Part of the problem of modern medicine is that physicians are primarily trained to treat disease, while patients experience illness; focusing on the former while failing to consider the latter may lead not only to misdiagnosis and inadequate therapy, but also, almost certainly, to deep dissatisfaction on the part of the one seeking help.

What are the nonbiomedical reasons that bring patients to the physi-

Religion and Medicine: The Physician's Perspective

cian? A. J. Barsky has identified three major motivational categories: (1) emotional response to stress, (2) social isolation, and (3) informational needs. (Psychiatric disorders were considered a fourth category, but I prefer to classify these as biomedical.)

The relationship between *stress and illness* is complicated. At the simplest level, the patient may frankly recognize that the primary problem is emotional and that nothing is physically wrong ("The kids are making me a nervous wreck"; "I just lost my job and I can't sleep"; "My wife has died and I'm falling to pieces"). On the other hand, severe stress may manifest itself in physical complaints[6] which mimic those of true disease and may be equally debilitating. Discernment that an illness is functional and not organic may require considerable skill, a fair amount of objective testing, and the passage of time. Finally, the presence of organic disease may itself induce stress which then worsens the expression of the physical illness in a kind of vicious circle. Indeed, fear and worry prompted by sickness may cause the patient more difficulty than the primary symptoms (and consume more of the physician's time). Most patients with primary or secondary problems due to stress desire relief of symptoms (i.e., want to get well), but this is not always so. Sometimes there is a hidden desire to be declared sick and to remain so. The gain is that by being certified ill one may garner sympathy, avoid work, escape responsibilities, or even manipulate friends and family.

Social isolation implies the absence of significant others in the life of an individual. It is a phenomenon that is increasingly common—accompanying widespread disintegration of families, a mobile society, economic or social stereotyping, and aging of the population. If a person feels of no value, lonely, or unloved, it becomes critical to find an anchor—someone who cares and will listen. It is not uncommon for the physician to fill that role. If the physician reacts as expected, the patient is able to express feelings, obtain advice, receive consolation, and be physically touched during examination to the extent that a sense of personal value and belonging is produced. Even in a day when medicine is considered depersonalized, such social transactions are extraordinarily common. It is remarkable that social isolation can also be addressed through relationships with medical institutions. The teaching hospital where I work (Parkland Memorial Hospital) cares for the medically indigent of Dallas. It has all the characteristics of a university-associated metropolitan hospital: excellent medicine and limited niceties. The clinics are overcrowded, and a visit to the physician may easily consume four to six hours by the time prescriptions are filled. Moreover, since resident physicians leave after a three- to four-year training period, the patient receives a new doctor periodically, unless his or her physician is a faculty member. Yet loyalty to the hospital is intense. Many of the patients, covered by Medicaid or Medicare, could be cared for by a private physician. I can recall only one or two leaving. When asked why the loyalty, the response almost always is, "Because Parkland knows me"; that is, the institution and its personnel, for all the problems, have somehow conveyed a sense of community and personhood. It is not only that the patient has a record (thus an identity) and knows nurses, clerks, and doctors, but also that there are thousands of others in the same boat. In this sense both the individual physician and the institution express the priestly function: conferring values and affirming worth.[7]

The third major nonbiomedical reason for visiting the physician has been designated *informational*, but might better be called *informational-confessional*. Informational requests may be straightforward or complex. For example, a parent whose child has been exposed to hepatitis at school may visit the physician simply to find out the chances of contracting disease or whether gamma globulin should be given. Similarly, a person with valvular heart disease may wish to know the mortality associated with surgical replacement of the involved valve. On the other hand, a person with a vague new abdominal pain for which there is no ready explanation may come to the doctor not primarily for treatment of that pain, which may be minor, but because he or she fears cancer may be the cause. In such a case the information sought is not facts or statistics but the assurance that nothing serious is wrong.

The confessional component is illustrated in a case cited by Barsky:

> A married electronics repairman presented with dysuria [painful urination] and penile discharge. He criticized both the internist and urologist whom he had consulted within the last week. Although they reported negative cultures of his urine and discharge, the patient complained that they had not been thorough enough to rule out all possible venereal disease. A more detailed history revealed that the patient had recently had sexual relations with a prostitute. He felt so guilty about his infidelity that he was convinced he had contracted venereal disease, almost as though it were a deserved and fitting punishment. His real reason for coming was not to obtain yet another culture but rather for the opportunity to confess to something about which he felt guilty.[8]

I do not know how common this type of confession is in ordinary medical practice, but if my experience is any indication, I suspect it is frequent. There seems to be a need in many patients to reveal the dark side. Sometimes confessions are blurted out and sometimes they are told haltingly with great pain. I have become so used to hearing troubling secrets that every time I take a history I try to make available the opportunity for sharing of socially or religiously forbidden thoughts or actions which may have produced physical symptoms, guilt, or fear. Formally religious people are particularly prone to have guilt in the sexual area—sometimes over acts, but often simply over fantasy. They also tend to feel that they and no others are thus afflicted. Frequently, because of shame, they do not want their pastor to know, and so they convert the physician into confessor. The list of confessional needs is unlimited: fear, anger, jealousy, marital discord, use of illicit drugs, secret alcoholism, sexual dysfunction, even criminal activity have all been expressed by patients under my care.

Failure to recognize the hidden priestly needs of patients may introduce confusion in diagnosis and therapy. Refusal to accept the priestly role will likely impair the return to health or, at the very least, render the course more difficult than it need be.

ILLNESS AND THE SERIOUS QUESTIONS

It is probably safe to say that most people spend relatively little time contemplating philosophical matters, and certainly not life or death.[9] Obviously, if the nation is at war or some great natural disaster strikes, the general society may have its attention diverted to questions of meaning and fate, but in day-to-day intercourse such issues remain submerged at the subconscious level. Ordinarily we expect to live for a good period of time, even as we age, and therefore we utilize our time for work and pleasure rather than for a consideration of meaning. Even when we hear of tragedy, we assume that it is something that happens to someone else and not ourselves. We may feel sympathy or shock, but not risk; others die but we live. A presumption of personal immunity is not unusual even in scholars whose job it is to think, speak, and write about finitude-mortality (philosophers, theologians) or by professionals regularly exposed to death (physicians, nurses, and their colleagues). Perhaps this is a necessary adaptation to allow us to exist in a constantly threatening universe, seeking our daily needs and pursuing some modicum of happiness. The problem is that things have a way of breaking in and diverting our focus from the ordinary to the extraordinary. One of the most common of the reorienting events is illness in oneself or a significant other. The degree to which ordinariness is disrupted by illness usually correlates with its seriousness (or perceived seriousness); one is not likely to ponder fate in response to a cold but may well do so when faced with a cancer (or fear that one might have a cancer).

The questioning process induced by illness tends to progress through three distinct phases. While these phases often develop sequentially, this is not necessarily so; questions in all three phases may arise simultaneously. The process may also abort at any stage. Phase-one questions are *informational*. The initial query is almost always the same: "What's wrong with me?" Fortunately this question can usually be answered, sometimes immediately, sometimes only after extensive tests or passage of sufficient time to allow the disease to reveal itself. If no disease is found or the diagnosis is trivial, treatment is unnecessary and questions fade away. On the other hand, diagnosis of nontrivial sickness induces emotions that range from mild concern to frank fear and prompts additional questions of the informational type. How does the disease manifest itself? What can I expect? Is there treatment? What are the risks of treatment? How long do I have to live? Answers to these questions usually come from the science of medicine and do not in and of themselves require anything but knowledge ("If one has diabetes, one is at risk for long-term complications involving the eyes, kidneys, nerves, and blood vessels—on average seventeen to twenty years after onset"). Priestliness in phase one has two requirements: to deliver facts, especially bad facts, with gentleness, and to perceive and address unspoken anxieties in a way that is supportive and not destructive (blunt recitation of odds and prognosis is usually not a virtue).

Second-phase questions are *behavioral* in nature. They are much more likely to remain unexpressed than those of phase one. The words and thoughts behind them vary, but the tone is unmistakable. Can I go through with what I have to go through? Do I have courage? Will I be able to finish with dignity (if my disease is irreversible)? Such questions cannot be answered for another by the physician or anyone else. Answers come only as the illness is experienced and runs its course. Even in the same person answers may differ depending upon the circumstance. The courage required to undergo a major surgical procedure with a known operative mortality of 2 percent but the possibility of immediate relief of symptoms (as in coronary artery bypass surgery for angina pectoris) may be entirely distinct from that required to face a chronic debilitating disease (as in multiple sclerosis or progressive muscular dystrophy).

Third-phase questions might best be termed *religious*, utilizing the definition of "religious" offered at the beginning of this chapter. They have to do with matters of first importance. They have to do with meaning and destiny. They tend to be asked when the disease to be dealt with is fatal or potentially fatal, or when it is chronic and debilitating, although they may arise with any illness requiring alteration in life-style. There are three general questions, though they be posed in a variety of ways: Why did this happen to me? What can I learn about life and about myself from this experience? For what may I hope? Answers depend upon what one believes.

The belief structure of an individual may be latent, with no conscious impact on behavior, or it may be dominant in life. Whatever its nature before, it inevitably faces examination after serious illness comes, especially if death or incapacity threaten early appearance relative to age or responsibilities. Once a dread diagnosis is made, the response almost inevitably begins "Why me?" followed quickly by "It isn't fair!" This requires activation of a personal theodicy. It is not enough to have a general explanation for pain, suffering, and death in the world; what is needed is an understanding of my own pain, suffering, and death. Peter Berger has stated it well: "It is possible to argue that the human condition, fraught as it is with suffering and with the finality of death, demands interpretations that not only satisfy theoretically but give inner sustenance in meeting the crisis of suffering and death."[10] Neither general nor specific theodicies are easy.

The spectrum of personal theodicies is very broad, ranging from the view that life is simply chance ("That's the breaks") all the way to the belief that every event (including illness) is divinely orchestrated. The latter is extremely difficult to deal with if illness is interpreted as God's judgment on personal sin, a very common and ancient response as exemplified by the question to Jesus: "Rabbi, who sinned, this man or his parents, that he was born blind?" (John 9:2). It is not my purpose here to attempt a discussion of various theodicies, but I do want to say that both physician and patient need to avoid facile answers. The physician should make every effort to explain "whys" in scientific terms while remaining agnostic as to cosmic reasons (which probably do not exist). Thus one might say to the questioning patient with an unrelenting hepatitis that will lead to destruction of the liver and death, "You contracted the hepatitis virus by way of the blood that had to be transfused when your ulcer was bleeding. Most people recover from transfusion hepatitis. Why yours did not reverse I don't know. It happens." This recommendation is really one of necessity. One is agnostic about the question "Why me?" because one has to be.

If "Why me?" is fundamentally unanswerable, it is intrinsically of little value. On the other hand, it becomes extraordinarily useful if it drives one to the second question: "What can I learn from this experience (what can I know beyond mere existence)?" Such a question is really about ultimate things. It is about the possibility of God and the meaning of life. It asks such subquestions as: Why is there something and not nothing? Where did it all start? Who or what is behind life? Where did humans come from? Where do they go? What is reality? How do I fit into it? Is there something beyond time, space, substance, and causality—the philosophical categories of existence? What does life mean and what does death mean? As Hans Küng has said: "They are questions not only for the dying but for the living." And they are, to use his phrase, all or none in nature. The problem is that the living, even though they are always in the process of dying, may never pose them. Recognizing this, one may dare to say that serious illness can bring an undeniable gift: the induction of primal questions the answer to which is God. Religion states that in the midst of tragedy, in illness, in loneliness, in dying, there is something that sustains, "something stable in all change, something unconditional in all that is conditioned, something absolute."[11] To discover that is to have a theodicy even as one has moved beyond questions of theodicy. It is my judgment that illness-forced consideration of primal queries represents a gift even if the answers one derives are negative or indeterminant. To conclude that there is no answer after struggle is better, it seems, than never to have given the alternative a chance. It may even give the sort of peace that comes from having tried.

The third of the serious questions, normative for the sick, deals with the possibility of hope. It has both secular and religious components. At the most basic level a patient hopes to get well or, failing recovery, that pain, suffering, and disability will be limited. Whether that hope is realistic can usually be answered with fair accuracy by the physician, since the course and outcome of most diseases are known within broad statistical bounds. All prognoses should be identified as tentative, however, since a given individual may deviate widely from the statistical norm. Moreover, inexplicable things happen in clinical practice, including reversal of presumably incurable disease (even cancer). Apart from the rare experience of seemingly miraculous cure, it should be emphasized to each patient that medicine changes continually (research goes on) and that disease beyond the reach of science today may not be so tomorrow. In short, secular hope should not be denied even in the most seriously ill.

Having said this, in the end it is not medical care or prognosis or postponement of death that must be addressed by the question of hope. It is the problem of a finitude that has been made visible by serious illness, transported from the time frame of a vague someday to the immediate present. In bare essential it is the cry of Job: "If a man die, shall he live again?" (Job 14:14). Do I cease to be with death, or is there hope that beyond the limits of physical life I am? It is a profoundly religious question, but it is asked by religious and nonreligious alike. Such a question cannot be answered by facts; it can only be approached in that tentative human endeavor called faith. There are no proofs. Yet it is a matter of intense interest to me that human beings seem to be constitutionally religious and concerned with life beyond death. Tomb evidence in multiple unrelated civilizations attests to this and clearly indicates that from early times the idea was prevalent that death was somehow coupled with judgment on the quality of one's temporal life. To cite one example, W. B. Ober has pointed out that moral standards and the concept of judgment of the dead are integral to the Egyptian Book of the Dead (1500 B.C.).[12] These notions radically differentiated it from earlier and contemporary primitive magical codes. According to the Book, after the soul entered the afterworld and made "negative confession" (the recital of shortcomings during life), the heart was weighed on a balance against "the feather of truth," symbol of Maat, the goddess of truth, justice, and cosmic order, to determine worthiness to enter the blessed company of Osiris. Such views were not limited to ancient Egypt. Massive archaeologic evidence in widely divergent cultures unequivocally supports the idea that humans, through much of their history, have suspected that life does not end with death.

Whether one wishes to attribute the idea of gods (God) and judgment after death to wishful projections of the human mind (in the manner of Ludwig von Feuerbach) or is inclined to consider the pervasiveness of such formulations as impressive evidence of an underlying Reality that prompts consideration of itself (revelation), it must be admitted that even in the modern world thoughts of life, death, and life after death continually arise. They are powerfully motivating and require respect whether one agrees or disagrees with their truth. For those who are able to believe that there awaits at death a beneficent and loving God, hope becomes real, fear is diminished, and calm is restored.

THE PHYSICIAN'S BELIEF AND PATIENT CARE

In the first section of this chapter the influence of patients' beliefs on medical care was briefly covered. Here the reverse will be considered, namely, the influence of the physician's personal beliefs on the patient during the encounter with illness. Not at issue is the type of quiet religious faith that renders a physician more kind, compassionate, and caring. Nor is it considered a problem when belief influences medical recommendations, as long as those beliefs are openly held but not pressed. One would not likely consult a Roman Catholic obstetrician to obtain birth control pills, but one would presumably not be offended if as a matter of principle he or she did not prescribe them. The problems of concern are those that may arise when the patient has strong religious beliefs and the doctor has none (or different ones) or, conversely, when the physician is highly religious and the patient is not. In either situation the potential for conflict is real and the physician must take care to avoid unseemly or even unethical behavior. A broader issue is whether religion should ever be overtly addressed in the patient-doctor relationship and, specifically, whether the physician's personal beliefs should be identified or discussed.

The problems that arise when the patient has strong beliefs not shared by the physician have already been discussed. The most difficult situation arises when religious faith interdicts medical care, as in the case of the child with meningitis cited earlier. It must be reiterated that rejection of the patient because of religion, or attempts to dissuade belief, are unacceptable, although it is reasonable to urge the proper medical course on scientific grounds. It is not always easy to avoid scorn, ridicule, or intolerance under these circumstances, but it is absolutely necessary to do so. The chief aim is to help the patient, not to win arguments.

A second scenario, increasingly common in the United States, involves a physician with fervent religious beliefs who feels the need to impose those beliefs on his or her patients, especially if those patients are seriously ill or facing death. It is a phenomenon almost exclusively

Religion and Medicine: The Physician's Perspective

limited to physicians belonging to the evangelical wing of Christianity. (Some other religions, including a variety of sects particularly attractive to young people, actively proselytize, but they have essentially no representation in the ranks of orthodox medicine.) Aggressive evangelistic behavior among Christians is based on two understandings: (1) that they are commissioned to preach the gospel and baptize in this world and (2) that one who dies without accepting Christ as Savior from sin misses the chance to experience the eternal presence of God that is symbolized by the word "heaven." In my experience most such physicians are highly idealistic, genuinely interested in their patients, and motivated to share that which has brought them peace and happiness. The problem is that the faith tends to be offered under inappropriate conditions, cast in terms of "you ought to believe this" rather than "this is what I believe." Often there is a coercive element, even when it is not intended, simply because the physician is directing medical care and the patient is, of necessity, in a dependent posture. Thus a discussion which might be appropriate between equals in good health may be totally inappropriate when one partner to the dialogue is handicapped by sickness, weakness, dependence, or even fear. Stated simply, use of illness to manipulate the religious beliefs of another is unethical, immoral, and totally unacceptable even when motives are good and pure. (History is rife with examples of bad things done in the name of good religion.)

Thus far I have indicated that the personal beliefs of the physician have the potential to cause harm to the patient either because, being negative, they undermine a sustaining faith or because, being positive, they lead to manipulation and domination in an area where acquiescence in faith, to be valid, must be offered from a background of free choice (true faith comes when one chooses to believe, not when one is caused to believe). The question then must be asked: Is religion a forbidden subject between patient and physician? It is clear that one's answer to this question will be influenced by one's view of religion in general. An excellent illustration is provided by a lively exchange recently published in the *Journal of Consulting and Clinical Psychology*. A. E. Bergin opened the dialogue with a carefully stated but nonetheless sharp attack on the functional exclusion of religion from psychotherapy.[13] He noted that an "examination of thirty introductory psychology texts turned up no references to the possible reality of spiritual factors" and pointed out that the words "God" and "religion" were conspicuously absent from indexes. "Psychological writers," he wrote, "have a tendency to censor or taboo in

Medical Perspectives

a casual and sometimes arrogant way something that is sensitive and precious to most human beings." Bergin particularly objected to the concept that exclusion of religion and religious discussion leads to value-free therapy, when in fact those who exclude religious factors often establish goals that are not neutral but actively hostile to theistic systems of belief. He found this a peculiar situation when all the evidence points to the fact that a majority of the American population, at least, is theistically oriented. He concluded that "religion is at the fringe of clinical psychology when it should be at the center." G. B. Walls and A. Ellis immediately responded with vigorous disagreement. Walls wrote: "His [Bergin's] suggestion that there be 'acceptance of [divine] authority' in making value judgments is a potentially dangerous notion that could result in the assertion of absolutes without justification."[14] Ellis argued strongly against any consideration of religion in psychotherapy (and presumably medicine in general), stating:

> The emotionally healthy individual is flexible, open, tolerant, and changing, and the devoutly religious person tends to be inflexible, closed, intolerant, and unchanging. Religiosity, therefore, is in many respects equivalent to irrational thinking and emotional disturbance. . . . Since it is their [people's] biological as well as sociological nature to invent absolutes and musts, they had better minimize these tendencies, even if they cannot totally eliminate them. The less religious they are, the more emotionally healthy they will tend to be.[15]

As indicated by these papers, the role of religion and the appropriateness of allowing religious dialogue between patient and physician is controversial,[16] perhaps more so in the case of psychological or psychiatric problems than with physical illness. Having acknowledged this, I want to state that in my opinion such dialogue is not only permissible but on occasion nonoptional if serious disease is present, if the patient is experiencing the sort of primal questions alluded to earlier, and if the whole person rather than the disease is to be dealt with. Patients have fears and anxieties, and those fears and anxieties in the seriously ill are often about death. If they are felt but not expressed, they tend to be more debilitating and terrifying than if they are discussed, even when the discussion provides no final answers. A fairly recent experience from my own medical service may illustrate:

> A young woman was admitted with a distended abdomen stretched tight with fluid. Such an accumulation of fluid is most often due to cirrhosis of the liver secondary to alcoholism or previous hepatitis, but hers was not.

Religion and Medicine: The Physician's Perspective

She had a rare disease called "paroxysmal nocturnal hemoglobinuria" in which there is an abnormality in the oxygen-carrying molecule (hemoglobin) of the red blood cell. For complicated reasons that need not be detailed, this abnormality had caused clotting of blood in the veins draining the liver, with the result that fluid oozed from its surface into the abdominal cavity. Treatment of this condition is ineffective and the outlook is grim. The facts had been conveyed to her in a general way. Each day on rounds I found her crying and depressed but unwilling to talk. One afternoon when I came she had a visitor who was dressed in a postal worker's uniform. She introduced him as her pastor. He said to me: "She's having a hard time dealing with this happening to *her*." To which, almost without thinking, I responded: "The rain falls on the just and the unjust." The postman-pastor's face lit up and said: "Hark! Did I perceive a Scripture?" After I acknowledged that I knew something about the Bible, the patient said, "I thought you might be one of them" and then began, without restraint, to identify her fears of death and the means of her dying. She further explained that she had been reluctant to voice her fears before, thinking that as a doctor I wouldn't understand her need to talk about death, death-anxieties, and God. The important thing is not that she found out that I was "one of them" (Christians), glad as I was that she had suspected it, but that her defenses against self-revelation became unnecessary when it was perceived that she would be heard with sympathy. Her disease was not changed by this discourse; it still proceeds inexorably. But her illness is lighter as a result, and she is now more well even as she continues sick. Fear is no longer her sole emotion.

In regard to specific religious dialogue between physician and patient, I suggest the following guidelines. First, such dialogue may take place but does not have to take place (either physician or patient may be unequipped or unready to enter in). Second, dialogue must be invited by the patient, not imposed by the physician (in the case just cited a clue was picked up by the patient from the physician's conversation; the questions verbalized in response constituted the invitation). Third, the physician must be open, nonjudgmental, and honest. He or she will often be required to say "I don't know." He or she may share their own religious beliefs as being personally valuable and helpful but must not insist that those beliefs be considered ultimate truth by the one with whom they are shared. Nonreligious physicians may enter into religious dialogue (and help) simply by caring and listening, whether they consider the patient's thoughts, questions, and beliefs rational or irrational. Fourth, whatever its nature, the purpose of the dialogue should be burden-lifting or burden-sharing, not burden-producing. One cringes to hear, no matter how well-meaning, a statement like "If you have faith enough, you'll get well." It is tough enough to be sick without having to consider as a cause inadequacy or failure in the realm of personal religious belief. The foundation rule of medical practice also applies to religious discussion: *primum non nocere* (first, do no harm).

NECESSITIES

For the reasons outlined earlier it seems that religion and medicine can be separated only by a conscious and massive effort. That is because the religious dimension is inherently present whenever there is suffering or when finitude is made visible by life-threatening disease. It is present whether physician or patient is religious or areligious. It is not defined by any particular set of religious beliefs, although as already indicated particular beliefs can have powerful influence on treatment and outcome. The religious dimension can be ignored, but it is ignored only with loss to both patient and physician. I believe it is this point that was being addressed in a sparse editorial entitled "The Fourth Book" by Samuel Vaisrub in the *Journal of the American Medical Association*.[17] He pointed out that the three "books" by which God is revealed according to Western Christian culture—nature, conscience, Bible—were presently of little consequence to most as mediators of the divine will. He suggests that the divine will must now be read, by physicians at least, in a fourth book, whose influence cannot be ignored:

> Dictates of the physician's conscience may not coincide with the enjoinders of the Holy Writ as perceived by its exegetes. His ethical choices may be no easier than those of the dissenting scientists and theologians of the past. Might he not wish that God would express His will more explicitly in yet another book? Perhaps the Book as been already written. It may have been inscribed on the faces of the sick whose silence is more eloquent than words.

If one is to accept silent requests (sometimes cries) for help precipitated by illness in a human being, what are the necessities? Put another way, what are the religious demands that must be met by physicians whether or not they personally are religious? My own judgment is that the following comprehend the minimal requirements: The physician must (1) be trustworthy, (2) treat the person as a person, (3) be kind, (4) maintain hope, and (5) assist in discovering what it really means to live.

It is clear to me after twenty-five years in medicine that patients want their physician, almost above all else, to be *trustworthy*. This does not mean simply that he or she tell the truth, important as that is and as carefully as that must be done. It means also that the patient must be able to rely on the physician to provide help when it is needed, to be available and not to hide. Doctors with unlisted telephone numbers are one of the sadnesses of our time. To know that when you call I will come is to have a sense of mooring in the frightening sea of serious illness.

A second powerful need of patients is to be *dealt with as a person*. On the surface this would seem obvious, but there are complications. That is because at one level it is necessary that the physician be in an authoritative stance, with the patient a dependent recipient of advice and guidance. This follows from the fact that the physician has knowledge and experience in medicine not shared by the patient, requiring that the physician have greater input into the medical decision-making than the one who is sick. An egalitarian approach wherein the patient decides the course of his or her own care is not ideal because competence is not equivalent. Even when medical knowledge is profound, one needs a guide who can say, "This is what I think we ought to do." The late Dr. Franz Ingelfinger emphasized this point compellingly. Even though he was one of the world's leading experts on function and disorders of the esophagus, ironically he developed and died from a cancer of that organ. When his illness became known, friends from all over the world contacted him with advice regarding treatment. He described the result as follows:

> At that point I received from physician friends throughout the country a barrage of well-intentioned but contradictory advice. The question of prophylactic radiotherapy was particularly moot. As a result, not only I but my wife, my son and daughter-in-law (both doctors), and other family members became increasingly confused and emotionally distraught. Finally, when the pangs of indecision had become nearly intolerable, one wise physician friend said "What you need is a doctor." He was telling me to forget the information I already had and the information I was receiving from many quarters, and to seek instead a person who would dominate, who would tell me what to do, who would in a paternalistic manner assume responsibility for my care. When that excellent advice was followed, my family and I sensed immediate and immense relief. The incapacity of enervating worry was dispelled, and I could return to my usual anxieties, such as deciding on the fate of manuscripts or giving lectures like this.[18]

The recognition that there is not an equality of medical competence does not require authoritarian attitudes. In regard to personhood, collegiality should be full. This means that the patient should be considered worthy of dialogue between equals and be provided sufficient information to understand the illness and participate in decisions when options are available. Shared information should include both risks and benefits of participating or not participating in a given therapeutic regimen together with the physician's judgment about the best course to take. Implicit is the right of refusal on the part of the patient without jeopardy to the professional relationship. To illustrate, the physician does not do a patient with hyperthyroidism (overactivity of the thyroid gland) a favor by saying, "There are three forms of treatment—drugs, surgery, or radioactive iodine. Which do you prefer?" Rather, collegiality is activated by explaining the benefits and risks of each therapy, following which a recommendation is given together with the reasons. Thus for a fifty-six-year-old woman with hyperthyroidism and no concurrent disease, a recommendation for treatment with radioactive iodine might be offered, with the explanation that the procedure is simple, that genetic risk is not operative because the patient is beyond the child-bearing age, and that many years of experience show that such therapy does not place the subject at risk for developing cancer of the thryroid. An opportunity for questioning would then be provided. If the patient still chooses therapy with antithyroid drugs because of fear that "radioactivity causes cancer," the physician may legitimately address those fears in an attempt to channel therapy in the direction considered optimal. If the argument fails, the doctor should proceed with the patient's wishes cheerfully and helpfully, not attempting to punish her emotionally for not following advice. The same principles apply if there is only one form of therapy and the choice is simply to treat or not to treat. Every person has the right to refuse medical intervention. It is unethical, however, to prescribe harmful therapy even if the patient wishes it. This is a surprisingly common problem. For example, many patients request penicillin for a cold even though antibiotics do not work against viruses and can lead to dangerous allergic reactions or superinfections with resistant organisms. In my opinion the same applies to euthanasia. The physician may covenant with the patient not to use extraordinary means of therapy in hopeless situations, but it is unacceptable to end the life by a positive action such as the administration of a lethal drug, even if begged to do so.

To summarize this tricky area, one might say that the problem from the physician's standpoint is to avoid transference of legitimate authority, based on medical knowledge, into illegitimate authoritarianism, based on the patient's dependence.

The third requirement for meeting needs is so obvious that one hesitates to write it: *be kind*. That means, very simply, to be sympathetic, friendly, gentle, tenderhearted, and generous in word and deed. Having recently gone through a prolonged and eventually fatal illness with my father, I was struck again by how utterly important it is to experience caring and gentle sympathy from the physician as an illness runs its course. We were fortunate to have an internist who was both competent and kind, and we looked forward to his twice-daily comings, even though we knew what lay ahead. He simply made us feel better. In ancient times when Jacob was received with kindness unexpectedly by his estranged brother Esau, he exclaimed, "Truly to see your face is like seeing the face of God, with such favor have you received me" (Gen. 33:10). Kindness is like that.

Providing *hope*, particularly if the situation looks hopeless, is more difficult. I have already touched on this in the earlier section on illness and serious questions. I wish to emphasize here three avenues of hope. First, the physician can assure that all possible help and comfort will be provided during the illness and that there will be a medical companion. Second, as mentioned earlier, it can be emphasized that medical science does not stand still. What is incurable today may well be curable tomorrow, even dread disease like cancer, multiple sclerosis, or cystic fibrosis. Space precludes recitation of hope-providing current research, but exciting things are going on in a wide variety of diseases. The aim is to be realistic regarding prognosis while holding open the possibility of change. Experience teaches that such advances can be dramatic and rapid, redeeming large segments of the ill. Who would have thought a decade ago that 50 percent of acute lymphoblastic leukemias in children could now be cured by chemotherapy, even though the root cause of the disease remains undefined? Or that patients with kidney failure could receive a transplanted kidney and be well? Or that smallpox would be eliminated? Yet all this has happened, and there is more to come. Third, for some at least, it is possible to offer hope beyond hope, the experience of the presence of God. Whether that comes and how it comes will not be discussed in these brief remarks, except to say that if it comes it is a special gift, even an ultimate gift, for which the only response is thanks.

Medical Perspectives

The last necessity, perhaps only rarely achieved, is to help the patient learn, in the midst of an illness which may lead to death, *what it really means to live*. Somehow the best physicians have a way of helping it happen. They seem to be able to convey four bedrock lessons that are at once simple and profound:

1. *Life must be lived day by day, and ordinary life has the potential of fulfilling beauty.* It is a common problem for people to live in the past (when things were better), or for the future (when problems will disappear), and to miss the present. Serious illness makes clear what most of us keep hidden: the fact that our days are numbered. It has a way of making each day precious in its ordinariness and of allowing the assignment of true values. The fun and games, what Mr. Sammler called "the confusion and degraded clowning of this life through which we are speeding,"[19] are seen for what they are: trivial and nonlasting. Life and relationships become preeminent, the only things that count. Alice Stewart Trillin, writing about her experience with cancer, caught that truth as follows:

> It astonishes me that having faced the terror, we continue to live, even to live with a great deal of joy. It is commonplace for people who have cancer—particularly those who feel as well as I do—to talk about how much richer their lives are because they have confronted death. Yes, my life is very rich. I have even begun to understand that wonderful line in *King Lear*, "Ripeness is all." I suppose that becoming ripe means finding out that none of the really important questions have answers. I wish that life had devised a less terrifying, less risky way of making me ripe. But I wasn't given any choice about this.
>
> William Saroyan said recently, "I'm growing old! I'm falling apart! And it's very interesting!" I'd be willing to bet that Mr. Saroyan, like me, would much rather be young and all in one piece. But somehow his longing for youth and wholeness doesn't destroy him or stop him from getting up in the morning and writing, as he says, to save his life. We will never kill the dragon. But each morning we confront him. Then we give our children breakfast, perhaps put a bit more mulch on the peas, and hope that we can convince the dragon to stay away for a while longer.[20]

The dragon will come. The trick is not to waste the days before the appointment.

2. *Courage in human life is not extraordinary but ordinary.* This is an experiential statement, not an abstract one. Many years ago I was surprised when I saw bravery exhibited in the face of suffering and death by those who would not have judged themselves or been judged by

others *a priori* as brave. I now take it for granted. People by and large face what they have to face and do what they have to do and take what they have to take with quiet dignity and resignation. I don't mean that there are not tears or a sense of sadness and loss, or even fear. I do mean that these are dealt with, almost always, without whimpering or emotional disintegration. And that is what courage and grace are all about. I try to convey this message early to the seriously ill: You can go through with that which you have to go through. And I will help you.

3. *Illness can sensitize one to the problems of others.* A fundamental characteristic of contemporary society seems to be unconcern for the problems of others. Manifestations vary from an emotional and material acquisitiveness which precludes sharing of self or resources with those in need, all the way to the "Genovese syndrome," the refusal to come to the aid of one in imminent danger of injury or death. (The latter refers to the several dozen people who watched a young woman named Kitty Genovese being murdered over a half-hour period in New York City without attempting rescue or calling the police.) Illness tends to remove the hardness. The experience of suffering somehow makes it easier to see the suffering of others and to want to help. It is observed in the hospital all the time—one patient helping another in a dozen different ways, even though as strangers before sharing illness no words might have been exchanged on passing in the street. In the same manner women who have had mastectomies visit those who are about to, and subjects with colostomies form clubs to help those soon to face it. Sometimes one first learns to care in the midst of one's own need for caring. It is a life-expanding experience.

4. *Death is not the worst thing in life.* On the face this seems a peculiar statement. Most of us do not want to die, even as we know that some day we must. And certainly we do not want to die prematurely. Death is a friend for only a few: suicides in their despair, those with unrelieved suffering, the imprisoned and tortured, perhaps some of the very aged in their loneliness. We hate death because of what it causes us to lose or miss (family, friends, fun, achievement), but it is more than that. There is also for most of us an element of fear. We not only fear the act of dying, we fear our postdeath fate. The act of dying is fear-inducing because it is unknown and none of us has gone through it before. Our worry about destiny usually takes one of two directions: either there is nothingness (with death I cease to be) or there is judgment (in which I fear I will be found wanting). I have written about these matters

elsewhere[21] and have pointed out that the act of dying, once actually entered, appears to be a nonfearful event if near-death visions have any validity. Questions of divine judgment and ultimate fate are beyond address by experience or science; they can only be approached in religious terms, which of necessity are statements of faith rather than fact. Different answers have been given, varying from the Christian concept of continued life as recognizable essence after death ("resurrection of the body") with judgment dependent upon one's response to the Christ, to the Hindu view of cycling reincarnations (*samsara-karma*) influenced by human actions. It is not my purpose to discuss the various answers or to provide a personal assessment of probabilities. I only want to say that the absence of an answer to death is worse than death. Put in another way, death is not the worst thing in life; fear of death is. The writer to the Hebrews understood this when he asserted that to fear death was to be a slave all of one's life (see Heb. 2:15). Whether the physician can relieve that fear is problematical. Even if the physician holds such beliefs as to take away or alleviate fear of death in the personal life, that may not be transferable to the patient under care. What can be conveyed is the lesson which says that one can never really live until one is prepared to die.

RELIGION AND MEDICINE—A PERSONAL NOTE

In this chapter, I have tried to give some thought to the relationship between religion and medicine from the perspective of a physician who cares for sick people. The focus has been on the patient, the needs made manifest by the impact of illness, and how the physician interacts with those needs. I would like to close with a word about the role of religion in my personal life as a physician, independent of any relationship with a particular patient. I was lucky enough to have a sufficiently adequate mind to function well in the academic world, where I am a professor of medicine. Some honors have come my way, my research has gone well, I write in textbooks, edit scientific journals, and advise the government on the research it should support. I love all of it. But in the end, the thing that means the most to me is taking care of a sick human being and trying to help not just with the disease but, as far as possible, with the patient's personal struggle. Perhaps it is because I see in the patient's fight, my fight. Certainly it is because I follow One (or try to) who, though called the Christ, identifies with the woundedness of the world. With time, the sense of inadequacy grows. Answers, which once seemed easy, come harder. The things that sustain are two: people are important (worth all the effort), and God is everything (even seen through a glass, darkly). So one appropriates the prayer attributed to Maimonides:

> I begin once more my daily work. Be thou with me, Almighty, Father of Mercy, in all my efforts to heal the sick. For without thee, man is but a helpless creature. Grant that I may be filled with love for my art and for my fellow man. May the thirst for gain and the desire for fame be from my heart. For these are the enemies of Pity and the ministers of Hate. Grant that I may be able to devote myself body and soul to the children who suffer from pain.
>
> Preserve my strength, that I may be able to restore the strength of the rich and the poor, the good and the bad, the friend and the foe. Let me see in the sufferer the man alone. When wiser men teach me, let me be humble to learn; for the mind of man is so puny, and the art of healing is so vast. But when fools are ready to advise me or find fault with me, let me not listen to their folly. Let me be intent upon one thing, O Father of Mercy, to be always merciful to thy suffering children.
>
> May there never arise in me the notion that I know enough, but give me strength and leisure and zeal to enlarge my knowledge. Our work is great, and the mind of man presses forward forever. Thou hast chosen me in thy grace, to watch over the life and death of thy creatures. I am about to fulfill my duties. Guide me in this immense work so that it may be of avail.

I find that prayer beautiful. It grasps the oneness of religion and medicine. It speaks to the priestly function. In the best moments it is what one prays—and from time to time tries to live.

NOTES

1. I. E. Redlener and C. S. Scott, "Incompatibilities of Professional and Religious Ideology: Problems of Medical Management and Outcome in a Case of Pediatric Meningitis," *Social Science and Medicine*, 13B (1979): 89–93.

2. T. F. Ackerman, "The Limits of Beneficence: Jehovah's Witnesses and Childhood Cancer," *Hastings Center Report* 10 (1980): 13–18.

3. "Back to Middletown," *The Public Interest* 63 (1981): 135–36.

4. A. Kleinman, L. Eisenberg, and B. Good, "Culture, Illness, and Care: Clinical Lessons from Anthropologic and Cross-culture Research," *Annals of Internal Medicine* 88 (1978): 251–58.

5. A. J. Barsky, III, "Hidden Reasons Some Patients Visit Doctors," *Annals of Internal Medicine* 94 (1981): 492–98.

6. While emotional stress may produce symptoms suggesting organic disease

in the absence of any biologic disturbance, the evidence is now very suggestive that life stress confers vulnerability to organic disease. Put simply, emotional trauma predisposes a person to physical sickness. The physician can be easily misled in this circumstance, attributing illness to the precipitating stress when in fact disease is present.

7. It is obvious that physicians and institutions by attitude and action can also devalue and depersonalize.

8. Barsky, "Hidden Reasons."

9. As with all generalizations there are major exceptions. It is entirely possible to think about ultimate problems under noncrisis conditions. Religious people are wont to do so naturally from time to time, as are other contemplative types. Intuitively and experientially, however, I believe the overall construct developed here to be correct.

10. Peter L. Berger, *A Rumor of Angels: Modern Society and the Rediscovery of the Supernatural* (Garden City, N.Y.: Doubleday & Co., 1969), p. 31.

11. Hans Küng, *On Being a Christian*, trans. Edward Quinn (Garden City, N.Y.: Doubleday & Co., 1976), p. 76.

12. W. B. Ober, "Weighing the Heart Against the Feather of Truth," *Bulletin of the New York Academy of Medicine* 55 (1979): 636–51.

13. A. E. Bergin, "Psychotherapy and Religious Values," *Journal of Consulting and Clinical Psychology* 48 (1980): 95–105.

14. G. B. Walls, "Values and Psychotherapy: A Comment on 'Psychotherapy and Religious Values,'" *Journal of Consulting and Clinical Psychology* 48 (1980): 640–41.

15. A. Ellis, "Psychotherapy and Atheistic Values: A Response to A. E. Bergin's 'Psychotherapy and Religious Values,'" *Journal of Consulting and Clinical Psychology* 48 (1980): 635–39.

16. A. E. Bergin, "Religious and Humanistic Values: A Reply to Ellis and Walls," *Journal of Consulting and Clinical Psychology* 48 (1980): 642–45.

17. Samuel Vaisrub, "The Fourth Book," *Journal of the American Medical Association*, 244 (1980): 1362.

18. Franz J. Ingelfinger, "Arrogance," *New England Journal of Medicine* 303 (1980): 1507–11.

19. Saul Bellow, *Mr. Sammler's Planet* (Greenwich, Conn.: Fawcett Publications, 1971), p. 286.

20. Alice Stewart Trillin, "Of Dragons and Garden Peas: A Cancer Patient Talks to Doctors," *New England Journal of Medicine* 304 (1981): 699–701.

21. Daniel W. Foster, *A Layman's Guide to Modern Medicine* (New York: Simon & Schuster, 1980), pp. 371–78.

PART SIX

Pastoral Perspectives

11

The Congregation: Place of Healing and Sending

F. DEAN LUEKING

It is the Sabbath. People are gathering for worship. A family files into the sanctuary. They are much at home there, but this time it is different. The mother is absent. She is in a nearby hospital, awaiting surgery on the day following. Familiar phrases in hymns, prayers, and Scripture that have been heard a hundred times before have a new and deeper ring of meaning as they think of the one missing from the family circle and what awaits her the next day.

Across the aisle sits a man who can walk into the building and sit down without limping or wincing with pain as he takes his place in the pew. A year ago he underwent surgery for the rebuilding of a hip badly deteriorated by degenerative arthritis. Around him in the congregation are familiar faces for whom he has extra appreciation. These are people who visited him during his hospital stay and provided transportation to and from the hospital for his wife during the first hectic days he spent there.

Halfway back sits a middle-aged woman about to stifle a yawn. She came to worship straight from her shift as a nurse in the intensive-care unit of the hospital where she works. This time she stayed two hours past her regular shift, helping with a critical case. A four-week-old child nearly died of heart-defect problems. The nurse, herself a mother, took extra time to explain to the distraught parents that the occasional and ominous sounds from the oxygen machine were not danger signals but part of the functioning of the equipment vital to the normal breathing of the child.

Under the balcony near the exit, at his regular place, sits a doctor. His

273

beeper is quiet at the moment. He is on call, ready to be interrupted from his worship by a hospital call in connection with several of his patients who are battling resistive, baffling ailments.

Such a scene is real rather than imagined; the people and their circumstances are those I know from experience and can be repeated in thousands of congregations throughout the United States and beyond on any given Sunday morning or Friday evening at twilight.

The particular urgencies of body, mind, and spirit which belong to these four groups of people are but a microcosm of the much wider world of problems of those who are sick and those who are working at their care. Sick people and their families who watch and wait with them, and doctors and nurses and other health-care practitioners who offer professional medical care for them, are the focus of this chapter. To be sure, the world of the well and the ill includes many who do not profess religious faith or participate in congregations. But the attention here is on those who do and the difference it makes.

The congregation has certain unique resources to bring to people in illness and health and all who care about them in varied ways. What these are and what they mean for an inquiry into religion and medicine is before us now.

The hospitalized mother, absent from the family gathered for worship, is in a position to widen and deepen her spiritual life as she passes through an episode of illness which takes her to the hospital. What she has been taught from the earliest time of her spiritual formation now comes to bear upon her life in ways not known to her in times of health.

Like health, sickness in the life of a person of religious conviction has a spiritual context. That is another way of stating a truth expressed in the opening chapter of this book: that in the religious perspective, health and illness must be endowed with meaning. In congregations of the Christian and Jewish tradition, the biblical truth is taught that God created humans in the divine image and blessed men and women with a wholeness and harmony with God, with other people, with nature, and with the self that is implicit in the rich biblical word *shalom*. In such a view, illness is a sign that a disruption has occurred in that harmonious relationship. Disease comes as an intrusion. It bears witness to the reality of sin in life. The fall of humankind into sin is the underlying and alien circumstance in which sickness and death occur. That may be taught as an abstraction, but it is experienced as no abstraction at all when the body and spirit are assaulted by fever and pain. The biblical truth proclaims the good news that God intervenes with care and healing and purpose amid the onslaught of that which attacks the crown of God's creating work—the human being. One interesting New Testament word for that saving work of God was taken directly from the day. *Hygeia* (literally "health") is what the apostle Paul brought into the Christian vocabulary as soundness and wholeness of life and belief in response to the grace of God (see 1 Tim. 1:10; 2 Tim. 4:3; Titus 1:9). The root meaning is "health," not only bodily health, but the drawing of the whole being of the person, mind, and spirit as well, back into right relationship with God, with people, with the self.

Thus that hospitalized mother, absent from her family and congregation because of illness, has a spiritual context in which to accept her new surroundings. The veil of mystery that lies over the experience of becoming ill and the unsettling fears that accompany it are so threatening. Questions that come naturally to people beset by illness ("How did I get this way?" "What's going to happen to me?") are given a setting in which answers may be formed. It is not as though religious conviction enables the patient to draw a straight line from this illness to that sinful act or thought. We see through a glass darkly, and all that lies behind illness is not made clear. But the conviction that all humans share the mortal destiny of a fallen humankind, that all have sinned and fall short of the glory of God, helps a person lying ill to find bearings and grounding for what is going on.

That spiritual context makes something else possible that counts in times of illness: illness cannot be denied. Strong currents in popular culture further the illusion that one need not give much thought to illness, need not prepare for that inevitable experience. There will always be some pill, some medical prevention, some technological magic of the doctor and hospital that will fix it quickly. That denial of the inevitability of illness and the unpreparedness to face it play mean tricks on people when the illusion is shattered and sickness sets in. I recall visiting a man in a hospital who told me of his astonishment over what had taken place in his hospital room shortly before I entered. His roommate had gotten out of bed, dressed, and left the hospital for home, so trapped was he in panic at the reality of illness that had invaded his life.

Not all religious people keep the essential biblical truth in mind when sickness strikes, nor do we meet that dilemma with flawless serenity. Clergy serving ill people know of them what we know of ourselves. We need support, instruction, assurance, admonition, and the promise of divine grace when life is upended by sickness and injury. The faith we hold upholds us in the face of fears, frustrations, and anger at illness.

The power of faith in the living God does make a difference. It brings us a humbling awareness that all of us belong to the human family in which sin leaves its mark in the experience of disease. Getting sick is an unavoidable sign of that membership. One is not alone in illness; therefore one is not being singled out for punishment. One is not exempt from the burden of having to lay things aside. Capable, vigorous, busy people must learn to adjust schedules, to defer otherwise important activities, to accept the immediate matter at hand: a body that is hurting and needing help. God is near with help. God's promise of mercy, care, and wisdom in leading all people, God's responding to prayer, God's providing varied ways of healing all come to sharper focus when that mother, and her faithful counterparts all over the world every day and night, is in the hospital. The good news of divine love comes through as truly good news in such moments and hours. The stage is set to hear anew, and this time really to hear, the ancient words which have inspired hope and courage in so many: "God is our refuge and strength, a very present help in trouble" (Ps. 46:1), and "Humble yourselves therefore under the mighty hand of God. . . . Cast all your anxieties on him, for he cares about you" (1 Pet. 5:6–7). That mother in the hospital is part of a family network of care; she also belongs to the larger community of the congregation of people who care.

The act of informing one's pastor or rabbi of an illness is in itself an expression of special trust between lay person and clergy. It says much more than "I'm going into the hospital." It lifts up and makes tangible an affirmation, a bonding, an appeal. What is affirmed is the bond of mutual trust between clergy and lay person that both are called to serve each other with faith and love. God puts the divine Word into the words of trust, comfort, and reassurance that are spoken back and forth, as well as in the words of confession, doubt, and dismay that surface from the deeper regions of the spirit. People do not always speak aloud their inner misgivings about facing illness; often the announcement of going into the hospital is shorthand for that, however. Informing clergy is a way people have of expressing their need for what God offers. It is a moment of opening toward new levels of belonging and growing in the community of faith.

No one knows the larger purposes God accomplishes in times of pain

The Congregation: Place of Healing and Sending

and crisis. Both patient and clergy can regard the moment as not only one to be endured but also a new opening toward things undreamed of. What comes to mind is the circumstance in a hospital room of a person I recall visiting years ago. My attention was to the ill person of our congregation, but in the next bed lay a man whose ears were open to every word being said. On return visits he kept on listening but saying nothing. One late evening, before both men were asleep, he asked his hospital roommate about his religious affiliation. Leaving the hospital with the promise of continuing recovery gave the man more to think about than when he entered. He found his way to a very different life in time, recovering the spiritual base from which he had drifted and enlarging that base to exercise a widespread influence for lasting good in so many lives around him. It all seemed to start again for him in circumstances so unpromising: crisis, illness, worry, pain. Such forces are stern teachers, but that was what he needed to come to a penitent awareness that the vital spiritual foundation for life was neglected. Humility and faith in the redeeming love of God is health-giving. This man's experience is one witness among countless others who found, in the worst of times, the best of gifts.

Relationships in the religious community become far more open and purposeful in a hospital room. In the church or synagogue it is understandable that people are for the most part on their "religious behavior." Our clothes, our manners, our mutual niceties are not to be scorned as hypocritical. That is the way it is, and we cannot live all our congregational moments at the flashpoints of passionate religious intensity. But in the hospital emergency room at 3:00 A.M. the scene is very different. The externals of ritual and tradition must now deliver the core of the faith. The heart of all the reasons why we dress, speak, and do as we do in the formal occasions of worship is now laid bare. If there is no Word that can speak directly to horrendous pain or brutal death, that emptiness becomes clear at such a time and place.

Conversely, when the power of God does not depend upon religious surroundings and traditional settings but breaks forth in all its naked efficacy, both the person who delivers it and the one receiving it stand in awe. Directness, brevity, and fidelity in ministry are called forth in clergy and laity when the extremity of the human need has cleared the air. Early in my pastoral ministry I was called to an emergency ward just before dawn. I did not know the parishioner well but began to unfold to him the whole counsel of God from Genesis on. He stopped me in the middle of one of my sentences, took me firmly by the arm, and told me to get down on my knees and in *one sentence* of prayer beg God for the mercy he needed to get through that hour. I did, and God responded. Many clergy and lay visitors of the sick have had some similar experience in which the lesson learned was that of directness, brevity, and trust that the efficacy of the Word does not depend on the volume of our words.

There are times when the Word has been at work in a patient's life in such a way that our words are not needed at all; the communication of deep care and love finds channels other than verbosity. There are many variations on this theme, but here is the essence of the matter expressed by a young pastor ministering to a black congregation in Indiana:

In the second year of my ministry at Grace, Joselyn Fields fell sick. In spring they diagnosed a cancer. In summer they discovered it had metastasized dramatically. But autumn she was dying. She was 47 years old.

Spring, summer, and autumn, I visited the woman.

Well, I didn't know what to say, nor did I understand what I had the *right* to say. I wore out the Psalms; they were safe. I prayed often that the Lord's will be done, scared to tell him, or Joselyn, what his will ought to be; and scared of his will anyway.

One day when she awoke from surgery, I determined to be cheerful, to bring life unto her and surely to avoid the spectre that unsettled me—death.

I spoke brightly of the sunlight outside, vigorously of the tennis I played that morning, sweetly of the flowers, hopefully of the day when she would sit again at the organ, reading music during the sermon. . . .

But Joselyn raised a black bony finger, pointed squarely at my nose, and said, "Shut up!"

I learned so slowly . . . and Joselyn Fields taught me . . . I, who had thought to give her the world she didn't have, was in fact taking away the only world she *did* have. I had been cancelling her serious, noble, faithful, and dignified dance with death.

I shut up. I learned. I kept visiting her. And then the autumn whitened into winter, and Joselyn became no more than bones, her rich skin turned ashy, her breath filled the room with a close odor which ever thereafter has meant dying to my nostrils. . . .

I entered her room at noon one day, saying nothing. I sat beside her through the afternoon, until the sun had slanted into darkness, saying nothing. She lay awake, her eyelids paper-thin and closed, drooping, watchful eyes, saying nothing. The evening took us, and with the evening came the Holy Spirit. For the words I finally said were not my own. . . . I said, "I love you." And Joselyn opened her eyes . . . and she hugged me. She whispered "I love you, too."

The Congregation: Place of Healing and Sending

> And that was all we said. But that was the power from on high, cloaking both of us in astonished simplicity, even as Jesus had said it would! For in a word that I did not know I knew, a need had found not only its expression, but its solution, too! Joselyn died. And I did not grieve.[1]

An entire lifetime of experience in faith lies behind that black woman's last illness. The rich heritage of divine grace and truth that had nurtured her through her years had a final flowering that helps us see the difference it makes when that grace and truth are known and shared. She was part of a community in which she was teacher as well as learner.

I have searched in vain for statistical data on the difference it makes that people carry into illness a lively faith in God and partnership in a congregation of such faith. It is probably wrong to start out assuming that any such data exist. These are matters beyond the researcher's poll and the computer's tally. The generalization stands, however, that when people encounter serious disease with firm religious grounding and in the fellowship of caring people, it does make a difference for good. People are equipped to face the reality of illness, to accept dire changes in their lives and schedules with humility, to trust that God works for good in circumstances that are not good, that the core of their faith is tested and not found wanting, that new directions and focused values can emerge from the crucible of suffering, and that recovery can mean more than the body restored—the spirit deepened as well. That generalization is documented each time people of religious commitment put that commitment to work in times of health problems. Day after day throughout the land, people find strength from God in prayer, reflection upon God's Word, belief in God's promises, and support from God's people. They do so because of rituals and traditions of faith which touch their lives powerfully before and after, as well as during the onset of illness.

Among the circumstances of life which make people highly susceptible to a disruption of health is the death of a spouse or someone close in the family or circle of friends. Thus it is particularly beneficial and literally health-giving when religious practice affords people the needed means for meeting the stressful demands of grief. I recall a situation in which a husband in the prime of life died in an instant at his dining room table. His wife was stunned to the core of her being by this totally unexpected loss. She meant well by planning a backyard picnic immediately after the burial service just three days after her husband's death before her eyes. But with her plans of good food and laughter as a fitting tribute to her husband's life, she failed to take into account the necessity of facing the loss and sorrow side of that experience. She firmly resisted even talking about that, viewing it somehow as gloomy and negative and unwelcome. Within three months she was in the hospital herself with a severe abdominal ailment which did not surprise those responsible for her medical and spiritual care. The fierce buildup of tension, grief, bewildering new responsibilities, and anger over the sudden loss of a spouse contributed directly to her becoming seriously ill. Then, finally, she began to come to terms with unresolved matters in her life and to appreciate what the Christian faith said to her.

She and all of us with her can benefit from the long tradition of Judaism and the God-given instincts of Jews neither to ignore the One who shepherds us through the dark valley of death nor hurry through the shadowed days and weeks which follow without learning the deeper lessons. It was the unique vocation of faithful Jews to deal with death and dying long before it became almost faddish to map out the contours of that experience. Today as well as a thousand years ago—yes, three thousand years back!—the people of the first covenant teach and live these rituals in the congregation which minister to the health of the living as they cope with the loss that death imposes. First comes *aninut*, the period between death and burial. Then follows *shivah*, a period of seven days; then *sheloshim*, the thirty days following the burial. In the case of the death of a parent, the religious prescription for mourning extends over an eleven-month time. The graduated steps of liturgical observance give the bereaved person a path back to normal functioning. A sense of order and security is offered in the midst of chaos and disorientation. The Jew has a tradition to tell him or her what to do and what to expect. Closure is provided; the surrounding community of the congregation is helped to know and perform its therapeutic role.

Picture this scene: Some weeks have passed since a wife lost her husband in an airplane crash. The shock has worn off; the pain of that loss is at its peak. The widow is present in the Friday evening service. She is invited to reflect, with the whole congregation, upon these words:

> When cherished ties are broken and the chain of love is shattered, only trust and the strength of faith can lighten the heaviness of the heart. At times, the pain of separation seems more than we can bear, but if we dwell too long on our loss we embitter our hearts and harm ourselves and those about us.
>
> The Psalmist said that in his affliction he learned the law of God. And in

truth, grief is a great teacher, when it sends you back to serve and bless the living. We learn how to counsel and comfort those who, like ourselves, are bowed with sorrow. We learn when to keep silence in their presence, and when a word will assure them of our love and concern.

Thus, even when they are gone, the departed are with us, moving us to live as, in their higher moments, they themselves wished to live. We remember them now; they live in our hearts; they are an abiding blessing.[2]

Then she is asked to rise, along with all others who are moving through their time of bereavement. Her husband's name is spoken as the *kaddish* prayers are offered. After the synagogue service is completed, she goes into the adjoining hall for *onegg shabat*, a time for conversation, for words of care and friendship, for all the heartening reminders to her that she is part of the congregation that cares and helps her be the same consoling influence for others. All of that ministers to the health of people in a time of particular vulnerability. Life goes on with the spiritual support of people who embody a tradition that has stood the test of the centuries.

In the Christian celebration of the Eucharist there are provisions of spiritual care which minister directly to the well-being of people who know their need of spiritual foundations for staying well or coming through a time of illness. The bread and the wine of the meal of Christ are visible signs to Christians of that inward power of divine grace which is cherished for the good news it brings in life's bad situations. In the Christian congregation at worship, too, those who have died are named in the prayers of remembrance. In the liturgy of Holy Communion, people who feel keenly the absence of a family member or friend are reassured that as Christians gather to receive in the Eucharist the risen Christ, they do so "together with angels and archangels and the whole company of heaven." The "together with" phrase opens up to grieving persons that wider mystery of the eternal dimension of God's grace. The burden of loneliness is lifted as people of faith sense the surrounding cloud of witnesses with whom the praise of God is shared. Such spiritual force serves the well-being of people who need that healing gift to find their momentum in wholesome and purposeful living again. Christians are given the bread and wine of Holy Communion in hospitals when they cannot join the community at worship because of illness. From the earliest days of the church the sacramental bread and wine are taken to the sick and the infirm, reminding each recipient of the bonds of faith and love which still unite them with the church on earth and the faithful who rest in God beyond this life. The communion is a sign, symbol, and seal of Christ's promise to be present with his people always. Our mealtimes are essential for health and life; the meal of Christ takes that truth to deeper spiritual realms of Christian experience.

Another liturgical moment among Christians which addresses the loneliness problem in modern life is an ancient practice now finding a widespread restoration in Roman Catholic and Protestant congregations. Simply a handshake, sometimes an embrace, and words spoken such as "Christ's peace!" "the peace of God," "Christ's grace be with you," give people access to one another at a level deeper than ordinary greetings. Even though formalized and thus often carried out with an awkwardness, people are doing something healthful for each other. I have seen couples in troubled marriages begin to find each other with communication as the peace is passed in public worship. I have seen family members, particularly youth with elders and vice versa, cross over unseen barriers of generation gaps in such moments. I have seen strangers begin to sense the deeper spirit of divine acceptance, as well as their place in a new congregation, through such moments of hands clasped and faithful words spoken with genuineness.

Where else in our society do such things occur? On buses or commuter trains, at sports arenas, concerts, or office coffee breaks? The congregation is a unique place of bringing isolated and alienated people back into a circle of belonging in which acceptance, recognition, mutual purpose, love for one another, and the worship of God work together to make life whole instead of crippled in isolation. The measure of such formalized events in the congregation is not only that they happen there. It is measured in what they set in motion in attitudes and actions with people during the week between worship service, the inner spirits bolstered, the love engendered and shared, the wholesome and enlarging contacts they initiate out beyond the place of worship. Such forces for human well-being can never be measured in the statisticians' count; yet they exist and play their healing part beyond our knowledge.

The congregation is the setting for the practice of traditions which speak to the heart of human alienation from God and which lead people back into the fellowship with God and with one another that God intends for fullness of life. Their relevance and power are experienced especially in times when the threatening problems of illness, stress, or death are heavy. Again this week in the world, Catholic priests will anoint ill parishioners in the sacramental rite which before the Second Vatican Council two decades ago was regarded as the last rites before death rather than a ministry to all ill persons. In this week also, lay ministers among Baptist, Episcopal, Pentecostal, Reorganized Latter-day Saints, Mormon, Adventist, and other groups within Christendom will come home from their secular jobs and find time to go to hospitals, homes for the aged, and private residences for the purpose of carrying out the apostolic injunction "Is any among you sick? Let him call for the elders of the church, and let them pray over him, anointing him with oil in the name of the Lord; and the prayer of faith will save the sick man, and the Lord will raise him up; and if he has committed sins, he will be forgiven" (James 5:14, 15).

In congregations of Jews and Christians again this week special groups of trained laity will offer counsel to people in crisis situations of job stress or loss of work altogether, marital and family problems, alcoholism and drug dependency, and other problems of life that wear humans down and render them more vulnerable to the dysfunctioning of body, mind, and spirit. Such a cadre of paraprofessional lay counselors at Valley Beth Shalom Synagogue in Encino, California, is a modern expression of serving groups in earlier centuries of Judaism, the visitors of the ill (*bikkur holim*) and those who helped bereaved families with the burial of the dead (*kaddisha*). Within Christian congregations as well, such intercongregational training programs as the Stephen Series have equipped thousands of lay Christians across the land to grow in the skills of care and service to people in need. The traditions of help reach beyond the conventional religious practices. Not long ago one of the nurses in our congregation told of the interest aroused among the intensive-care staff of the children's hospital in which she works. The child of a gypsy family was critically ill; the hospital lobby was the gathering place for several dozen gypsies who were waiting anxiously while other gypsies were sacrificing live chickens and conducting other unusual rituals in a room the hospital administration had set aside for them!

Congregations are always just at the edges of their full potential for recognizing and applying the fullness of religious tradition to the well-being of human life. In spite of the assumption that everybody who has had an operation wants to talk about it, many regard illness as a private affair and guard it accordingly. It is almost as if becoming ill were an embarrassment, a taboo. While people have every right to the manner and measure of their opening up about illness, the gift of health and the burden of disease cannot be kept in isolation according to the biblical faith. Why not program more directly into congregational life occasions when people who have something to say can say it? The list only begins with the following:

- Having lay people visit as well as clergy support in a crisis time during a hospital stay.

- Having a congregation mobilize a group of its members to help the household of an ill person to continue to function through a time of acute or prolonged illness.

- Offering assistance by donating blood, sorting through the maze of paper work incurred in Medicare and other insurance coverage, and sometimes assisting the family in meeting the emergency financial problems brought on by illness.

- Helping people allay their fears of medicine and hospital procedures by explaining what happened, how they felt when going through it, and the appreciation for skilled and caring doctors and nurses, as well as the benefit of medical research and equipment in hospitals.

- Helping well people realize the vitality of the spiritual resources drawn upon when health gives way to illness, envisioning the hospital as a place where the providence of God is present. Helping people to cope with their unreal expectations from doctors and hospitals as well as to report serious malpractice problems without regarding litigation as the only means of such protest.

- Drawing in to congregation programs physicians and nurses, hospital administrators, and volunteers to speak of what they see at the juncture of religion and medicine. Providing a forum of intelligent concern and interest for medical professionals to express the dilemmas of modern health care with which they struggle.

- Encouraging clergy to visit their congregation members who are health-care professionals at their places of work. Glimpsing their daily vocation with greater understanding and empathy for what goes into their accomplishments and failures, fulfillments and frustrations, and joining them in seeing the interconnections between religious tradition and modern medical practice.

The Congregation: Place of Healing and Sending

When such initiatives are undertaken from within the congregation, clergy and laity awaken to the striking emphasis from hospitals in the past two decades to join congregations in such educational ventures. Lutheran General Hospital in Park Ridge, Illinois, has pioneered such programs, which are designed to put the hospital and the congregation in closer contact with each other and to help each discover how each needs the other so that both can serve people more adequately. Such cross-walks of cooperation are already functioning between congregations and hospitals that are under direct religious sponsorship and support. The National Opinion Research Center in Chicago, Illinois, reports that there are 728 such hospitals in the United States today, 10 percent of the total number. A more relevant statistic is the 190,609 beds provided by these hospitals, which is 14 percent of the total in the United States.[3] Many of the nation's hospitals were begun under direct religious auspices but are no longer so identified, supported, or controlled. This is not to exclude them, however, from the scope of this chapter. An essential part of biblical belief is that God works for good far beyond the institutions under the direct control of religious groups, and that conviction gives a religious perspective to every hospital where the work of healing and care is offered. I am aware of an increasing number of hospitals which have no specific religious orientation and yet offer an expanded chaplaincy program and cooperative arrangements with local congregations. An example is the practice of a nearby hospital over the past ten years of simply informing our church office when someone of our congregation enters, or someone entering who has no religious affiliation but who indicates an interest in religious contact. The trend is growing, to the benefit of all involved.

The Sunday morning or Friday evening congregation scene envisioned at the opening of this chapter included a doctor and nurse. They suggest the part which religious commitment has in the lives of those who take care of us medically. Again, I have found no statistics on a comprehensive national basis which shed light on the numbers of health-care professionals who identify themselves as people of religious commitment. The American Medical Association, to which approximately 70 percent of the doctors in the United States belong, has no religious category in their identifying criteria of membership. Neither does the federal government statistical record. The absence of that category, particularly in the former organization, is a fact to ponder. The institutions responsible for accrediting men and women for the care of something as precious as health and human life itself does not regard the religious question as relevant. That is, perhaps, one more reason why studies of this type are necessary. The distance between the two disciplines, which were intertwined intimately in earlier centuries, has been a separation beneficial to neither.[4] Particularly in this day when medical and biological research has touched upon the mystery and miracle of life itself, as in the developments in recent years in recombinant DNA, the gaps and mutual misunderstandings on both sides must be remedied.

Coming at the issue from another side, however, it is possible to say that medicine and religion have been in close contact all along in recent decades. I am speaking of the presence of medical professionals in congregations as faithful, active members along with plumbers, sales people, bus drivers, housewives, and parishioners from all walks of life. Doctors, nurses, and those who administer the multifaceted responsibilities of a modern hospital have basic spiritual needs no different from others. In my ministry to medical people, I have worked at finding the right attitude for their vocation that affords proper respect without unwarranted deference. They share the same need of the forgiveness of sins dear to us all. As is the case in any other specific vocation, however, the medical profession has certain aspects that deserve attention and understanding by clergy and laity. Over the past twenty-seven years of the pastorate I have learned that—

- People expect the superhuman of doctors and nurses. By virtue of their access to modern medical technology, we expect them to do wonders every time. The doctor is the visible, tangible sign of what all that vaunted scientific accomplishment is going to do for us when we hurt all over and fear for our lives.

- The modern hospital can be viewed as the temple of technology where our natural idolatries may run wild. Even though the doctor may not have an answer, somewhere in that huge complex of stainless steel and miracle equipment will come the answer that will deliver us back into the physical health commonly spoken of as "the most important thing we have."

- Doctors especially, but nurses and administrators as well, are not only idolized. They are bitterly resented and increasingly attacked via litigation when they do not deliver what we commonly expect:

positive results. They know something we do not know, they talk in terms most of us cannot even pronounce, let alone spell. They charge outrageous fees. Some are arrogant (as uppity as some clergy) with little feeling for the patient as a person.

- Competition for entrance into medical school is extraordinary and potentially crippling of the moral sense as candidates will do anything to gain entrance into that system, which appears to them as an elitist, lucrative life.

- Once into medical school and ensuing residencies, the demands upon medical students are among the most unhealthful in the land, jeopardizing not only their bodies but the minds, souls, and marriages of those who journey through the mine fields of preparation for the medical profession.

All this says that religious ministry and congregational functions have all the more relevance for those in medicine and those working hard to get in.

It may be that ours is not a typical congregation. I am not sure that many church or synagogue choirs have a chief of surgery, a dermatologist, a neurosurgeon, a general practitioner, an obstetrician, and two nurses in the choir. There they are, week after week, for an evening of rehearsal and a full Sabbath morning schedule of singing plus Bach cantatas on seven more Sunday afternoons of the year. Again, it is not remarkable that medical people sing in choirs and participate actively in the congregation. Together with them, people from all walks of life receive and give spiritual nurture, and are thus equipped to think and act with distinctive motives in their daily vocation. Let me illustrate.

Among the physicians in the choir, there come to mind two who help me understand the meaning of the congregation for people who function well in the face of formidable pressures each day. Some years ago one was assisting the other with a patient undergoing surgery. The attending surgeon, knowing that his younger colleague was interested in music, invited him to a church concert. The invitation was offered while the last stitches of a thoracic surgery were put in. That almost casual invitation was more timely than the surgeon realized. His partner across the operating table had just been through a searing personal problem which was causing him to do what many of us do when the bottom drops out of life—pour ourselves into our work without the balancing which keeps us humane. The assisting physician accepted the invitation and more. He found a new beginning in his worship life by joining the congregation. New friendships, new opportunities to trust people and be entrusted with wider responsibilities, encouragement, support, experiencing the love of God in the company of a congregation—all these flowed together to change greatly the course of his life at a critical juncture. The spiritual nurture and values he had learned in his family early in his life were revived. His daily rounds as a neurosurgeon bring him face to face with people struggling with major, life-threatening problems. Few people go to neurosurgeons with less than calamitous health problems. From before dawn until after dusk on most days this surgeon is working with people in crisis. Having found his own place in a congregation again, he is equipped to meet these demands in ways he did not have before.

The experience of this surgeon helps to lift up the biblical theme of vocation. Coming together in the church or synagogue for the worship of God so that he can live out that truth in the course of the week in the work that he does—such is the rhythmic picture of life under God in the fellowship of God's people for the serving of people in the world. A key New Testament source for this theme among Christians is this passage: "And his gifts were that some should be apostles, some prophets, some evangelists, some pastors and teachers, to equip the saints for the work of ministry . . ." (Eph. 4:11–12). "Saints"—the standard New Testament term for believers—means people like the surgeon or the charwoman scrubbing down the hospital hallway floor, people doing their daily work with a consciousness of serving God as people are served. Clergy and all the functions of the congregation are intended to equip and deliver people into the daily rounds of life with the empowering love of God as the motivating force in their attitudes and actions.

In Judaism a similar biblical theme is conveyed in key words such as *halakah* (a life of holiness), *zedakah* (righteousness in living), and *shlemut* (wholeness, the consistency of self in worship with the self in daily life). The congregation is the generating community in which these divine truths are celebrated, taught, and prayed for. This is one essential criterion for the integrity of faith and worship, that it equip men and women for the serving of others in the power of the love which has come into their lives from God.

There are some 64,000 men and women in the 125 medical schools of the nation today. What motivates them to work so hard and sacrifice so much in order to enter medicine? There is no single answer, of course. But the religious sense of vocation is one strong motive that is being inculcated among all those who are finding in the congregation what I know to be true in the lives of our own doctors and nurses who enrich our parish by their faithful participation. Watching highly trained people in medicine handle the pressures of their vocation, and seeing them deepen inwardly as they grow professionally, is to see the process whereby technically competent people become true partners with God in the larger meaning of healing. Their vocational sense with its deeply religious roots is marked by their humility in the face of what they do not know, care for patients as people, and their daily work as a *diakonia*, a service to God as people are being served. That *halakah*, holiness of life, creates deep reservoirs of the spirit which enable a physician to be thoughtful and caring for the patient long after the normal reserves of human interest are depleted. Doctors face strong countercurrents of other motives which have little to do with God-given service. The congregation and clergy need to see how much it can mean for people called to be healers of others to find healing themselves.

Doctors and nurses, no less than people in other callings, need a place where they can get their bearings as they come to terms with the failures, misjudgments, and problems peculiar to their work. All along the line in the medical profession the fact of failure poses a special threat. It can mean exclusion from medical school, or the lesser ranks when it comes to the more choice internships or residencies. It can mean the health or the life of a patient in a critical moment. A surgeon-parishioner tells of an experience in which his colleague let a surgical tool slip in an extremely delicate procedure. The resulting crisis was so devastating that the surgeon suddenly walked out of the operating room, leaving his colleague with a patient whose life was in the balance. At this particular hospital the surgical staff meets regularly under the guidance of the chief of surgery to provide a setting in which those crisis moments are reviewed. Such a regular practice is salutary and supportive in great measure, as well as a time of instruction and prevention of the repetition of such dilemmas.

But when no colleague can fully understand the failure and no supportive experience of other doctors can assuage the guilt and self-doubt caused by some failure in helping a patient recover and live, the congregation has a place where the doctor can join everyone else in laying before God the burdens that no human can bear. Little do we clergy realize what it means to bear the responsibility of decisions and actions day after day which have to do with the health and life of fellow human beings. Charles Bosk's book on the handling of medical failure has the interesting title *Forgive and Remember*.[5] Its case-study presentation of the pressures that build among surgeons and the ways they find to handle them is useful reading for anyone ministering to doctors. The realities of that world of the operating room accentuate the relevance of the words with which many worship services of congregations begin: "Almighty God, to whom all hearts are open, all desires known, and from whom no secrets are hid; cleanse the thoughts of our hearts by the inspiration of your Holy Spirit, that we may perfectly love you and worthily magnify your holy name." It is not enough that the physician's conscience is the only guide and thus the patient's only protection. The physician's conscience as well as his or her mind and body need divine mercy, encouragement, refreshment, and the affirmation which comes in the community of faith. Thus medical professionals will find in the grace of God and the fellowship of God's people what we all find, that we can outlive our failures and grow through them instead of becoming their victims.

The congregation is a place where the separated worlds of religion and medicine are not so separated. People of religious conviction and medical vocation gather there; they embody the juncture of religion and medicine and represent an underestimated aspect of the subject of this book. For medical people who are participants in congregations, the issues of religion and medicine are real rather than abstract. They are a front-line resource in drawing the two realms ever closer. The worst thing would be that their potential would never be recognized because religious leadership was too dull or preoccupied with lesser things, or that people of religious commitment in medicine saw their daily work only as a job instead of a profoundly meaningful vocation. The further we go in the challenges and perplexities and the excitement of these times, the more we must avoid missing our destiny. As we attend to the riches of our faith tradition and stay close to people in need, the best thing will continue to happen. God will be served as people are served with medical skill and religious devotion. The congregation will ever be a vital gathering place for people to hold fast to that vision of service and help one another impart it effectively to a world that may be more interested than we dreamed.

NOTES

1. Walter Wangerin, "The Time in the City," Commencement Address, Christ Seminary–Seminex, St. Louis, *Together* 7 (July 1981): 3–6.

2. *Gates of Prayer: The New Union Prayerbook* (New York: Central Conference of American Rabbis, 1975), p. 623.

3. I am indebted to Dr. William McCready for these data; he is a staff person of the National Opinion Research Center, Chicago, Illinois.

4. The subject is explored thoughtfully by Kenneth Vaux, *This Mortal Coil: The Meaning of Health and Disease* (New York: Harper & Row, 1978).

5. Charles L. Bosk, *Forgive and Remember: Managing Medical Failure* (Chicago: University of Chicago Press, 1979).

12

The Hospital Chaplain Between Worlds

LAWRENCE E. HOLST

A hospital chaplain walks between the worlds of religion and medicine. He is both pastor and clinician, theologically educated and clinically trained, endorsed by both church and hospital.* A hospital chaplain is of the church but not in the parish. He is nobody's pastor but everybody's pastor. His salary is from the hospital, his mandate from the church. By history and tradition he is closer to his colleagues in the parish ministry, but his daily interactions are with physicians and nurses. In many hospitals the chaplain's garb is a white or blue clinical coat inscribed with a cross—symbols of medicine and religion. Often these two worlds are complementary, but sometimes they are contradictory. Always their interaction requires exploration.

To move between these two worlds that are so markedly different, and yet were at one time united, creates tension. The tension can be painful, confusing, exciting, creative. Like many tensions it is never fully resolved and perhaps never will be or should be. Each world has its own domain, problems, and mission. Each needs the support of, but independence from, the other.

The hospital chaplain moves between the two worlds of religion and medicine. By having legitimacy in both worlds, the hospital chaplain is a strategic person in the attempt to effect greater reconciliation between religion and medicine. The hospital chaplain has much to contribute to and receive from an inquiry into medicine and religion, providing the inquiry does not remove itself from that most vital place where the issues

*Chaplains are of both genders, but the male term will be used to simplify style.

293

of medicine and religion dynamically interact: the bedside of the suffering patient.

THE CONTEXT OF THE HOSPITAL FOSTERS
"IN-BETWEENNESS"

Most hospital chaplains began their ministry somewhere in a parish. It was a setting where they had primacy and where most of their pastoral care was rendered to people of a similar faith who held membership in that single congregation. They can well recall that a formal installation service on a Sunday morning suddenly provided them with pastoral authority and responsibility. A covenant was established; mutual claims were affirmed.

The hospital chaplain can also recall from his parish ministry spending much time in groups: public worship, Bible classes, board and committee meetings. Ministry to individuals was supported by the formal structures of worship and usually included elements from those structures: prayer, Scripture reading, confession-absolution, the administration of the sacraments. It was a natural, expected transition. Why not re-create together in the solitude of a hospital room what the two of them had shared together with the worshiping community Sunday after Sunday?

Recalling those days in the parish, the hospital chaplain remembers how gracefully his ministry was accepted, how minimal was the role confusion. Now the chaplain finds himself not in the parish but in the hospital. Instead of chancels and pulpits, he finds himself at bedsides, in postsurgical recovery and emergency rooms. Now he may spend more time reading patient charts than he does the Bible. He feels little primacy in this world. He is not treated with the reverence and favor to which he had grown accustomed in the parish. It is a much lonelier world, one without the mutual claims and support of a worshiping community. In a setting where tasks are so carefully delineated and precisely measured, he feels out of his element. No longer is his role assumed. It is questioned and challenged. "What are you going to do for my patient, chaplain?" is not an uncommon question.

Nor does the chaplain have unilateral access to the patient. He shares that access with many: physicians, nurses, social workers, nutritionists, physical-occupational-speech therapists. Who does what to whom, and when, needs to be defined—and scheduled. Gone is the homogeneity of membership in a single parish. The chaplain's "congregation" comes from a variety of backgrounds, representing a broad spectrum of faith, or no faith. Gone too is the familiarity of a prior relationship with his parishioners. The hospital chaplain begins his ministry from scratch. Gone too is the authority bequeathed through installation. The chaplain has no claim upon the patient and can assume no authority, except perhaps a symbolic one. He doesn't admit the patient to the hospital. Nor will he treat, medicate, or discharge the patient. What he does with and for the patient will be by consent.

Patients come into the hospital seeking medical care not pastoral care. It is the physician they have "installed" and imbued with authority. It is to the physician that the patient raises his most immediate and urgent questions: What is wrong with me? Is it serious? What can you do about it? Will it hurt? Will I get better? The chaplain has little impact upon those issues.

The hospital chaplain cannot presume a religious motivation in the patient. In fact, if he serves a large metropolitan hospital he will learn that under 50 percent of the patients hold current membership in a parish, and a considerably smaller percentage are active members. The chaplain cannot draw comfortably upon the traditional faith resources since they may be neither welcome nor meaningful to the patient. This means that much time must be spent getting acquainted, developing a feel for the religious needs and meanings of the patient.

Time is important in hospital ministry. Hospitalization averages seven to ten days. Indeed, the chaplain's is a parenthetical ministry. Yet during that week in a person's life the chaplain has the rare opportunity to focus his energies upon relationship. Just as the chaplain is spared the myriad of organizational-administrative responsibilities of the parish pastor, so he is spared the technical demands of medical management within the hospital. He carries no equipment; he takes nothing into or out of the patient's room; he has no responsibilities to inject or extract, to weigh, count or measure anything. Nor does he even have to chart. Hospital accrediting bodies tend to ignore him and his services.

Hence the hospital chaplain is one of the few people in the pressurized, urgent, regimented clinical world who can wander the corridors, move in and out of patient rooms (invited or not), pull up a chair and visit. Here the chaplain can listen to "the voice of illness." And a rich, meaningful voice it is—a voice that cries out in anguish, that rebels against the boundaries and vulnerabilities, that rejoices over recovery, that grieves over losses. To engage that voice, with all its variations and nuances, is the rich privilege of listening. The vagueness and impreciseness of the chaplain's role opens the door for many diverse and creative encounters.

The confinement of ministry to the parenthesis of illness also offers some advantages to the chaplain. As the chaplain encounters the patient, there is no debris from prior contacts, no obligations for the future. Their encounter is for the present. Images do not need to be maintained. This is important, because illness unmasks people, frequently exposing raw, primitive emotions. In the relative anonymity of a chaplain-patient relationship, these can be unashamedly expressed. The possibilities for candor are rich; the potential for posthospital embarrassment is minimal. The two of them (chaplain and patient) are not likely to meet again.

Of course it is not all so simple. The context of anonymity alone is not sufficient to guarantee openness. It requires sensitive listening, accurate empathy, nonpossessive warmth on the part of the chaplain, and the capacity to trust and risk on the part of the patient.

In a sense, the chaplain walks in that interim in a patient's life between a preillness state for which the patient yearns and a posthospital state the patient may fear. That interim provides the patient his first exposure after the tumor, the coronary, the biopsy, the colitis, the malignancy have been confirmed. It can be a crucial time, a time when appearances are altered, future plans revised.

Such is the ministry of the hospital chaplain: extemporaneous, informal, casual, conversational. It seems so out of character in the frenetic, pressurized world of the hospital. The chaplain sits and visits; yet he does it differently from a neighbor or relative. He counsels with patients; yet he is not a certified psychotherapist. He ministers to patients, but often without the familiar accouterments of Word and Sacraments. In many ways the chaplain is an enigma to both the church and the hospital. The physician may question the chaplain's role and relevance; the parish pastor may question the chaplain's identity and commitment. Such is the "in-betweenness" fostered by the context of the hospital.

THE TRAINING OF THE CHAPLAIN FOSTERS "IN-BETWEENNESS"

Prior to the 1940s there was no formal training for institutional chaplaincy. Such positions often went to older pastors who could no longer tolerate the rigors of parish ministry. Some did well, but few claimed professional peership with a clinical team. Two factors changed this: the advent of a clinical training process for clergy in 1925 and the development of organizations to certify hospital chaplains in the 1950s.

Like that of the parish pastor, the hospital chaplain's preparation for ministry occurred in a seminary, with a major emphasis upon biblical theology, dogmatics, church history, philosophy, and the arts and humanities. The educational process was didactic, cognitive, and deductive. But his preparation for chaplaincy occurred in a hospital, with a major emphasis upon psychology, psychodynamics, psychopathology, and individual and small-group counseling. That educational process was inductive, experiential, and clinical. Each preparation was vital though different.

Clinical pastoral education began in 1925 in a state mental hospital in Worcester, Massachusetts. In part it grew out of dissatisfaction with traditional theological education of that day, which was considered by many to be too abstract, too removed from life, too divorced from the practical tasks of ministry. C.P.E. (Clinical Pastoral Education) was an effort to get theological students out of their classrooms and chapel into the wards and clinics that house suffering people. As one of its founders, Anton Boisen, a Congregational minister, said on the occasion of that movement's twenty-fifth anniversary in 1950:

> This movement has no new gospel to proclaim; we are not seeking to introduce anything into the theological curriculum beyond a new approach to some ancient problems. We are trying, rather to call attention back to the central task of the church, that of saving souls, and to the central problem of theology, that of sin and salvation. What is new is the attempt to begin with the study of the living human documents rather than with books and to focus attention upon those who are grappling desperately with the issues of spiritual life and death.

In some ways that statement by Boisen is conservative, he was not introducing new subjects. But in another respect it was radical; it proposed a clinical method of learning that challenged the basic structures of theological education.

Boisen and others in the C.P.E. movement attempted to stimulate pastors to explore their own inner world in order to become more sensitive companions for others in their struggles with the vital issues of life. C.P.E. boldly attempted to link the external and internal world of the learner, the cognitive with the emotive, theory with practice, theology with psychology. At least four major philosophic streams provided the intellectual context and impetus for C.P.E. in the 1920s and 1930s:

1. *Theological liberalism*, which saw itself as a reaction against the

authoritarianism, the sterile dogmatism of religion. Optimistic in its view of human nature, social in its outlook, liberalism focused upon the internal authority of one's personal religious experience, rather than the external authority of church dogma and upon the autonomy of human reason.

2. *Philosophic pragmatism,* which espoused a scientific, empirical method of learning that focused more upon function than theory. Its approach was clinical and inductive; its goal was to increase functional competency. In juxtaposition to the formation of C.P.E., the American Bar Association was being organized, the American Medical Association was being reorganized, and an accrediting agency in public education was being formed. In addition, the professions of social work and public health were taking root. It was an era of professionalism. The pastor, once the most learned person in the community, was now perceived as professionally inferior to these other professions.

3. *Freudian psychology,* which held that neuroses were due to the repression of the dark, irrational drives, passions, and impulses seething just beneath consciousness. It was a grim challenge to a world that assumed behavior was totally under rational control. Less optimistic about human nature than theological liberalism, it called for a careful study and analysis of the individual, particularly of one's competing-conflicting intrapsychic forces. It introduced a new vocabulary: id, superego, repression, displacement, libido, cathexis, transference, defense mechanisms. Freudian psychology brought a clinical, quasi-scientific sophistication to the field of psychotherapy.

4. *Religious existentialism,* which like Freudian psychology was individual in its orientation and like theological liberalism was anti-authoritarian. It blended optimism and pessimism. It viewed humans as free and responsible to make life's decisions, but without benefit of objective standards and without certainty as to the outcome of those decisions. Man is both self-authenticating and lonely. Likewise, existentialism—somewhat akin to theological liberalism—placed more emphasis upon religious experience than upon the nature of God.

From each of these philosophic movements, C.P.E. borrowed certain emphases:

- From *theological liberalism* came the emphasis upon individual experience

- From *philosophic pragmatism* came the emphasis upon the empirical-clinical method of learning
- From *Freudian psychology* came the emphasis upon the inner world
- From *religious existentialism* came the emphasis upon individual freedom and responsibility to authenticate one's decisions.

No doubt the borrowing was selective, and no doubt there were other forces and influences. How and why C.P.E. developed as it did is a matter of conjecture. That it has had a profound impact on theological education and hospital chaplaincy is beyond debate. By participating in this process and experiencing its double impact upon education and pastoral care, the hospital chaplain again finds himself "in-between."

THE INFLUENCE OF PSYCHOLOGY HAS FOSTERED "IN-BETWEENNESS"

No doubt a primary criticism of hospital chaplaincy has been its seeming uncritical embracing of psychology. Rather than informing his theology, many feel psychology has become the chaplain's theology. Without conceding or refuting the charge, it is understandable how such a strong influence occurred. Psychology has been a vital part of the chaplain's preparation and has supplied him with skills that were readily discernible and marketable in the clinical world. Psychology has provided fresh insights into humankind's existential estrangement. While theology has historically portrayed the human race as in a state of sinful rebellion, psychology has pictured the chaos graphically: humanity enmeshed in a biological order that includes primitive, conflictual forces not always within conscious control; humanity struggling to gratify instincts within the prohibitions of society and making the necessary displacements of psychic energy.

What has been important in all this is that the chaplain has been helped by psychology to more profoundly understand the internal dynamics of human beings. In so doing, he has been challenged to rethink certain traditional means and methods of ministry. As psychology has raised critical issues of ministry for the chaplain, he has in turn raised critical issues for religion.

Perhaps the challenge has come most forcefully through psychology's understanding of personality development. While psychology certainly does not know all there is to know about personality, it has postulated some very important axioms which, if taken seriously, raise some critical questions about ministry:

- That the broad foundations of personality are larger than consciousness
- That one's personality structure is formed early in life, possibly within the first five to six years
- That reactive patterns to one's early environment, learned in childhood, carry over with minor modifications into adulthood
- That differences in personality have to do with genetic endowment and the early influences, particular those of parents (or parent substitutes)
- That our most basic early learning comes through relationships, transmitted more nonverbally than verbally, more by experience than by precept.

Long before the child can speak, psychology informs us, the child has experienced the full gamut of emotions: love-hate, acceptance-rejection, trust-mistrust, order-chaos, pleasure-pain, reward-punishment. In other words, long before the child learns the word to identify the experience, the child has already had the experience.

There are those whose early experiences were emotionally rich and positive. These children were surrounded by warm, consistent, emotionally generous people who were able to communicate those qualities and provide a trustworthy environment. Finding one's surroundings trustworthy and relatively consistent, it was more possible for these children to trust others and themselves.

Unfortunately there are those whose early experiences have been destructive, whose early human ties were so damaging and inconsistent as to severely block their capacity to trust others, their environment, or themselves. As a result their self-image is so impoverished, their need for nurturing so great, their fear of rejection so profound that it is virtually impossible for them to enter into mature, reciprocally rewarding relationships.

That personality development occurs in fairly predictable stages and sequences is a matter of general agreement within the field of psychology. How fixed these developmental patterns become, as well as the possibility and degree for later modification, is a matter of debate within the field of psychology.

What does this have to do with pastoral care in a hospital, or ministry anywhere? As the chaplain, under the influence of psychology, began to probe more deeply into the intricacies and idiosyncrasies of his own and others' internal lives, he was intrigued, troubled, challenged. As was previously stated, the C.P.E. process encouraged such pursuit. Self-awareness, introspection, is seen by that process as vital to ministry. As this process occurred—sometimes with the aid of personal psycho-therapy—the chaplain began to raise more and more questions about his ministry and that of the church. Most particularly he began to challenge ministry's heavy reliance upon verbal proclamation. It seemed too broad, too intellectual, too removed from the dynamic lives of people he encountered.

It was becoming increasingly apparent to him, or so he thought, that senders and receivers of messages are influenced by many factors, many of which are unconscious. It was becoming equally apparent to him, or so he thought, that the message sent was not necessarily the message received, not because of any deficiency in the message or any fault of the sender, but because of the predisposition of the receiver. Psychology had demonstrated to the chaplain through his training that words are symbols. What they symbolized will be determined not alone by the message or the sender, but more so by the experiences, associations, and perceptions of the *receiver*.

This being so, the chaplain (under the influence of psychology) came to see that words identify an experience, but they don't create the experi-ence. The words "I love you" do not create love in a relationship; rather, they identify a quality that one hopes is present in that relationship. If love is not there, the words themselves will probably make little differ-ence. How each person in that relationship has experienced love—what each of them brings to it experientially out of the past—will determine the meaning of that word in the present. Of course, without broad agree-ments on words like "love," without some commonality of experiences, communication would be impossible. Yet despite those broad, con-sensually validated experiences, there are also unique peculiar meanings and experiences each of us brings to the word. This is even more so with words that are emotionally charged, like "love." Therefore we can never fully know how the messages sent are being received until and unless we come to know the internal reference of the receiver.

The communication principle that derives from personality develop-ment is that one moves, or proceeds, from the personal experience to the concept. In a sense we project onto concepts our associations and meanings. Where our personal experience is somewhat congruent with the consensually validated meaning of the concept, effective communication is likely to occur. That is, the message sent is the message received. On the other hand, where there is a marked incongruence between our personal experience and the consensually validated meaning of the concept, communication will be distorted and confused. Between those two extremes there are many shades of variation in communication effectiveness.

Symbols have always been very important in the religious community. Most of the traditional Christian symbols are relational in nature. In that sense they are dynamic and interpersonal. Again, people will project onto those symbols their own associations and experiences, their own internal reality. Carroll Wise, an early leader in C.P.E. and pastoral counseling, once said: "The only way any formulation of faith can vitally affect personality is for the inner dynamics of personality to become harmonious with the ideas presented." Wise's statement is a sharp challenge to the church: to be more in touch with the inner dynamics of people and to work at helping those dynamics to become more congruent with the gospel.

If, as psychology informs us, dynamic learning proceeds from the experience to the concept (or formulation), and that the major vehicle for such learning is through warm, consistent, loving relationships, then the church's mandate to proclaim the gospel takes on some new and bold dimensions. Inherent in Wise's statement is also an implied criticism of a church that has tended for too long to overrely upon verbal proclamations and creedal formulations as the primary means of communication.

The hospital chaplain has taken seriously the insights of psychology and has attempted to incorporate them into his ministry, particularly those that help him get more fully into the inner world, into the inner dynamics of "the living human documents." Perhaps he has overlearned. Some would say so. In attempting to bring a corrective to what he perceived to be ministry's overreliance upon verbal proclamations, the clinically trained hospital chaplain went to the opposite extreme and underutilized the traditional resources of the church. In his concern for the subjective perceptions of the individual, he came at times perilously close to reducing religion to those subjective perceptions. Like the religious existentialist, he tended to become more absorbed in people's *experience* of God than in the *nature* of God. Or, to put it another way, in his retreat from what he considered to be an overobjectification of faith (e.g., dogma for dogma's sake), he was drawn into an oversubjectification of faith. Like theological liberalism (one of C.P.E.'s many roots), it was a faith marked by individualism and antiinstitutionalism and validated only by the feelings and experiences of that individual at that moment.

So the chaplain encountered the tension: Just as dogma without personal experience renders dogma empty and sterile, likewise personal experience without the structure and durability of dogma detaches that religious experience from history, tradition, and the religious community. The chaplain walks within that tension, between those objective-subjective dimensions of religion, between proclamation and experience. Both are important. The chaplain represents a faith community that transcends the individual and this moment in time. That community—through the Spirit of God and by consensus—has formulated doctrines and symbols and words that have survived countless generations. They have nurtured, enriched, edified, and strengthened the individual, and they can in the future. They can and do shape faith. Sitting in a darkened hospital room with a solitary patient, momentarily separated from those symbols and from that community, the chaplain is a symbolic link to that faith and its resources. If we miss that sense of history and community, if we reduce religious faith alone to subjective experiences of the moment, we lose its authentic, transcendental character.

Yet we also realize that each individual will subjectively perceive and incorporate those ancient formulations and doctrines and symbols. That is, it is vitally important to so realize if our ministry is to have relevance for that individual.

Yet each person's perception of truth does not make it truth, in religion or anything else. We do not have to assume or pretend that it does, any more than a psychotherapist equates a severely depressed, guilt-ridden person's self-image as "reality." The therapist accepts that self-image as "reality" for that client for that moment. But at the same moment the therapist brings another reality—a reality consensually validated by society—namely, that this depressed person is of infinitely more value than his or her own self-image can or will allow. For the therapist to know his client's "reality" is important, but for his behavior to be determined alone by that "reality" would be foolish.

The chaplain walks between (1) a *faith assumption* that the gospel he proclaims has validity and reality despite how, or even whether, it is internally appropriated by the patient and (2) a *clinical assumption* that this faith will have dynamic, functional value for that patient only when the internal realities become consistent with the message. The chaplain knows from clinical experience that there is a vast difference between *being* forgiven and *feeling* forgiven; between *being* loved and *feeling* loved. To lay hold of both sides of the tension is important if the chaplain is to effect some synthesis between the theological and clinical worlds.

CONFLICTING VIEWS OF HEALTH HAVE FOSTERED "IN-BETWEENNESS"

While the strong influence of psychology upon ministry has fostered tension between the hospital chaplain and the church, conflicting views of health have tended to put him in tension with medicine. Until the era of scientific medicine, health and illness were seen essentially as religious issues. The Bible spends much time with the problem of suffering. Much of the focus is upon political suffering, that is, the suffering inflicted by humans upon humans, because most of the Bible was written by a persecuted minority, during times of captivity and martyrdom. No doubt that fact has skewed the Bible's view of suffering.

However, regardless of the source, suffering was seen in relationship to God. Either God sent it (as retribution) or God allowed it (for our discipline and growth). There is no single biblical view of suffering. There are many views posited by a variety of writers who confronted a variety of circumstances over that thousand-year period. No doubt the most primitive and enduring (but by no means only) theory has been retribution (the Latin word *retribere* means literally "to give back"). The motif assumes personal responsibility. The recurring question in a hospital room, "Why did this happen to me?" usually contains the hidden assumption "I must have done something." Our word "pain" comes from the Latin word *poena*, which means punishment or perfection. While not a comforting theory, retribution does compel the sufferer to reflect upon the message of illness: What is it telling me—about myself, my life, God? What must I now do? The world is just; God is in control. The suffering must be deserved.

However, as the Israelites' suffering increased both in intensity and duration, it seemed to them that the punishment exceeded "the crime." Somehow retribution works best when the suffering is light, brief, or someone else's. To the Hebrew, retribution now seemed too narrow, too simplistic to explain all suffering.

Other theories emerged, not so much to explain suffering but to help people to endure it. Suffering could be redeemed, put to good use, be a means of discipline, growth, insight, maturity, faith. But always suffering is seen in relationship to God. The Lament Psalms, with their protests and arguments directed at God, are tacit reminders of that fact.

Jesus' attitude toward suffering was a curious blend of passivity and aggression. He healed people, and no doubt there were many of his healings not recorded in the New Testament. We do not know fully why he healed or why he did not heal more. But it seems that Jesus did not allow his time and energies to be totally consumed with healing diseases, of which there were a considerable number in his day. Preaching and teaching were fully as important to him.

Nowhere does Jesus suggest that the removal of suffering was his primary mission. Nor does he anywhere hint that the banishment of suffering is anything we should expect as believers. Indeed sin, not suffering, was his primary concern. The healing power was there and on occasion was aggessively employed. His miracles were an active defiance of enemies: he stilled a storm, cast out demons, fed five thousand on morsels, raised Lazarus from the dead. He fought nature, sickness, hunger, and death head on—and he won!

But that kind of aggressive power was not consistent with Jesus. In his personal suffering, he was more passive, acquiescent. He endured, he transcended. But he made it abundantly clear that suffering is inevitable, even more so for a follower. His temptations in the wilderness (to turn stones into bread, to leap from the pinnacle of the Temple, to win a kingdom without the cross) were inducements to use power for his own ends. It became clear to him that there were no shortcuts to "Canaan," but that it would be reached by way of a cross!

The cross was a nonviolent response to violence. It met suffering by bearing and enduring. Because the entire New Testament was written over a brief period of time which was entirely filled with martyrdom, there is in it an urgent, almost desperate expectancy not so characteristic of the Old Testament. So with regard to "the sufferings of this present time," there was the future hope of peace and justice. Not now but soon: "We *shall* inherit the kingdom," "we *shall* be comforted." Again, suffering is not to be explained; it is to be endured and redeemed—faithfully and courageously. In Jesus we have a companion-sufferer. He knows, hears, cries, and dies with us.

No doubt one of the great strengths of the religious (biblical) response to suffering is its reflectiveness. "What does it mean—about life, about

God, about me?" However, it is a more passive approach. The early hospices and hospitals founded by the Christian church offered more spiritual comfort than physical relief.

Scientific inquiry could no longer write off illness as the working of some obscure spiritual force. It became necessary to find empirical causes. Illness was an enemy to be conquered, not endured. It has no moral message. It is a vicious power that ravages and destroys. Modern medicine began an aggressive attack upon it. The battle raged. The medical arsenal to do battle grew in numbers and power: potent drugs, antibiotics, surgery, radioactive therapy, chemotherapy, nuclear medicine, electroconvulsive therapy, cardiopulmonary resuscitation, computerized diagnoses, CAT scans, ultrasound (intraabdominal and intracranial), monitoring equipment (cardiomonitoring, intraarterial monitoring, pulmonary-venous monitoring). Enemies were uncovered: bacteria, viruses, rickettsia, protozoa, worms.

The aggressiveness paid off. Victories were won, particularly with regard to infectious diseases. True, other allies joined the fight: improved sanitation, purer drinking water, better nutrition, vaccines, higher standards of living, improved housing and working conditions. Little matter which "weapons" did the most. The tide had turned. Smallpox, diphtheria, cholera, tuberculosis, polio, Bright's disease, rheumatic and scarlet fevers, and measles were either eliminated or prevented.

One of the unfortunate by-products of the successful war on disease was that it drove a wedge between religion and medicine. There were other losses. There was more focus on the illness than on the ill person. The human was compartmentalized, as were those who treated him. Our views of illness became more narrow and physical. Health was defined in functional terms, as "the absence of illness."

The hospital chaplain was there—between religion and medicine. He was willing to join the fight against disease, though in a lesser rank. It was hard to fit him in. What could he do to aid the medical enterprise? Encourage people when they get discouraged? Boost their morale? Help them smile through it? Help uncooperative patients to cooperate and to take treatment? The only clear shot the chaplain had at the patient was when he was dying or dead. Death represented the failure of medicine. It was a battle lost. The chaplain played an accommodating role. There was not much of a role in a setting that primarily treated disease and defined disease in narrow, physical terms.

How could you quantify the chaplain's efforts? What difference did it really make in the functional recovery of a patient to know that his or her sins were forgiven, that the forces of evil are submissive to God's ultimate will, that the sting of death has been removed in the resurrection of Jesus Christ?

The chaplain found himself in a dilemma back in the 1930s, 1940s, and early 1950s. He wanted acceptance in the clinical world, but his heart wasn't really in it. He realized that functional health is a state only partially (not fully), only temporarily (never permanently) attained. He realized from Scriptures that health was defined more fully as *shalom*: peace, joy, serenity, faith, trust, forgiveness. It was a view that was more relational than functional, for one did not need a sound body to experience *shalom*. The chaplain realized from Scripture that salvation had more to do with deliverance from sin and death than it did from physical suffering, so the tension continued.

The chaplain began to see and confront the tension more directly. However, there began to occur another important phenomenon which changed not only the role of the chaplain but also the role of the hospital. After the early medical victories, new illnesses began to take their place. Many of them were harder to pin down and destroy: heart attacks, hypertension, depression, addictions, accidents, emotional and physical violence. These new illnesses have fuzzy edges. They don't lend themselves to microscopes and vaccines. They seem more related to stress, pressure, life-style, relationships. Now the battleground is not so clearcut, the enemy not so neatly defined, the medical arsenal not so potent.

Where do we start? Though the new battle has brought frustrations and fewer victories than before, it has caused the medical world to rethink its concepts of health and illness. At Lutheran General Hospital, where Project Ten began, this rethinking has produced a statement of Human Ecology: "The understanding and treatment and care of human beings as whole persons in light of their relationships to God, to themselves, to their families, and to their society." This is a broad view which sees illness as a complex interaction between the biologic-psychological-social-mental-spiritual forces within people, as well as the interplay of heredity, environment, decisions, life-styles, diet, exercise, values, faith, meaningful commitments.

Indeed, the Latin word *casus* (from which comes our word "case") means "a fallout of harmony." Illness represents a disharmony on many fronts. This means we suffer on many dimensions simultaneously. To seek and to explore those various dimensions of disharmony within each person and family is the monumental task of today's hospital, but it needs to be done if we are to be as effective in this "second war" as we were in the first.

But as illness is multidimensional, so are the resources for health. There are physical, social, emotional, spiritual capacities and strengths within people which need to be mobilized and channeled. Patients have become more active participants in their own health as we continue to discover the vital links between habits, life-styles, values, and health.

There is the increased effort to help people find fullness of living, which includes among other things self-affirmation, effectively relating to others, trusting in God's continuous love, and experiencing peace, joy, and the courage to live. There has also come an increased recognition of the need for interdisciplinary understanding and interaction. As illness is seen in more complex terms, so has the recognition come that no one profession or method or service can independently or exclusively meet all the forces of illness. Many hospitals today seek to foster a milieu in which each profession has the opportunity to employ its own unique skills, perspective, and goals in the care of people, but where each discipline is also charged with responsibility to critically assess its contribution to optimal patient care.

There are still tensions. Functional health is still the predominant goal in most hospitals. There are patients who prefer a more limited, physically oriented approach to their bodily ailments without, as one put it, "the frills and fancy stuff." But among many there is the growing recognition that we cannot fight these "new illnesses" with the "old weapons." Because of this and the changing views of health and the role of hospitals, religion and medicine have never been closer than they are today.

CONCLUSION

The chaplain walks between two powerful, influential worlds: religion and medicine. Each world has its own ethos, vocabulary, methodology, and mission. Because of the similarities between the fields, the chaplain has identified with both worlds; because of the differences between them, he has stood apart from each world. Partly due to the chaplain's effectiveness in relating to both worlds, but probably due to the changing nature and scope of illness today, religion and medicine find themselves in a more serious engagement than at any time in the past century.

In this regard, the timing of Project Ten is fortunate. To put the resources of both worlds together in this common effort holds great promise. The hospital chaplain has more than a mild interest in this venture. From it he has two major hopes:

1. *A renewed sense of history.* Absorption in the clinical world can distort perspective. Getting in touch with one's traditional roots can renew the chaplain's sense of the ongoing, unfolding history of pastoral care, toward which he has made and is making a significant contribution.

2. *A reinforced prophetic role.* In individual pastoral care, bringing comfort to those "casualties" of our society (a *priestly function*) has led to some forfeiture of a *prophetic role*. To help people struggle with the newly emerging medical-moral issues will be a need and expectation of "prophetic" pastoral care in the future. The chaplain will discover that his clinical training and experience will not be sufficient to meet those needs in a sufficient and competent manner. This project will help the chaplain identify and fulfill that prophetic task.

The chaplain also has two concerns about the project:

1. *That religious traditions be explored with discernment.* Any study of history must consider context—the issues and circumstances of the period under study. Historical movements in the faith traditions, like any historical movement, were human responses to perceived needs. As in any movement, there were excesses, overreactions, "truths" that were culturally bound. It is necessary to explore the wisdom of traditions critically and discriminately if such wisdom is to serve us today. Because it is historical, belonging to faith traditions, does not *necessarily* mean it will or should be relevant to us today.

2. *That the project not become an exercise in historic scholarship— interesting, but irrelevant.* It is extremely important that the project maintain that critical balance between past and present, theory and practice, library and sick room, scholar and clinician. To fail in that balance could result in driving a deeper wedge between religion and medicine.

Without question, the need for and the promise of such an ambitious project remains clear and compelling.

Epilogue

DAVID T. STEIN

**Life can only be understood backwards: but it must be lived
forwards.**

—Kierkegaard

Most books need no postscript, afterthought, addendum, or epilogue.
This book deserves one. I had planned to write something entirely different, but life's events have a way of authoring their own story.

I remember the pathos of the moment, her first postoperative seizure.
She was with her husband, who was chairing a conference of internationally respected scholars. I ran for the house doctor in the Caribbean
hotel. The doctor was "not in." One of the conference consultants who is
chairman of the hematology section at the University of Illinois Medical
Center advised that she be taken to the island hospital. I called for the
ambulance. It arrived without flashing light or siren.

Two hours later she returned to the hotel. Her bills for ambulance
service and outpatient care totaled twenty-five dollars, fifteen for the
ambulance and ten for her medical care. The same afternoon she sat by
the pool, enjoying the balm and breeze of the Caribbean. We had dinner
together that evening in a lovely French café—Elsa, Marty, Beverly,
Dean, Judi, and I.

That was seven months ago. Last Sunday, the eleventh day of October,
Annus Christi 1981, we sang at Elsa Marty's memorial service:

> Lord, let at last thine angels come,
> To Abr'ham's bosom bear me home,
> That I may die unfearing;
> And in its narrow chamber keep
> My body safe in peaceful sleep
> Until thy reappearing.

Epilogue

And then from death awaken me,
That these mine eyes with joy may see,
O Son of God, thy glorious face,
My Savior and my fount of grace.
Lord Jesus Christ, my prayer attend,
My prayer attend,
And I will praise thee without end!

The congregation stood to sing this closing chorus of Bach's Passion According to St. John—Elsa's choice for her memorial service. There was not a dry eye or a depressed heart. There was celebration in the sound, and victory in the song.

"Life can only be understood backwards; but it must be lived forwards." Project Ten: Health/Medicine and the Faith Traditions was struggling for intellectual and conceptual birth, being debated and discussed and shaped as the struggle for life went on in Elsa's fight with cancer.

She was a testimony of courage and determination. She did not surrender to the past; she fought bravely and boldly for life, God's good gift. She lived forwards. But finally she knew that all the clinical care, postop therapy, and medical and scientific interventions would not succeed. In that awareness, she did not retreat from life for a moment. Elsa's tradition and her faith were anchored in the victory of the Lord of life and death. It is indeed remarkable that the first chapters of this book were written during the days of these events.

But the Epilogue is not complete. Another "she" is this day in Room 817 at Lutheran General Hospital. She is recovering from brain surgery. She has fought the disease of cancer for more than seven years. Each medical intervention and effort for healing have enjoyed at least partial success. Dorothy knows so much better than anyone else the sustaining presence of her God during these months and years of illness. Her husband Larry Holst, Division Chief of Pastoral Care at Lutheran General Hospital, authors the last chapter of this book.

I remember Dorothy and Elsa discussing their experiences one evening while sitting together on a couch looking over the emerald blue waters of Nassau Bay. Those who stood around these two remarkable women as they shared their private stories were more than impressed. They tucked into their hearts that night a reverence for such faith to face the presence and ugliness of a disease like cancer. "Life can only be understood backwards; but it must be lived forwards."

Epilogue

The end of this volume is the beginning of a major project which is intended to embrace the endless contradictions, conflicts, and dilemmas of the worlds of medicine and religion. I have seen miracles happen through modern medicine. I have also seen miracles happen in spite of modern medicine. Project Ten: Health/Medicine and the Faith Traditions is the contribution of many people who believe in the value of the debate, the discussion, the disputation—those who dedicate their time and effort to study the past, assess the present, and give tomorrow a legacy of careful, scholarly, and usable knowledge. But more than knowledge, we seek the wisdom to apply our learning, for wisdom means nothing unless our own experience gives it meaning.

Bibliography

MARY-CARROLL SULLIVAN

The following list is in no way all-encompassing. It merely serves to alert readers to the variety of literature available along traditional axes and thematic axes. The disparity of perspectives (theoretician, practitioner, professional, lay person) provides a comprehensive though not exhaustive presentation of the breadth and depth of interfacing facets in the fields of religion and health. Many of the authors listed have written extensively in the area in which they are cited and have treated correlative topics as well. These references should be regarded as a starting point for further investigation. They are presented in the categorical models outlined by Martin E. Marty and Kenneth L. Vaux in Chapters 1 and 7 of this book.

Religion and Medicine

Alexander, Rolf. *The Doctor Alone Can't Cure You*. St. Paul: Macalester Park Publishing Co., 1949.

Allen, D. F. "The Ethical Responsibility of the Physician: A Judeo-Christian Perspective." *Yale Journal of Biology and Medicine* 49, no. 5 (November 1976): 447–54.

"AMA Journal Establishes Medicine-Religion Department." *Journal of the Medical Association of the State of Alabama* 36, no. 11 (May 1967): 1333–35.

Amundsen, Darrel W. "Casuistry and Professional Obligations: The Regulation of Physicians by the Court of Conscience in the Late Middle Ages." *Transactions and Studies of the College of Physicians of Philadelphia* 3 (1982): 22–39, 93–112.

Bibliography

_____."Medical Deontology and Pestilential Disease in the Late Middle Ages." *Journal of the History of Medicine* 32 (October 1977): 403–21.

_____."Medieval Canon Law on Medical and Surgical Practice by the Clergy." *Bulletin of the History of Medicine* 52, no. 1 (Spring 1978): 22–44.

_____."Visigothic Medical Legislation." *Bulletin of the History of Medicine* 45 (1971): 37–60.

Applied Religion. Vols. 1–9. Edited by J. L. Jones. Cleveland: Temple Press, 1923–32.

Ardene, Jean Paul de Rom d'. *Lettres intéressantes pour les médecines de profession, utile aux ecclésiatiques qui veulent s'appliquer à la médecine, curieuses pour tout lecteur*. Avignon: Chez L. Chambeau, 1759.

Austin, P. "Medicine and Religion." *Virginia Medical Monthly* 93, no. 1 (January 1966): 7–11.

Avicenna. *Canon Medicinae*. Translated by Gerard of Cremona. Venice: Apud Juntas, 1952.

Baker, Joseph J. "A Physician's View of Man." In *Man, Medicine, and Theology*, pp. 65–76. New York: Lutheran Church in America, Board of Social Ministry, 1967.

Ballinger, M. B. "The Physician and the Protestant Religion." *Illinois Medical Journal* 132, no. 6 (December 1967): 843–44.

Banks, R. "Health and the Spiritual Dimension: Relationships and Implications for Professional Preparation Programs." *Journal of the School of Health* 50, no. 4 (April 1980): 195–202.

Barbour, Ian G. *Christianity and the Scientist*. New York: Association Press, 1960.

Barton, Richard Thomas. *Religious Doctrine and Medical Practice*. Springfield, Ill.: Charles C. Thomas, 1958.

Bauer, John E. "The Health Seekers in the Westward Movement." *Mississippi Valley Historical Review* 46 (June 1959): 91–110.

Belgum, David R., ed. *Religion and Medicine: Essays on Meaning, Values, and Health*. Ames, Iowa: Iowa State University Press, 1967.

Black, John. *The Dominion of Man*. Edinburgh: Edinburgh University Press, 1970.

Blishen, Bernard R. *Doctors and Doctrines: The Ideology of Medical Care in Canada*. Toronto: University of Toronto Press, 1969.

Brendle, Thomas Royce, and Unger, Claude W. *Folk Medicine of the Pennsylvania Germans: The Non-occult Cures*. New York: A. M. Kelley, 1970.

Bromiley, G. W., ed. *Zwingli and Bullinger*. Library of Christian Classics 24. Philadelphia: Westminster Press, 1953.

Broughton, Leonard Gaston. *Religion and Health*. New York: F. U. Revell, 1909.

Calian, C. S. "Theological and Scientific Understandings of Health." *Hospital Progress* 59, no. 12 (December 1978): 45–47, 61–62.

Bibliography

Cameron, J. M. "The Bible and Legal Medicine." *Medicine, Science, and the Law* 10, no. 1 (January 1970): 7–13.

Carstairs, G. Morris. "Medicine and Faith in Rural Rajasthan." In *Health, Culture, and Community*. Edited by Benjamin D. Paul, pp. 107–34. New York: Russell Sage Foundation, 1955.

"A Contemporary Bibliography on Psychiatry and Religion." *International Psychiatry Clinics* 5, no. 4 (1969): 305–13.

Convocation on Medicine and Theology, Mayo Clinic and Rochester Methodist Hospital. *Dialogue in Medicine and Theology*. Edited by Dale White. Nashville: Abingdon Press, 1968.

Cope, Oliver. *Man, Mind, and Medicine: The Doctor's Education*. Philadelphia: J. B. Lippincott Co., 1968.

Debreyne, Pierre J. C. *La théologie morale et les sciences médicales*. 6th ed. Edited by Ange E. A. Ferrand. Paris: Poussielque frères, 1884.

Doniger, Simon, ed. *Religion and Health: A Symposium by Paul Tillich and Others*. New York: Association Press, 1958.

Edmunds, Vincent, and Scorer, Charles Gordon, eds. *Ideals in Medicine: A Christian Approach to Medical Practice*. London: Tyndale Press, 1958.

Heinecken, Martin J. "Medicine and Theology." In *Man, Medicine, and Theology*, pp. 7–46. New York: Lutheran Church in America, Board of Social Ministry, 1967.

Hiltner, Seward. *Religion and Health*. New York: Macmillan Co., 1943.

Marty, Martin E. *A Nation of Behavers*. Chicago: University of Chicago Press, 1976.

Poole, Robert, and Hiltner, Seward, eds. "Human and Religious Values in Medical Practice." Multilith. Chicago: American Medical Association, 1978.

Shriver, Donald W. *Medicine and Religion: Strategies of Care*. Pittsburgh: University of Pittsburgh Press, 1981.

Szasz, Thomas. *The Theology of Medicine: The Political-Philosophical Foundations of Medical Ethics*. Baton Rouge: Louisiana State University Press, 1977.

Tillich, Paul. "The Relation of Religion and Health: Historical Considerations and Theoretical Questions." *The Review of Religion* 10 (May 1946): 348–84.

World Council of Churches. *The Healing Church: The Tübingen Consultation*. Geneva: World Council of Churches, 1965.

Judaism

Aboab, Isaac (d. 1492). *Menorat HaMaor*. Jerusalem: Mosad Kook, 1961.

Adler, Mark. "Religious Commitment in Medical Practice: A Jewish Perspective." *Yale Journal of Biology and Medicine* 49, no. 3 (July 1976): 295–300.

Alpert, Rebecca T. "From Jewish Science to Rabbinical Counseling: The Evaluation of the Relationship Between Religion and Health by the American Reform Rabbinate, 1916–1954." Ph.D. dissertation, Temple University, 1978.

Bibliography

Appel, John. "Christian Science and the Jews." *Jewish Social Studies* 31 (April 1969): 100–121.

Assia: Original Articles, Abstracts, and Reports on Matters of Halacha and Medicine. Edited by Abraham Steinberg. Jerusalem: The Falk Schlesinger Institute for Medical Halachic Research at Shaare Zedek Hospital, 1972.

Bakan, David. *Sigmund Freud and the Jewish Mystical Tradition.* Boston: Beacon Press, 1975.

Baron, Salo W. *A Social and Religious History of the Jews.* 2d ed. Philadelphia: JPSA, 1958.

Baruch, J. Z. "[Maimonides as Physician]." *Tijdschrift Voor Ziekenverpleging* 23, no. 3 (February 1970): 143–50.

Belkin, Samuel. *Philo and the Oral Law: The Philonic Interpretation of Biblical Law in Relation to the Palestinian Halakah.* Cambridge, Mass.: Harvard University Press, 1940.

Berkowitz, P., and Berkowitz, N. S. "The Jewish Patient in the Hospital." *American Journal of Nursing* 67, no. 11 (November 1967): 2335–37.

"Beyond the Science: III, Prayer of a Hebrew Physician." *Journal of the American Osteopathic Association* 74, no. 5 (January 1975): 369–70.

Birnbaum, Ervin. *The Politics of Compromise: State and Religion in Israel.* Cranberry, N.J.: Fairleigh Dickinson University Press, 1970.

Bloom, M. S. "Some Aspects of Judaism and Dentistry." *New York State Dental Journal* 56, no. 5 (May 1976): 166.

Buchler, Adolf. *Studies in Sin and Atonement in the Rabbinic Literature of the First Century.* 1928. Library of Biblical Studies. New York: Ktav Publishing House, 1967.

Carmoly, Eliakim. *Histoire des Médecins Juifs.* Brussels, 1844.

Chavel, C. *Kit 'vei HaRamban.* Jerusalem: Mosad HaRav Kook, 1965.

Cowen, D. L. "A Late Medieval Yiddish Manuscript on Bloodletting." *Clio Medica* 10, no. 4 (December 1975): 267–76.

Cronbach, Abraham. "The Psychoanalytic Study of Judaism." *Hebrew Union College Annual* 8–9 (1931–32): 605–731.

Ebied, Rifaat Y. *Bibliography of Medieval Arabic and Jewish Medicine and Allied Sciences.* London: Wellcome Institute, 1971.

Ebstein, Wilhelm. *Die Medizin im Neuen Testament und im Talmud.* Stuttgart, 1903.

Friedenwald, Harry. *The Jews and Medicine: Essays.* 2 vols. Baltimore: Johns Hopkins Press, 1944.

Gross, Louis. *What Is Jewish Science?* Brooklyn: Jewish Science Centre of Union Temple, 1928.

The Jewish Patients' Bill of Rights. Pamphlet. New York: Agudath Israel of America, n.d.

Bibliography

Roman Catholicism

Abbott, Walter M., ed. *The Documents of Vatican II*. New York: America Press, 1966.

Anselm, Saint. *Book of Meditations and Prayers*. London: Burns & Oates, 1872.

————. *Cur Deus Homo*. Edinburgh: John Grant, 1909.

Antonelli, Guiseppe. *Medicina pastoralis in usum confessariorum et curiarum ecclesiasticarum*. 3 vols. Rome: F. Pustet, 1906.

Antony-Schmitt, Marie Madeleine. *Le cult de saint Sebastien en Alsace: Médecine populaire et saints guerisseurs; Essai de sociologie religieuse*. Strasbourg: Librairie Istra, 1977.

Aquinas Institute of Philosophy and Theology, Institute of Spiritual Theology. *Sex, Love, and the Life of the Spirit*. Chicago: Priory Press, 1966.

Arbesmann, Rudolph. "The Concept of 'Christus Medicus' in St. Augustine." *Traditio* 10 (1954): 70–93.

Ashley, Benedict M., and O'Rourke, Kevin D. *Health Care Ethics: A Theological Analysis*. St. Louis: Catholic Hospital Association, 1978.

Augustine, Saint. *Writings of Saint Augustine*. Vol. 15: *Treatises on Marriage and Other Subjects*. The Fathers of the Church: A New Translation 27. Edited by Roy Joseph Defarrari. New York, 1955.

Curran, Charles E. *Contemporary Problems in Moral Theology*. Notre Dame: Fides Publishers, 1970.

Haring, Bernard. *Morality Is for Persons*. New York: Farrar, Straus & Giroux, 1971.

The Human Body: Papal Teachings, Selected and Arranged by the Benedictine Monks of Solesmes. Boston: St. Paul Editions, 1960.

Kelly, Gerald. *Medico-Moral Problems*. St. Louis: Catholic Hospital Association, 1958.

Overkage, P., and Rahner, K. *Das Problem der Homonisation*. Questiones disputatae 12/13. Freiburg, 1961.

Rahner, Karl. *On the Theology of Death*. New York: Herder & Herder, 1961.

Reich, Warren. *Medico-Moral Problems and the Principle of Totality: A Catholic Viewpoint*. Washington, D.C.: Veterans Administration Hospitals, 1967.

Lutheranism

American Lutheran Church. *Christian Faith and the Ministry of Healing*. New York: American Lutheran Church, 1965.

Beintker, Horst. "Die Bedeutung der Tradition bei Luther und im Luthertum." *Kairos: Zeitschrift für Religionsurssenschaft und Theologie* 21, no. 1 (1979): 1–29.

Blakely, R. G. "God—Concepts of Lutheran Deaf Adults." *American Annals of the Deaf* 113, no. 4 (September 1968): 942–44.

Bibliography

Childs, James M. "A Theology for Lutheran Social Services." *Trinity Seminary Review* 1, no. 9 (Spring 1979): 9–15.

Goldammer, K. "[Diagnosis of Disease as Existence Analysis in Religious Symbolic Language]." *Neue Münchner Beitrage zur Geschichte der Medizin und Naturwissenschaften: Medizinhistorische Reihe* 7–8 (1978): 145–61.

Golder, Christian. *History of the Deaconess Movement in the Christian Church.* Cincinnati: Jennings & Pye, 1903.

Larsen, Donald H., with David E. Farley and Norman E. Minich. "Health and Healing in the Lutheran Church: Tradition and Practice." In *Health and Healing: Ministry of the Church.* Edited by Henry L. Letterman, pp. 43–59. Chicago: Wheat Ridge Foundation, 1980.

Lundeen, Lyman T. "Process Theology and Lutheran Priorities." *Currents in Theology and Mission* 7 (1980): 24–33.

Luther, Martin. "Der grosse Katechismus, 1529." In *Luthers Werke in Auswall.* Vol. 4: *Schriften von 1529 bis 1545.* 5th rev. ed. Edited by Otto Clemen, pp. 31–34. Berlin: Walter de Gruyter, 1959.

Preus, Herman A. "Luther on the Universal Priesthood and the Office of the Ministry." *Concordia Journal* 5, no. 2 (March 1979): 55–62.

Rohe, H. W. "A Denominational Executive Lutheran Church, Missouri Synod, Examines the Deaf Church and the Community." *American Annals of the Deaf* 113, no. 4 (September 1968): 934–35.

Schwarzwaller, Klaus. "Theologische Kriterien für politische Entscheidungen bei Luther." *Kerygma und Dogma* 26 (April–June 1980): 88–108.

Sherman, Franklin, ed. *Christian Hope and the Future of Humanity.* Minneapolis: Augsburg Publishing House, 1969.

Simonson, S. H. "An Ephphatha Services Chaplain Views the American Lutheran Church at Work with the Deaf in 1967." *American Annals of the Deaf* 113, no. 4 (September 1968): 893–95.

Tappert, Theodore G., ed. *Luther: Letters of Spiritual Counsel.* Library of Christian Classics 18. Philadelphia: Westminster Press, 1955.

United Lutheran Church. *Report of the Commission on Anointing and Healing.* 1962.

Wentz, Frederick K., and Witmer, Robert H. *The Problem of Abortion.* New York: Lutheran Church in America, Board of Social Ministry, 1967.

Islam

Akhavayni al-Bukhari, Abu Baker Rabi ibn Ahmad al. *Hiddayat al-muta'allimin fi al-tibb* [Direction of Teachers in Medicine]. Edited by Jalal Matini. Danishgah Intisharat, Meshed University Publications 9. Meshed, Iran: Meshed University Press, 1965.

Alwaye, Mohiaddin. "The Conception of Life in Islam." *Majallat al-Azhar* (Journal of al-Azhar University) 45 (March 1973): 56–88.

Bibliography

Avicenna (Husayn bin Abd-Ullah Hasan bin Ali bin Sina) (Ibn Sina) al-Qanun fi al-Tibb (11th Century). Edited and translated by Mazhar H. Shah as *The General Principle of Avicenna's Canon of Medicine*. Karachi: Naveed Clinic, 1966.

Barber, S. G., and Wright, A. D. "Muslims, Ramaden, and Diabetes Mellitus" (letter). *British Medical Journal* 2, no. 6191 (September 1979): 675.

Brandenburg, D. "[Alchemy and Medicine: Therapeutics in Ancient Times and in the Islamic Middle Ages (II)]." *Medizinische Monatsschrift* 29, no. 1 (January 1975): 25–28.

Coulson, Noel James. *A History of Islamic Law*. Islamic Surveys 2. (Edinburgh: Edinburgh University Press, 1964.

Guraya, Muhammad Yusuf. "The Importance of Health in Islam and in Islamic Countries." *Hamdard* 14 (1971).

Hamarneh, S. "The Physician and the Health Professions in Medieval Islam." *Bulletin of the New York Academy of Medicine* 47, no. 9 (September 1971): 1088–112.

Hamdard: Voice of Eastern Medicine (journal). Organ of Institute of Health and Tibbi Research. Karachi, 1957ff.

Haque, Maulana Muntakhabul. "Health and Islam." *Hamdard* 14, no. 3–4 (July–September 1971): 44–45.

Hashmi, K. Z. "Doctors and the Islamic Penal Code" (letter). *Lancet* 1, no. 8116 (March 1979): 614.

Husaini, I. M. "Islam and Modern Problems." *Majallat al-Azhar* (Journal of al-Azhar University) 45 (February 1973): 123–49.

Ibn Taymiyah, Ahmad Ibn 'Abd Al-Halim (Ibn Taymiyya). *Majmu' Fatawa* [Collection of Religious Opinions] vol. 10: *Kitab' Ilm al-Suluk* [Book on the Science of Behavior] Riad, 1381–83, 1961–63.

Levey, Martin. "Medical Deontology in Ninth Century Islam." *Journal of the History of Medicine and Allied Sciences* 21 (1966): 358–73.

Said, Hakim Mohammed. "Al-Tibb al-Islami." *Hamdard* 19, nos. 1–6 (January–June 1976): 1–119.

————. "HE Is the Healer." *Hamdard* II, no. 13 (January–March 1968): 29–31.

Schacht, Joseph. *An Introduction to Islamic Law*. Oxford: Clarendon Press, 1964.

Schacht, Joseph, and Bosworth, C. E., eds. *The Legacy of Islam*. 2d ed. Oxford: Clarendon Press, 1974.

Mainline Protestant (Presbyterian, Anglican, Methodist)

Anglican-Clerical and Medical Committee of Inquiry into Spiritual Faith and Mental Healing. *Spiritual Healing*. London, 1914.

Anglican Diocese of Toronto, Committee on the Church's Ministry to the Sick." *Handbook*. Toronto, 1964.

Baragar, C. A. "John Wesley and Medicine." *Annals of Medical History* 10, no. 1

Bibliography

(March 1928): 59ff.

Beall, Otho T., Jr., and Shryock, Richard T. *Cotton Mather*. Baltimore: Johns Hopkins Press, 1954.

Bieler, André. *L'homme et la femme dans la morale calviniste: La doctrine reformée sur l'amour, le mariage, le célibat, le divorce, l'adultère et la prostitution, considerée dans son cadre historique*. Geneva: Labor & Fides, 1963.

Church of England, Church Information Office. *On Dying Well: An Anglican Contribution to the Debate on Euthanasia*. London, 1975.

Crowlesmith, John. "Spiritual Healing in the Methodist Church." *London Quarterly and Holborn Review* 181 (May 1960): 103–32.

_____, ed. *Religion and Medicine: Essays by Members of the Methodist Society for Medical and Pastoral Psychology*. London: Epworth Press, 1962.

Gusmer, Charles W. "Anointing of the Sick in the Church of England." *Worship* 45, no. 5 (May 1971): 262–72.

Hill, Alfred Wesley. *John Wesley Among the Physicians: At Study of Eighteenth-Century Medicine*. London: Epworth Press, 1958.

Jackson, Samuel M., ed. *Selected Works of Huldreich Zwingli (1484–1531), the Reformer of German Switzerland*. Philadelphia: University of Pennsylvania, 1901.

McAdoo, Henry R. *The Spirit of Anglicanism: A Survey of Anglican Theological Method in the Seventeenth Century*. New York: Charles Scribner's Sons, 1965.

The Methodist Church and Problems of Medical Care: Report on a Research Seminar by Lee Ranck. Washington, D.C.: Methodist Church (U.S.) Board of Social Concerns, Division of Temperance and General Welfare, n.d.: (1960s?).

Ott, Philip W. "A Corner of History: John Wesley and the Non-naturals." *Preventive Medicine* 9 (1980): 578–84.

Taylor, Jeremey. *The Rule and Exercises of Holy Dying*. London: R. Royston, 1951.

United Presbyterian Church in the U.S.A. *The Relation of Christian Faith to Health*. New York, 1960.

_____. General Assembly. *Sexuality and the Human Community*. Philadelphia, 1970.

Wesley, John. *Primitive Remedies*. Santa Barbara, Calif.: Woodbridge Press, 1973.

White, Dale, ed. *Dialogue in Medicine and Theology*. Nashville: Abingdon Press, 1967.

Eastern Christianity

Athenagoras. *Embassy for the Christians and the Resurrection of the Dead*. Translated by Joseph Hugh Crehan. Westminster, Md.: Newman Press, 1956.

Bibliography

Constantelos, Demetrios J. *Byzantine Philanthropy and Social Welfare*. Rutgers Byzantine Series. New Brunswick, N.J.: Rutgers University Press, 1968.

_____. *Marriage, Sexuality, and Celibacy: A Greek Orthodox Perspective*. Minneapolis: Light & Life Publishing Co., 1975.

Exetastes. *Contemporary Issues: Orthodox Christian Perspectives*. New York: Greek Orthodox Archdiocese Press, 1976.

Dionysiatou, Gabriel. *Malthousianismos: To Englema tes Genoktonias* [Malthusianism: The Crime of Genocide]. Volos: Holy Mountain Library, 1957.

Keenan, Sister Mary Emily. "St. Gregory of Nazianzus and Early Byzantine Medicine." *Bulletin of the History of Medicine* 9, no. 1 (January 1941): 8–30.

Service Book of the Holy Orthodox-Catholic Apostolic Church (the Euchologion). Compiled, translated, and arranged by Isabel Florence Hapgood. Rev. ed. with endorsement by Patriarch Tikhon. New York: Association Press, 1922.

Evangelical (Baptist, Fundamentalist, Pentecostal)

Abundant Life. Oral Roberts Evangelistic Association, Tulsa, Okla.

American Friends Service Committee, Family Planning Committee. *Who Shall Live? Man's Control over Birth and Death*. New York: Hill & Wang, 1970.

Blair, H. J. "Spiritual Healing: An Enquiry." *Evangelical Quarterly* 30 (July–September 1958): 147–51.

Blanco, R. L. "The Diary of Jonathan Potts: A Quaker Medical Student in Edinburgh (1966–67)." *Transactions and Studies of the College of Physicians of Philadelphia* 44, no. 3 (1977): 119–30.

Bourgeois, M., and Broustra, J. "Hysteria and Pentecostism (Ritual Possession and Hystero-Demonophthic Trance)." *Annales Medico-Psychologiques* 1, no. 1 (January 1974): 106–12.

Bragg, E. A., Jr., and Plotkin, S. A. "Fundamentalist and Eschatologic Approach to Ethics." *New England Journal of Medicine* 287, no. 4 (July 27, 1972): 205.

Cross, H. E., et al. "Cancer of the Cervix in the Amish." *Transactions of the Association of American Physicians* 80 (1967): 133–41.

Guyther, J. R. "Medical Attitudes of the Amish." *Maryland State Medical Journal* 28, no. 10 (October 1979): 40–41.

Innovative American Religions (Nineteenth Century: Christian Science, Mormon, Adventist, Jehovah's Witnesses)

This category refers to the distinctly American traditions which arose primarily in the nineteenth century and whose policy and polity addresses in a unique way the question of health as a pivotal issue.

Acherman, Terrence F. "The Limits of Beneficence: Jehovah's Witnesses and Childhood Cancer." *The Hastings Center Report* 10, no. 4 (August 1980): 13–18.

Bibliography

Amundsen, W. "Experience of the Seventh-Day Adventist Church in North America." *American Annals of the Deaf* 113, no. 4 (September 1968): 896–97.

Armstrong, Joseph. *The Mother Church*. Boston: Christian Science Publishing Society, 1911.

Bancroft, Samuel Putnam. *Mrs. Eddy as I Knew Her in 1870*. Boston: George H. Ellis Press, 1923.

Bates, Ernest S., and Dittimore, John V. *Mary Baker Eddy: The Truth and the Tradition*. New York: Alfred A. Knopf, 1932.

Bates, Joseph. *The Autobiography of Elder Joseph Bates*. Battle Creek, Mich.: Steam Press of the Seventh-Day Adventist Publishing Association, 1863. Reprint ed., Nashville: Southern Publishing Association, 1970.

Blake, John B. "Health Reform." In *The Rise of Adventism: Religion and Society in Mid-Nineteenth Century America*. Edited by Edwin S. Gaustad, pp. 30–49. New York: Harper & Row, 1974.

"Blood, Medicine, and the Law of God." *Watchtower*. Watchtower Bible and Tract Society of Pennsylvania, 1961.

"[Blood Transfusions and Jehovah's Witnesses]." *Nouvelle Presse Médicale* 4, 20 (May 1975): 1513–18.

Braden, Charles. *Christian Science Today: Power, Policy, Practice*. Dallas: Southern Methodist University Press, 1958.

Buckley, James Monroe. *Christian Science and Other Superstitions*. New York: The Century Co., 1899.

———. *Christian Science, Faith-Healing, and Kindred Phenomena*. New York, 1892.

Butler, Jonathan M. "Adventism and the American Experience." In *The Rise of Adventism*. Edited by Edwin S. Gaustad, pp. 173–206. New York: Harper & Row, 1974.

Canright, D. M. *Life of Mrs. E. G. White, Seventh-Day Adventist Prophet: Her False Claims Refuted*. Cincinnati: Standard Publishing Co., 1919.

Carver, Henry E. *Mrs. E. G. White's Claims to Divine Inspiration Examined*. 2d ed. Marion, Iowa: Advent and Sabbath Advocate Press, 1877.

Casale, F. "Blood Transfusions and Jehovah's Witnesses" (letter). *British Medical Journal* 1, no. 6180 (June 1979): 1796.

"Christian Science and Community Medicine." *New England Journal of Medicine* 290, no. 7 (February 1974): 401–2.

"Christian Science and Mind Cure in America: A Review Article." *Journal of the History of Behavioral Science* 11 (1975): 299–305.

Cleveland, S. E. "Jehovah's Witnesses and Human Tissue Donation." *Journal of Clinical Psychology* 32, no. 2 (April 1976): 453–58.

Defense of Eld. James White and Wife: Vindication of Their Moral and Christian Character. Battle Creek, Mich.: Seventh-Day Adventist Publishing Association, 1870.

Bibliography

DiPaolo, Vince. "Adventist Hospital Groups Get the Urge to Merge." *Modern Healthcare* 10 (October 1980): 56–62.

Ellen G. White Estate. *Medical Science and the Spirit of Prophecy*. Washington, D.C.: Review and Herald Publishing Association, 1971.

Enstrom, J. E. "Cancer and Total Mortality Among Active Mormons." *Cancer* 42, no. 4 (October 1978): 1943–51.

Ericksen, Ephraim E. *The Psychological and Ethical Aspects of Mormon Group Life*. Chicago: University of Chicago Press, 1922.

Eustace, Herbert W. *Christian Science: Its Clear Correct Teaching*. Berkeley, Calif.: Lederer, Street, & Zeus Co., 1934.

Flower, Benjamin O. *Christian Science as a Religious Belief and a Therapeutic Agent*. Boston: Twentieth Century Co., 1909.

Frankel, Lawrence S.; Damme, Catherine J.; and Van Eys, Jan. "Childhood Cancer and the Jehovah's Witness Faith." *Pediatrics* 60 (December 1977): 916–21.

Gaustad, Edwin S., ed. *The Rise of Adventism: Religion and Society in Mid-Nineteenth-Century America*. New York: Harper & Row, 1974.

Healing Through Spiritual Awakening. Boston: First Church of Christ, Scientist, 1955.

Jehovah's Witnesses and the Question of Blood. New York: Watchtower Bible and Tract Society of New York, 1977.

Loughborough, J. N. *Great Second Advent Movement: Its Rise and Progress*. Washington, D.C.: Review and Herald Publishing Association, 1909.

Nudelman, A. E., and Nudelman, B. E. "Health and Illness Behavior of Christian Scientists." *Social Science of Medicine* 6, no. 2 (April 1972): 499–513.

Numbers, Ronald L. *Prophetess of Health: A Study of Ellen G. White*. New York: Harper & Row, 1976.

Olsen, M. Ellsworth. *History of the Origin and Progress of Seventh-Day Adventists*. Washington, D.C.: Review and Herald Publishing Association, 1925.

Robinson, Dores E. *Story of Our Health Message: The Origin, Character, and Development of Health Education in the Seventh-Day Adventist Church*. 3d ed. Nashville: Southern Publishing Association, 1965.

Schwarz, Richard W. *John Harvey Kellog, M.D.* Nashville: Southern Publishing Association, 1970.

White, Ellen G. *Health: Or How to Live*. Battle Creek, Mich.: Steam Press of the Seventh-Day Adventist Publishing Association, 1965.

Eastern Religions

Ayurveda. In *Sacred Books of the East (Caraka Samhita)*. Edited by F. Max Mueller. Mystic, Conn.: Lawrence Verry, 1975.

Bibliography

Bocking, Brian. "Neo-Confucian Spirituality and the Samurai Ethic." *Religion* 10 (Spring 1980): 1–15.

Ichikawa, Akira. "Compassionate Politics: Buddhist Concepts as Political Guide." *Journal of Church and State* 21 (Spring 1979): 247–63.

Jones, Richard H. "Jung and Eastern Religious Traditions." *Religion* 9 (August 1979): 141–56.

Klunniar, Arthur, et al. *Medicine in Chinese Cultures: Comparative Studies of Health Care in Chinese and Other Societies.* Washington, D.C.: National Institute of Health, 1975.

Ling, Trevor O. "Philosophers, Gentlemen, and Anthropologists: Prolegomena to the Study of Religion." *Scottish Journal of Religious Studies* 1, no. 1 (Spring 1980): 26–39.

Matsugi, Nobuhiko. "A Contemporary Buddhist's Evaluation of Scientific Culture." *Japan Christian Quarterly* 46 (Spring 1980): 83–85.

Miyata, Mitsuo. "Die Verkundigung des Evangeliums in der japanischen Gesellschaft." *Zeitschrift für evangelische Ethik* 24 (April 1980): 130–43.

Porkert, Manfred. "Chinese Medicine: A Traditional Healing Science." In *Ways of Health*. Edited by David Sobel, pp. 147–72. New York: Harcourt Brace Jovanovich, 1979.

————. *The Theoretical Foundations of Chinese Medicine: Systems of Correspondence.* Cambridge: M. I. T. Press, 1974.

Ross, R. R. "Non-being and Being in Taoist and Western Traditions." *Religious Traditions* 2 (October 1979): 24–38.

Udupa, K. M., and Singh, Curmchan, eds. *Religion and Medicine.* Varanasi: Institute of Medical Sciences, Banaras Hindu University, 1974.

Weiss, Mitchell G. "Caraka Samhita on the Doctrine of Karma." In *Karma and Rebirth in Classical Indian Traditions*. Edited by W. D. O'Flaherty. Los Angeles: University of California Press, 1980.

Zimmer, Henry R. *Hindu Medicine.* Baltimore: Johns Hopkins Press, 1948.

Native Religions

Carmichael, S. "Medicine and Contemporary Cultism" (letter). *Canadian Medical Association Journal* 119, no. 8 (October 1978): 861.

Creson, D. L.; McKinley, C.; and Evans, R. "Folk Medicine in Mexican-American Sub-culture." *Diseases of the Nervous System* 30, no. 4 (April 1969): 264–66.

Gaviria, M., and Wintrob, R. M. "Supernatural Influence in Psychopathology: Puerto Rican Folk Beliefs About Mental Illness." *Canadian Psychiatric Association Journal* 21, no. 6 (October 1976): 361–69.

Hall, A. L., and Bourne, P. G. "Indigenous Therapists in Southern Black Urban Community." *Archives in General Psychiatry* 28, no. 1 (January 1973): 137–42.

Bibliography

Hand, Wayland D., ed. *American Folk Medicine: A Symposium*. Berkeley: University of California Press, 1976.

Kiev, Ari. *Curanderismo: Mexican-American Folk Psychiatry*, pp. 3–21, 33–47, 130–47. New York: Free Press, 1968.

————, ed., *Magic, Faith, and Healing*. New York: Free Press, 1964.

LaBarre, Weston. "Confession as Cathartic Therapy in American Indian Tribes." In *Magic, Faith, and Healing*. Edited by Ari Kiev. New York: Free Press, 1964.

Lubdhansky, I; Egri, G.; and Stokes, J. "Puerto Rican Spiritualists View Mental Illness: The Faith Healer as a Paraprofessional." *American Journal of Psychiatry* 127, no. 3 (September 1970): 312–21.

Luckert, K. W. "Traditional Navaho Theories of Disease and Healing." *Arizona Medicine* 29, no. 7 (July 1972): 571–73.

Marriott, Alice, and Rachlin, Carol K. *Peyote*. New York: Thomas Y. Crowell Co., 1971.

Middleton, John, ed. *Magic, Witchcraft, and Curing*. American Museum Sourcebooks in Anthropology. Garden City, N.Y.: Natural History Press, 1967.

Miller, S. I., and Schoenfeld, L. "Grief in the Navajo: Psychodynamics and Culture." *International Journal of Social Psychiatry* 19, no. 3 (Autumn 1973): 187–91.

Myerhoff, Barbara C. *Peyote Hunt: The Sacred Journey of the Huichol Indians*. Ithaca: Cornell University Press, 1974.

Nall, F. C., and Speilberg, J. "Social and Cultural Factors in the Responses of Mexican-Americans to Medical Treatment." *Journal of Health and Social Behavior* 8, no. 4 (December 1967): 299–308.

Snow, Loudell F. "Folk Medical Beliefs and Their Implications for Care of Patients: A Review Based on Studies Among Black Americans." *Annals of Internal Medicine* 81 (1974): 69–108.

————. "Sorcerers, Saints and Charlatans: Black Folk Healers in Urban America." *Culture, Medicine, and Psychiatry* 2, no. 1 (March 1978): 82–96.

Steiger, Brad. *Medicine Power: The American Indian's Revival of His Spiritual Heritage and Its Relevance for Modern Man*. New York: Doubleday & Co., 1974.

Well-being

Baumann, Barbara. "Diversities in Conceptions of Health and Physical Fitness." *Journal of Health and Human Behavior* 2 (1961): 39–46.

Besson, F. "[Health, That Modern Utopia]." *Praxis* 61, no. 6 (February 1972): 144–46.

Biersdorf, J. E., and Johnson, J. R., Jr. "Religion and Physical Disability." *Rehabilitation Record* 7, no. 1 (January–February 1966): 1–4.

Bissonnier, H. "The Mentally Retarded in the Plan of God." *Bulletin des Infirmières Catholiques Canadiennes* 36, no. 1 (January–February 1969): 3–10.

Bibliography

Breslow, Lester. "A Quantitative Approach to the World Health Organization Definition of Health: Physical, Mental, and Social Well-being." *International Journal of Epidemiology* 1 (1972): 347–55.

Carlson, Rick. *The End of Medicine*. New York: John Wiley & Sons, 1975.

Cooper, T., and Mitchell, S. C. "Preventive Medicine: The Approximation of Paradise." *Preventive Medicine* 1, no. 1 (March 1972): 15–19.

Coulter, Harris. *Homeopathic Medicine*. Falls Church, Va.: American Foundation for Homeopathy, 1972.

Dick, Russell Leslie. *Toward Health and Wholeness*. New York: Macmillan Co., 1960.

Dubos, René Jules. *Health and Disease*. New York: Time, Inc., 1965.

Gaylin, Ned L. "On Creativeness and a Psychology of Well-being." In *Innovations in Client-Centered Therapy*. Edited by David A. Wexler and Laura North Rice, pp. 343–44. New York: John Wiley & Sons, 1974.

Hagen, Kristofor. *Faith and Health*. Philadelphia: Fortress Press, 1961.

Hennes, James D. "Review Article: The Measurement of Health." *Medical Care Review* 29 (1972): 1269–88.

Herzlich, Claudine. *Health and Illness: Social Psychological Analysis*. London: Academe Press, 1973.

Hocking, William Ernest. *The Self, Its Body and Freedom*. New Haven: Yale University Press, 1928.

Hodson, Geoffrey. *Health and the Spiritual Life*. London: Theosophical Publishing House, 1930.

Hoffman, Hans. *Religion and Mental Health*. New York: Harper & Row, 1961.

Holinger, Paul C., and Tubesing, Donald A. "Models of Health and Wholeness." *Journal of Religion and Health* 18, no. 3 (1979): 203–12.

Holman, Charles. *The Religion of a Healthy Mind*. New York: Round Table Press, 1939.

Johns, Warren L., and Utt, Richard H., eds. *The Vision Bold: An Illustrated History of the Seventh-Day Adventist Philosophy of Health*. Washington, D.C.: Review and Herald Publishing Association, 1977.

Kosa, John, and Zola, Irving K., eds. *Poverty and Health: A Sociological Analysis*. Rev. ed. Cambridge, Mass.: Harvard University Press, 1975.

Lapsley, James N. *Salvation and Health: The Interlocking Processes of Life*. Philadelphia: Westminster Press, 1972.

Leavitt, Judith W., and Numbers, Ronald L., eds. *Sickness and Health in America*. Madison: University of Wisconsin Press, 1978. Pp. 433–41.

Lerner, Monroe. "Conceptualizations of Health and Social Well-being." In *Health Status Indexes*. Edited by Robert Berg, pp. 3, 6. Chicago: Hospital Research and Educational Trust, 1973.

Meserve, Harry C. "Guidelines for Health." *Journal of Religion and Health* 18, no. 3 (1979): 171–75.

Bibliography

Moses, Alfred Geiger. *Jewish Science: Psychology of Health, Joy, and Success, or the Applied Psychology of Judaism*. Mobile, Ala.: By the author, 1920.

Neale, Sister Ann. "The Concept of Health in Medicine: A Philosophical Analysis." Ph.D. dissertation, Georgetown University, 1976.

Nute, William L., Jr. "Health and Salvation: Definitions and Implications." *Study Encounter* 2, no. 3 (1966): 137–41.

Ott, Philip W. "John Wesley on Health: A Word for Sensible Regimen." *Methodist History* 18 (April 1980): 193–204.

Parker, Michael Wynne. *Healing and the Wholeness of Man*. New York: Regency Press, 1974.

Parkhurst, Genevieve. *Healing and Wholeness Are Yours*. St. Paul: Macalester Park Publishing Co., 1957.

Parsons, Talcott. "Definition of Health and Illness in the Light of American Values and Social Structure." In *Patients, Physicians, and Illness: A Sourcebook in Behavioral Science and Health*. 3d ed. Edited by E. Gartly Jaco. New York: Free Press, 1979.

———. "Definitions of Health in the Light of American Values and Social Structures." In *Social Structure and Personality*. New York: Free Press, 1964.

Rankin, W. W. "Concepts of Illness and Care of the Ill." *Ethics in Science and Medicine* 6, no. 4 (1979): 239–43.

Rather, Lelland J. *Disease, Life, and Man*. Stanford: Stanford University Press, 1958.

Russell, Leslie. *Toward Health and Wholeness*. New York: Macmillan Co., 1964.

Sandison, R. A. "Depression: Illness, Social Disease, or Natural State." *Lancet* 1, no. 762 (June 1972): 1227–29.

Sanford, John A. *Healing and Wholeness*. New York: Paulist Press, 1977.

Sobel, David S., ed. *Ways of Health: Holistic Approaches to Ancient and Contemporary Medicine*. New York: Harcourt Brace Jovanovich, 1979.

Tillich, Paul. "The Meaning of Health." In *Religion and Medicine: Essays on Meanings, Values, and Health*. Edited by David Belgum, pp. 3–12. Ames, Iowa: Iowa State University Press, 1967.

Van der Poel, C. J. "Healing Mission of the Church—a Search for Human Wholeness." *Hospital Progress* 57, no. 9 (September 1976): 84–88.

Vaux, Kenneth L. *This Mortal Coil: The Meaning of Health and Disease*. New York: Harper & Row, 1978.

White, R. W. "The Concept of Healthy Personality: What Do We Really Mean?" *The Counseling Psychologist* 4 (1973): 3–13.

Sexuality

Amelar, R. D., et al. "Male Infertility Practice and Orthodox Jewish Law." *Urology* 10, no. 2 (August 1977): 177–80.

Artificial Human Insemination: Report of a Commission Appointed by His Grace

Bibliography

the Archbishop of Canterbury. London, 1948.

Ashley, B. M. "From 'Humanae Vitae' to 'Human Sexuality': New Directions?" *Hospital Progress* 59, no. 7 (July 1978): 78–83.

Avortement et respect de la view humaine. Colloque du Centre catholique des médecins français (commission conjugale). Paris: Éditions du Seuil, 1972.

Bailey, Derrick Sherwin. *Homosexuality and the Western Christian Tradition*. Reprint of 1955 edition. Hamden, Conn.: Shoe String Press, 1975.

Baltazar, E. R. "Contraception and the Philosophy of Process." *Contraception and Holiness: The Catholic Predicament*. New York: Herder & Herder, 1964.

Barnhouse, Ruth T., and Holmes, Urban T., eds. *Male and Female: Christian Approaches to Sexuality*. New York: Seabury Press, 1976.

Batchelor, Edward, Jr., ed. *Homosexuality and Ethics*. New York: Pilgrim Press, 1980.

Bauer, Andrew, ed. *The Debate on Birth Control*. New York: Hawthorn Books, 1969.

Becker, W. "[Ethical and Legal Problems Around the Test-Tube Baby]." *Therapie der Gegenwart* 118, no. 3 (March 1979): 442–58.

Bergues, Helene, et al. *La prévention des naisances dans la famille: Ses origines dans les temps modernes*. Institut National d'Études Demographiques, Travaux et documents 35. Paris: Presses Universitaires de France, 1960.

Bleich, David. "Abortion in Halakhic Literature." *Tradition* 10, no. 1 (1968): 72–120.

Bleich, J. D., "Host-Mothers." *Tradition* 13 (Fall 1972): 127–29.

Bockle, Franz, and Pohier, Jean-Marie, eds. *Sexuality in Contemporary Catholicism*. New York: Seabury Press, 1974.

Bousquet, George Henri. *L'éthique sexuelle de l'Islam*. Rev. enl. ed. Vol. 14 of *Islam d'hier et aujourd'hui*. Edited by R. Brunschvig. Paris: G. P. Maisonneuve & Larose, 1966. 1st ed. (1953) titled *La morale de l'Islam et son éthique sexuelle*.

Braaten, Carl E. *The Ethics of Conception and Contraception*. New York: Lutheran Church in America, Board of Social Ministry, 1967.

Buck, Pearl. *The Terrible Choice: The Abortion Dilemma*. New York: Bantam Books, 1968.

Buckley, Michael J. *Morality and the Homosexual: A Catholic Approach to a Moral Problem*. Westminster, Md.: Newman Press, 1959.

Cabot, Richard Clarke. *Christianity and Sex*. New York: Macmillan Co., 1937.

Callahan, Daniel J. *Abortion: Law, Choice, and Morality*. New York: Macmillan Co., 1970.

————, ed. *The American Population Debate*. Garden City, N.Y.: Doubleday & Co., 1971.

Bibliography

Callahan, Sidney Cornelia. *Beyond Birth Control: The Christian Experience of Sex*. New York: Sheed & Ward, 1968.

Carmen, A., and Moody, H. *Abortion Counseling and Social Change*. Valley Forge, Pa.: Judson Press, 1973.

Carswell, R. W. "Historical Analysis of Religion and Sex." *Journal of School Health* 39, no. 10 (December 1969): 673–84.

Church of England. *Artificial Insemination by Donor: Two Contributions to a Christian Judgment*. London: Church Information Office, 1959.

Coffee, Patrick. "When Is Killing the Unborn a Homicidal Action?" *Linacre Quarterly* 43 (May 1976): 85–93.

Converse, T. A.; Buker, R. S., Jr.; and Lee, R. V. "Hutterite Midwifery." *American Journal of Obstetrics and Gynecology* 116, no. 5 (July 1973): 719–25.

Creighton, Phyllis, *Artificial Insemination by Donor: A Study of Ethics, Medicine, and Law in Our Technological Society*. Toronto: Anglican Book Centre, 1977.

————, ed. *Abortion: An Issue for Conscience*. Toronto: Anglican Church of Canada, 1974.

Curran, Charles E., ed. *Contraception: Authority and Dissent*. New York: Herder & Herder, 1969.

Dantine, W. "[Sterilization of the Woman from the Protestant Viewpoint]." *Deutsches Medizinisches Journal* 22, no. 20 (October 1971): 645–46.

Déclaration du Conseil de la Fédération protestante de France sur l'éducation sexuelle, la régulation des naissances et l'avortement. Paris: Bureau d'information protestant, 1973.

Diamond, E. F. "In Vitro Fertilization: A Moratorium Is in Order." *Hospital Progress* 60, no. 5 (May 1979): 66–68, 80.

Doherty, Dennis, ed. *Dimensions of Human Sexuality*. Garden City, N.Y.: Doubleday & Co., 1979.

Doniger, Simon, ed. *Sex and Religion Today*. New York: Association Press, 1953.

Duffy, Martin, ed. *Issues in Sexual Ethics*. Souderton, Pa.: United Church People for Biblical Witness, 1979.

Dyck, Arthur J. "Population Policies and Ethical Acceptability." In *Rapid Population Growth: Consequences and Policy Implications*. Prepared by a study committee of the Office of the Foreign Secretary, National Academy of Sciences. Baltimore: Johns Hopkins Press, 1971.

Eller, Vernard. *The Sex Manual for Puritans*. Nashville: Abingdon Press, 1971.

Epstein, Louis M. *Sex Laws and Customs in Judaism*. New York: Bloch Publishing Co., 1948; reprint, Ktav Publishing House, 1967.

Feldman, David Michael. *Birth Control in Jewish Law: Marital Relations, Contraception, and Abortion as Set Forth in the Classic Texts of Jewish Law*. Reprint of 1968 edition. Westport, Conn.: Greenwood Press, 1980.

Bibliography

————. *Marital Relations, Birth Control, and Abortion in Jewish Law*. New York: Schocken Books, 1974.

Foster, Lawrence. *Religion and Sexuality: Three American Communal Experiments of the Nineteenth Century*. New York: Oxford University Press, 1981.

Friedman, Benjamin. "Symposium on Artificial Insemination, the Religious Viewpoints: Jewish." *Syracuse Law Review* 7 (1955): 7–15.

"Genetic Engineering." *Assia* 15 (October 1976).

"Genetic Science and Man." *Theological Studies* 33 (September 1972): 332–51.

Genne, William H., ed. *A Synoptic of Recent Denominational Statements on Sexuality*. New York: National Council of Churches of Christ, Department of Educational Development, 1971.

Grace, James H., ed. *God, Sex, and the Social Project: The Glassboro Papers on Religion and Human Sexuality*. New York: E. Mellen Press, 1978.

Greenberg, Blu. "Abortion: A Challenge to Halakah." *Judaism* 98 (Spring 1976): 201–8.

Grimm, Robert. *Amour et sexualité: Essai d'éthique théologique*. Neuchâtel: Delachaux & Niestle, 1962.

Grisez, Germain G. *Contraception and the Natural Law*. Milwaukee: Bruce Publishing Co., 1964.

Gustafson, James M. "A Protestant Ethical Approach." In *The Morality of Abortion: Legal and Historical Perspectives*. Edited by John Thomas Noonan, pp. 101–22. Cambridge, Mass.: Harvard University Press, 1970.

Haeuber, A. "[Cesarean Section in Islamic Culture Tradition]." *Geburtshilfe und Frauenheilkunde* 29, no. 12 (December 1969): 1104–8.

Hamilton, Michael. "New Life for Old: Genetic Decision." *Christian Century* 86 (May 1969): 741–44.

Hathout, H. "Abortion and Islam." *Journal Medical Libanais* [Lebanese Medical Journal] 25, no. 3 (1972): 237–39.

Hellegers, A. E. "Fetal Development." *Theological Studies* 31 (March 1970): 3–9.

Heron, Alastair, ed. *Towards a Quaker View of Sex: An Essay by a Group of Friends*. London: Friends Home Service Committee, 1963; 2d rev. ed. 1964.

Igeret ha-Kodesh (English and Hebrew), *The Holy Letter: A Study in Medieval Jewish Sexual Morality, Ascribed to Mahmanides*. Translated and with an introduction by Seymour J. Cohen. New York: Ktav Publishing House, 1976.

Musallam, Basim F. "The Islamic Sanction of Contraception." In *Population and Its Problems: A Plain Man's Guide*. Edited by H. B. Parry. Oxford: Clarendon Press, 1974.

————. "Sex and Society in Islam: The Sanction and Medieval Techniques of Birth Control." Ph.D. dissertation, Harvard University, 1973.

Nazer, Isam R.; Karmi, Hasan S.; and Zayid, Mahmud Y., eds. *Islam and Family Planning*. 2 vols. Proceedings of the International Islamic Conference, Rabat,

Bibliography

Morocco, December 1971. Beirut: International Planned Parenthood Federation, Middle East and North Africa Region, 1974.

Patrinacos, Nicon D. *The Orthodox Church on Birth Control*. Garwood, N.J.: Graphic Arts Press, 1975.

Paul VI (Pope). "Humanae Vitae: On the Regulation of Birth (July 25, 1968)." In *The Gospel of Peace and Justice: Catholic Social Teaching Since Pope John*. Edited by Joseph Gremillion. Maryknoll, N.Y.: Orbis Books, 1976.

Policy Manual for Committee to Advise on Requests for Obstetrical/Gynaecological Sterilization Procedures. Rev. ed. London, Ont.: St. Joseph's Hospital, 1974.

Sacred Congregation for the Doctrine of the Faith. "Declaration on Certain Questions Concerning Sexual Ethics." In *The Pope Speaks* 21 (1976). Washington, D.C.: United States Catholic Conference, 1976.

Spitzer, Walter O., and Saylor, Carlyle L., eds. *Birth Control and the Christian: A Protestant Symposium on the Control of Human Production*. Wheaton, Ill.: Tyndale House, 1969.

"A Symposium: Fetal Research." *The Human Life Review* 1 (Fall 1975): Seymour Siegel, "I. A. Bias for Life: Abortion Does Not Justify Harmful Research," pp. 109–17; Harold O. J. Brown, "II. The Ethical Questions," pp. 118–28; David W. Louisell, "III. A Dissenting Statement," pp. 129–32; and Charles P. Kindregan, "IV. The Living Fetus and the Lay: The State's Role," pp. 133–56.

Wogaman, Philip J., ed. *The Population Crisis and Moral Responsibility*. Washington, D.C.: Public Affairs Press, 1973.

Wynn, John Charles, ed. *Sexual Ethics and Christian Responsibility: Some Divergent Views*. New York: Association Press, 1970.

Zaphiris, Chrysostom. "The Morality of Contraception: An Eastern Orthodox Opinion." *Journal of Ecumenical Studies* 11 (1974): 69–85.

Passages

Augustine, Saint. "The Good of Marriage *(De bono coniugali)*." In *Saint Augustinus Aurelius, Bishop of Hippo*. Washington, D.C.: Catholic University of America Press, 1969.

Baltensweiler, Heinrich. "Current Developments in the Theology of Marriage in the Reformed Churches." In *The Future of Marriage as Institution*. Edited by Franz Böckle, vol. 55 of *Concilium: Theology in the Age of Renewal*. New York: Herder & Herder, 1970.

Blazer, D., and Palmore, E. "Religion and Aging in a Longitudinal Panel." *Gerontologist* 16, no. 1 (February 1976): 82–85.

Callahan, Sidney, and Christiansen, Drew. "Ideal Old Age." *Soundings* 57 (Spring 1974): 1–16.

Evdokimov (Evdokimoff), Paul. *Sacrament de l'amour: Le mystère conjugal à la*

Bibliography

lumière de la tradition orthodoxe. Paris: Éditions de l'Epi, 1962. Greek ed.: *Mysterion tes agapes* [Mystery of love]. Translated by Serapheim Orphanos. Athens, 1967.

Falk, Ze'ev. *Jewish Matrimonial Law in the Middle Ages*. New York: Oxford University Press, 1966.

Francoeur, Robert T. *Utopian Motherhood*. New York: Doubleday & Co. 1970.

Greven, Philip J. *Child-rearing Concepts, 1628–1861*. Itasca, Ill.: Peacock Publishers, 1973.

Guinan, S. M. "Aging and Religious Life." *Gerontologist* 12, no. 1 (Spring 1972): 21.

Huber, R., and Mauris, R. "[Clergy's Viewpoint: Prolonging of Life, Ethics and Geriatrics]." *Zeitschrift für Krankenflege unt Clinische Therapie* 67, no. 8–9 (August–September 1974): 323–25.

Hunter, K.; Linn, M. W.; and Pratt, T. C. "Minority Women's Attitudes About Aging." *Experimental Aging Research* 5, no. 2 (April 1979): 95–108.

Kartmann, L. L. "Jewish Ethnicity and Its Relevance for Gerontological Practice." *Journal of Gerontological Nursing* 4, no. 1 (January–February 1978): 34–39.

Kurtzman, Joel, and Gordon, Philip. *No More Dying: The Conquest of Aging and Extension of Human Life*. New York: Dell Publishing Co., 1976.

McCormick, Richard A. "Conjugal Morality." In *Married Love and Children*, pp. 24–32. New York: American Press, 1966.

MacNabb, Vincent. *Casti Connubii: Encyclical Letter on Christian Marriage, with Commentaries*. London, 1933.

Meyendorff, John. *Marriage: An Orthodox Perspective*. Crestwood, N.Y.: St. Vladimir's Seminary Press, 1970. 2d ed. 1975.

Moberg, D. O. "Religion in Old Age." *Geriatrics* 20, no. 11 (November 1965): 977–82.

Montefiore, C. H. "Ethical Problems of Geriatrics." *Gerontologia Clinica* (Basel) 11, no. 2 (1969): 65–74.

Novak, Michael, ed. *The Experience of Marriage: The Testimony of Catholic Laymen*. New York: Macmillan Co., 1964.

Pacella, B. L. "The Mystical Tradition in Youth." In *Proceedings of the Rudolf Virchow Medical Society in the City of New York* 27 (1968–69): 135–42.

Rauf, M. A. "Muslim Marriage Customs." *Journal of the American Medical Association* 218, no. 3 (October 1971): 447–48.

Rosner, F. "Geriatrics in the Medical Aphorisms of Moses Maimonides." *Postgraduate Medicine* 55, no. 1 (January 1974): 229.

Schaneveldt, Jay D. "Mormon Adolescents' Likes and Dislikes Towards Parents and Home." *Adolescence* 8, no. 30 (1973): 171–78.

Zampella, A. D. "A Sampling of Attitudes Toward Aging." *Journal of the American Geriatrics Society* 17, no. 5 (May 1969): 488–92.

Bibliography

Dignity

Aitken, P. W. "The Right to Live and the Right to Die." *Medical Times* 95, no. 11 (November 1967): 1184–87.

Bakan, David. *The Quality of Human Existence: An Essay of Psychology and Religion*. Chicago: Rand McNally, 1966.

Clouser, K. D. "The Sanctity of Life: An Analysis of a Concept." *Annals of Internal Medicine* 78, no. 1 (January 1973): 119–25.

Downing, A. B., ed. *Euthanasia and the Right to Die*. Atlantic Highlands, N.J.: Humanities Press, 1970.

Fletcher, John. "Human Experimentation: Ethics in the Consent Situation." *Law and Contemporary Problems* 32 (1967): 620–49.

Freund, Paul Abraham, ed. *Experimentation with Human Subjects*. New York: George Braziller, 1970.

Gershuni, Y. "Heart Transplantation in the Light of Jewish Law." *Or ha-Mixrah* 18, no. 3 (April 1969): 133–37.

Gustafson, James M. "God's Transcendence and the Value of Human Life." *Christian Ethics and the Community*. Philadelphia: Pilgrim Press, 1971.

––––––. "Mongolism, Parental Desires, and the Right to Life." *Perspectives in Biology and Medicine* 16 (Summer 1973): 529–57.

Liebman, Joshua Loth. *Hope for Man: An Optimistic Philosophy and Guide to Self-Fulfillment*. New York: Simon & Schuster, 1966.

McFadden, Charles J. *The Dignity of Life: Moral Values in a Changing Society*. Huntington, Ind.: Our Sunday Visitor, 1976. First published as *Medical Ethics for Nurses*. Philadelphia: F. A. Davis Co., 1946; 2d ed. 1949; 6th ed. 1967.

May, William E. *Human Existence, Medicine, and Ethics*. Chicago: Franciscan Herald Press, 1977.

O'Rourke, K. D. "Rationale and Implications of Sanctity of Life Commitment." *Hospital Progress* 55, no. 2 (February 1974): 57–59.

Shannon, T. A. "Death with Dignity" (letter). *New England Journal of Medicine* 302, no. 2 (January 1980): 125.

Williams, Glanville H. *The Sanctity of Life and the Criminal Law*. New York: Alfred A. Knopf, 1957.

Morality

Augenstein, Leroy. *Come, Let Us Play God*. New York: Harper & Row, 1969.

Beauchamp, Tom, and Walter, LeRoy, eds. *Contemporary Issues in Bioethics*. Belmont, Calif: Dickenson, 1978.

Black, Peter McL. "Psychiatric Diseases, Informed Consent, Psychosurgery: A Reply to Dr. Thomas Szasz." *The Humanist*, (January–February 1978): 45–47.

––––––, and Szasz, Thomas S. "The Ethics of Psychosurgery." *The Humanist*

Bibliography

(July–August 1977): 6–11

Bleich, David. *Contemporary Halachic Problems*. Library of Jewish Law and Ethics 4. Edited by Norman Lamm. New York: Ktav Publishing House, Yeshiva University Press, 1977.

Bliss, Brian, and Johnson, Alan. *Aims and Motives in Clinical Medicine: A Practical Approach to Medical Ethics*. London: Pitman Medical Publishing Co., 1975.

Bok, Sissela. "The Ethics of Giving Placebos." *Scientific American* 231, no. 5 (November 1974): 18.

Bonhoeffer, Dietrich. *Ethics*. 1949. Reprint. Edited by Eberhard Bethge. New York: Macmillan Co., 1965.

British Council of Churches. *Sex and Morality: A Report to the British Council of Churches, October 1966*. London: SCM Press, 1966.

Calhoun, Cheryl. *Annotated Bibliography of Medical Oaths, Codes, and Prayers*. Washington, D.C.: Kennedy Institute, 1975.

Callahan, Daniel. *Ethical Issues in Genetic Counseling and the Use of Genetic Knowledge*. New York: Plenum Publishing Corp., 1973.

Carlton, Wendy. *In Our Professional Opinion: The Primacy of Clinical Judgment over Moral Choice*. Notre Dame, Ind.: University of Notre Dame Press, 1979.

Carmody, James. *Ethical Issues in Health Services: A Report and Annotated Bibliography*. National Center of Health Services Research Development, Report 70/32. Rockville, Md.: Department of Health, Education, and Welfare, Public Health Service, Health Services and Mental Health Administration, 1970.

Childress, James F. "Who Shall Live When Not All Can Live?" *Soundings* 53 (Winter 1970): 339–62.

Church of England, Church Information Office. *Decisions About Life and Death: A Problem in Modern Medicine*. London, 1965.

Crowder, Eleanor. "Manners, Morals, and Nurses: An Historical Overview of Nursing Ethics." *Texas Reports on Biology and Medicine* 32 (1974): 173–80.

Dyck, Arthur, and Reiser, Joel. *Ethics in Medicine: Historical Perspectives and Contemporary Concerns*. Cambridge: M. I. T. Press, 1977.

El-Qadi, Ahmad. "Professional Ethics: Ethics in the Medical Profession." *Journal of the Islamic Medical Association of the United States and Canada* 7, no. 2 (1976): 119–31.

Engelhardt, H. Tristram. "Ethical Issues in Aiding the Death of Young Children." *Beneficent Euthanasia*. Edited by Marvin Kohl. Buffalo, N.Y.: Prometheus Books, 1975.

Eshraghi, R. *Akhlaq-i-Pizishki* [Medical ethics]. Meshed, Iran: Meshed Medical School, 1969.

Fagley, Richard M. *The Population Explosion and Christian Responsibility*. New York: Oxford University Press, 1960.

Bibliography

Fletcher, Joseph Francis. *The Ethics of Genetic Control: Ending Reproductive Roulette*. Garden City, N.Y.: Doubleday & Co., 1974.

Gustafson, James. *The Contributions of Theology to Medical Ethics*. Milwaukee: Marquette University Press, 1975.

Haring, Bernard. *Ethics of Manipulation: Issues in Medicine, Behavior Control, and Genetics*. New York: Seabury Press, 1976.

Heller, P. "Informed Consent and the Old-fashioned Conscience of the Physician-Investigator." *Perspectives in Biology and Medicine* 20 (Spring 1977): 434–38.

Jakobovits, Immanuel. *Jewish Medical Ethics: A Comparative and Historical Study of Jewish Religious Attitudes to Medicine and Its Practice*. 1959. New enlarged ed. New York: Bloch Publishing Co., 1975.

John, W. de. "[Islam and Medical Ethics]." *Tijdschrift voor Ziekenverpleging* 23, no. 7 (March 1970): 359–61.

Jong, W. D. E. "[Islam and Medical Ethics]." *Nederlands Tijdschrift voor Geneeskunde* 114, no. 2 (January 1970): 63–65.

Last, G. "[Overpopulation and Islam]." *Therapie Der Gegewart* 117, no. 11 (November 1978): 1683–710.

Levey, Martin. "Medical Ethics of Medieval Islam with Special Reference to Al-Ruhawis' Practical Ethics of the Physician." In *Transactions of the American Philosophical Society*, vol. 25, pt. 3, pp. 13ff. Philadelphia: American Philosophical Society, 1967.

McCormick, Richard A. "Abortion and Moral Principles." In *The Wrong of Abortion*, pp. 1–13. New York: America Press, 1966.

————. *Ambiguity in Moral Choice*. Milwaukee: Marquette University Press, 1973.

————. *How Brave a New World: Dilemmas in Bioethics*. New York: Doubleday & Co., 1981.

O'Donnell, Thomas J. *Medicine and Christian Morality*. 3d revision; earlier editions titled *Morals in Medicine*. New York: Alba House, 1976.

Ramsey, Paul. *Basic Christian Ethics*. 1950. Reprint. Chicago: University of Chicago Press, 1980.

————. *Ethics at the Edges of Life: Medical and Legal Intersections*. 1978. Reprint. New Haven: Yale University Press, 1980.

Reiser, Stanley J.; Dyck, Arthur J.; and Curran, William J., eds. *Ethics in Medicine: Historical Perspectives and Contemporary Concerns*. Cambridge: M. I. T. Press, 1977.

Rosner, Fred, et al. *Jewish Bioethics*. New York: Hebrew Publishing Co., 1979.

Tendler, M.D., ed. *Medical Ethics: A Compendium of Jewish Moral, Ethical, and Religious Principles in Medicine Practice*. 5th ed. New York: Federation of Jewish Philanthropies, Committee on Religious Affairs, 1975.

Vaux, Kenneth. *Biomedical Ethics: Morality for the New Medicine*. New York: Harper & Row, 1974.

Bibliography

Weir, Robert F., ed. *Ethical Issues in Death and Dying*. New York: Columbia University Press, 1977.

Willis, Robert E. *The Ethics of Karl Barth*. Leiden: E. J. Brill, 1971. Pp. 367ff.

Madness

Allderidge, P. "Hospitals, Madhouses, and Asylums: Cycles in the Care of the Insane." *British Journal of Psychiatry* 134 (April 1979): 321–34.

Allison, J. "Adaptive Regression and Intense Religious Experiences." *Journal of Nervous and Mental Disease* 145, no. 6 (December 1967): 652–63.

Allport, Gordon. *Religion in the Developing Personality*. New York: New York University Press, 1960.

Altschule, M. D. "The Two Kinds of Depression According to St. Paul." *British Journal of Psychiatry* 113, no. 500 (July 1967): 779–80.

Apolito, A. "Psychoanalysis and Religion." *American Journal of Psychoanalysis*. 30, no. 2 (1970): 115–26.

Beit-Hallahmi, B. "Religion and Suicidal Behavior." *Psychological Reports* 37, no. 3, pt. 2 (December 1975): 1303–6.

_____ and Argyle, M. "Religious Ideas and Psychiatric Disorders." *International Journal of Social Psychiatry* 23, no. 1 (Spring 1977): 26–30.

Bergin, A. E. "Psychotherapy and Religious Values." *Journal of Consulting and Clinical Psychology* 48, no. 1 (February 1980): 95–105.

Berman, A. L., et al. "The Relation Between Death Anxiety, Belief in Afterlife, and Locus of Control." *Journal of Consulting and Clinical Psychology* 41 (October 1973): 318.

Black, M. S., and London, P. "The Dimensions of Guilt, Religion and Personal Ethics." *Journal of Social Psychology* 69, no. 1 (June 1966): 39–54.

Block, S. L. "St. Augustine: On Grief and Other Psychological Matters." *American Journal of Psychiatry* 122, no. 8 (February 1966): 943–46.

Blocker, F. "[Effects of Belonging to a Religious Denomination on Suicide and Suicide Attempt]. *Medizinische Welt* 14 (April 1971): 566–71.

Boisen, Anton. *The Exploration of the Inner World: A Study of Mental Disorders and Religious Experiences*. Philadelphia: University of Pennsylvania Press, 1971.

Bromberg, Walter. *From Shaman to Psychotherapist: A History of the Treatment of Mental Illness*. Chicago: Henry Regnery Co., 1975.

Diekman, A. J. "Sufism and Psychiatry." *Journal of Nervous and Mental Disease* 165, no. 4 (November 1977): 318–29.

Fehr, L. A., and Heintzelman, M. E. "Personality and Attitude Correlates of Religiosity: A Source of Controversy." *Journal of Psychology* 95 (January 1977): 63–66.

Fernando, S. J. "Aspects of Depression in a Jewish Minority Group." *Psychiatria Clinica* (Basel) 11, no. 1 (1978): 23–33.

Bibliography

Foucault, Michel. *Madness and Civilization: A History of Insanity in the Age of Reason*. 1965. Reprint. New York: Random House, 1973.

Frankl, Victor. *The Unconscious God: Psychotherapy and Theology*. New York: Simon & Schuster, 1975.

Freud, Sigmund. *Psychoanalysis and Faith: The Letters of Sigmund Freud and Oskar Pfister*. Translated by Eric Mosbacher. New York: Basic Books, 1964.

Galanter, M., and Buckley, P. "Evangelical Religion and Meditation Psychotherapeutic Effects." *Journal of Nervous and Mental Disease* 166, no. 10 (October 1978): 685–91.

Groesch, S. J., and Davis, W. E. "Psychiatric Patients' Religion and MMPI Responses." *Journal of Clinical Psychology* 33, no. 1 (January 1977): 168–71.

Guntrip, Henry James Samuel. *Psychotherapy and Religion*. New York: Harper & Row, 1957. First published as *Mental Pain and the Cure of Souls*. London: Independent Press, 1956.

Henderson, J. "Object Relations and the Psychotherapy of Sin." *Canadian Psychiatric Association Journal* 22, no. 8 (December 1977): 427–33.

Hoehn-Saric, R. "Transcendence and Psychotherapy." *American Journal of Psychotherapy* 28, no. 2 (1974): 252–64.

Jasperse, C. W. "Self-destruction and Religion." *Mental Health and Society* 3, no. 3–4 (1976): 154–68.

Kantor, R. E. "Schizophrenia and the Protestant Ethic." *Mental Hygiene* 50, no. 1 (January 1966): 18–23.

Katchadourian, H. "A Comparative Study of Mental Illness Among the Christians and Moslems of Lebanon." *International Journal of Social Psychiatry* 20, no. 1–2 (Spring–Summer 1974): 56–67.

Laing, R. D., and Esterson, A. *Sanity, Madness, and the Family*. 2d ed. New York: Basic Books, 1971.

Lewis, Helen B. *Shame and Guilt in Neurosis*. New York: International University Press, 1971.

Linn, Louis, and Schwartz, Leo. *Psychiatry and the Religious Experience*. New York: Random House, 1958.

Oates, Wayne E. *Anxiety in Christian Experience*. Philadelphia: Westminster Press, 1955.

Szasz, Thomas. *Manufacture of Madness: A Comparative Study of the Inquisition and the Mental Health Movement*. New York: Harper & Row, 1970.

Waldman, R. D. "The Sin-neurotic Complex: Perspectives in Religion and Psychiatry." *Psychoanalytic Review* 57, no. 1 (1970): 143–52.

Healing

Advent Christian Church, Committee on Divine Healing. *Introduction to the Ministry of Healing of the Church*. 1964.

Anderson, W. H., Jr. "Sacramental Healing." *Christianity Today* 5 (January

Bibliography

1961): 8–9.

Arnold, Dorothy Musgrave. *Called by Christ to Heal*. New York: Seabury Press, 1966.

Bailes, Frederick W. *Healing the Incurable*. 1949. Reprint. Marina Del Rey, Calif.: De Vorss & Co., 1972.

Banks, John Gayner. *Manual of Christian Healing*. San Diego: St. Luke's Press, 1959.

Barbanell, Maurice. *Saga of Spirit Healing*. London: Spiritualist Press, 1954.

Beers, R. F., Jr. "The Integrity of the Healing Process in the Relationship of the Patient, the Physician, and the Clergyman." *Johns Hopkins Medical Journal* 128, no. 5 (May 1971): 289–94.

Bilu, Y. "General Characteristics of Referrals to Traditional Healers in Israel." *Israel Annals of Psychiatry and Related Disciplines* 15, no. 3 (September 1977): 245–52.

Bishop, George. *Faith Healing: God or Fraud?* Nashville: Sherbourne Press, 1967.

Cassell, Eric. *The Healer's Art: A New Approach to the Doctor-Patient Relationship*. Philadelphia: J. B. Lippincott Co., 1976.

Chadwick, H. "Religion and the Healing Art." *Journal of the American Osteopathic Association* 65, no. 10 (June 1966): 1101–7.

Cowles, E. S. *Religion and Medicine in the Church: Report for the Joint Commission on Christian Healing*. New York, 1925.

Cunningham, Raymond J. "From Holiness to Healing: The Faith Cure in America, 1872–1892." *Church History* 43 (1974): 499–513.

Day, Albert E. *Letters on the Healing Ministry*. Nashville: Methodist Evangelistic Materials, 1964.

Dean, Paul William. *Effective Prayer Healing*. Los Angeles: De Vorss & Co., 1959.

Doniger, Simon, ed. *Healing, Human and Divine*. New York: Association Press, 1957.

Eddy, Mary Baker. *Christian Healing*. 1886. Reprint. Boston: Trustees of Mary Baker G. Eddy, 1936.

Ehrenreich, Barbara, and English, Deirdre. *Witches, Midwives, and Nurses: A History of Women Healers*. 2d ed. Glass Mountain Pamphlet 1. Old Westbury, N.Y.: Feminist Press, 1973.

Evans, Warren, Felt. *Healing by Faith, or Primitive Mind-Cure*. London: Reeves, 1885.

Kelsey, Morton T. *Healing and Christianity: In Ancient Thought and Modern Times*. New York: Harper & Row, 1973.

Kruger, Helen. *Other Healers, Other Cures: A Guide to Alternative Medicine*. Indianapolis: Bobbs-Merrill Co., 1974.

MacNutt, Francis. *Healing*. Notre Dame: Ave Maria Press, 1974.

Bibliography

Moses, Alfred Geiger. *Jewish Science: Divine Healing in Judaism*. Mobile, Ala.: By the author, 1916.

Ruiz, P., and Langrod, J. "The Role of Folk Healers in Community Mental Health Services." *Community Mental Health Journal* 12, no. 4 (Winter 1976): 392–98.

Scharlemann, Martin Henry. *Healing and Redemption*. St. Louis: Concordia Publishing House, 1965.

Caring

Beatriz de la Immaculada. "The Religious Nurse Opposite the Sick." *Epheta* 5, no. 14 (January–March 1966): 18–19.

Capellmann, Carl Franz. *Medicina pastoralis*. 4th ed. Aachen: Rudolph Barth, 1869. Translated by William Dassel as *Pastoral Medicine*. New York: F. Pustet, 1879.

Christian Medical Commission, World Council of Churches. "Position Paper on Health Care and Justice." *Contact* 16 (August 1973).

Christopher, W. I., Jr. "The Interdependence of the Hospital and the Religious Congregation." *Hospital Progress* 53, no. 10 (October 1972): 51–53 passim.

Dayringer, Richard. "The Religious Professional's Contribution to Health Care." *Religion and Health: Report of a Workshop*, pp. 39–57. Chicago: University of Illinois at the Medical Center, 1980.

Dayton, Edward R., ed. *Medicine and Missions: A Survey of Medical Missions*. Wheaton, Ill.: Medical Assistance Program, 1969.

Delaunay, Paul. *La médecine et l'église: Contribution à l'histoire de l'exercice médicale*. Paris: Éditions Hippocrate, 1948.

Dowling, Michael J. *Health Care and the Church*. Edited by Robert E. Koenig. New York: Pilgrim Press, 1977.

Flexner, J. M. "The Hospice Movement in North America—Is It Coming of Age?" *Southern Medical Journal* 72, no. 3 (March 1979): 248–50.

Galdston, Iago, ed. *Ministry and Medicine in Human Relations*. New York: Arno Press, 1955.

Hahn, J. A. "The Christian Administrator in a Secular Society." *Hospital Progress* 59, no. 9 (September 1978): 76–80.

Hiltner, Seward, ed. *Clinical Pastoral Training*. New York: Commission on Religion and Health, Federal Council of Churches of Christ, 1945.

Holoubek, J. E.; Black, C. L.; and Holoubek, A. B. "Cooperation of Physicians and Clergy in Treating the Whole Patient." *Journal of the Arkansas Medical Society* 69, no. 7 (December 1972): 216–18.

Houghton, Thomas. *Faith Healing Missions and the Teaching of Scripture*. London: C. J. Thyme & Jarvis, 1925.

Hume, Edgar Erskine. *Medical Work of the Knights Hospitallers of Saint John of Jerusalem*. Baltimore: Johns Hopkins Press, 1940.

Bibliography

Hume, Edward H. *Doctors Courageous*. New York: Harper & Bros., 1950.

Ingles, T. "St. Christopher's Hospice." *Nursing Outlook* 22, no. 12 (December 1974): 759–63.

Jacoby, George W. *Physician, Pastor, and Patient: Problems in Pastoral Medicine*. New York & London: P. B. Hoeber, 1936.

John Paul II (Pope). "Pope John Paul II: On the Health Care Apostolate." *Hospital Progress* 60, no. 11 (November 1979): 44–46.

Johnson, James T. *The Anglican Church: The Church's Ministry of Healing*. Report of the Archbishop's Commission. London, 1958.

Kagan, Henry E. "The Rabbi as Pastoral Counselor." *Synagogue Service Bulletin* (December 1951): 12–14.

Knights, Ward A., ed. *Pastoral Care in Health Facilities: A Book of Readings*. St. Louis: Catholic Hospital Association, 1977.

Kyle, William H., ed. *Healing Through Counselling: A Christian Counselling Centre*. London: Epworth Press, 1964.

Lambourne, R. A. *Community, Church, and Healing: A Study of Some of the Corporate Aspects of the Church's Ministry to the Sick*. London: Darton, Longman & Todd, 1963.

Letterman, Henry L., ed. *Health and Healing: Ministry of the Church*. Chicago: Wheat Ridge Foundation, 1980.

McGilvary, James C. "The Healing Ministry in the Mission of the Church." *Study Encounter* 2, no. 3 (1966): 122–28.

McMoran, S. R. "Religious in the Health Apostolate: Old Myths and New Realities." *Hospital Progress* 55, no. 11 (November 1974): 62–66.

Marcus, Jacob Rader. *Communal Sick-care in the German Ghetto*. Cincinnati: Hebrew Union College Press, 1947.

Martin, Bernard. *The Healing Ministry in the Church*. Richmond: John Knox Press, 1960.

Miller, Genevieve, ed. "Why Adventists Conduct a Health Work." *The Advent Review and Sabbath Herald* (August 11, 1949): 3–4; (August 18, 1949): 5–6; (August 25, 1949): 5–6.

Neely, T. D. "A Pastoral Ministry in a Mental Hospital." *Medical Annals of the District of Columbia* 41, no. 8 (August 1972): 520–22.

Oakes, J. "Pastoral Care of the Dying and the Bereaved." *District Nursing* 11, no. 12 (March 1969): 256–58.

O'Rourke, K. D. "Criteria for the Health Apostolate." *Hospital Progress* 58, no. 6 (June 1977): 56–59.

Parkhurst, Genevieve. *Healing the Whole Person*. New York: Morehouse-Barlow Co., 1968.

Pasha, Hakeem M. Azeez. "Establishment of Unani Hospitals in Islamic Countries." *Bulletin of the Institute of History of Medicine* (Hyderabad) 3 (1973): 69–78.

Bibliography

Polcino, M. R. "The Medical Mission Sisters, Their Founder, Mother Anna Dengel, M.D., and Their Role in the Historical Evolution of the Medical Mission Apostolate." *Transactions and Studies of the College of Physicians of Philadelphia* 35, no. 1 (July 1967): 1–25.

Presbyterian Church of England, Subcommittee on the Church's Ministry of Healing. *The Ministry of Healing in the Church: A Handbook of Principles and Practice with Contributions from Doctors and Ministers*. London: Independent Press, 1963.

Schmidt, H. "The Finnish Deaconess Sisters." *Schwester Review* 3, no. 6 (December 1965): 11–12.

Stoddard, Sandol. *The Hospice Movement: A Better Way of Caring for the Dying*. New York: Stein & Day, 1977.

Westberg, Granger E. *How to Start a Church-based Clinic*. Hinsdale, Ill.: Wholistic Health Center, 1974.

White, Ellen G. *Medical Ministry: A Treatise on Medical Missionary Work in the Gospel*. 2d ed. Mountain View, Calif: Pacific Press Publishing Association, 1963.

Young, Richard K., and Meiburg, Albert L., *Spiritual Therapy: How the Physician, Psychiatrist, and Minister Collaborate in Healing*. New York: Harper & Bros., 1960.

Suffering

Aquinas, Thomas. *Evil* 15, no. 2, "Utrum omnis actus luxuriae sit peccatum mortale" (Whether all sex acts are mortal sins). In *Questiones disputatae*, pp. 245–50. 5 vols. 7th ed. Vol. 2: *De malo*. Rome: Marietti, 1942.

Bakan, David. *Disease, Pain, and Sacrifice: Towards a Psychology of Suffering*. 1968. Reprint. Boston: Beacon Press, 1971.

Boros, Ladislaus. *Pain and Providence*. 1966. Reprint. New York: Seabury Press, 1975.

Bowker, John. *Problems of Suffering in the Religions of the World*. Cambridge: Cambridge University Press, 1970.

Buttrick, George Arthur. *God, Pain, and Evil*. Nashville: Abingdon Press, 1966.

Elphinstone, Andrew. *Freedom, Suffering, and Love*. London: SCM Press, 1976.

Fitch, Robert. *Of Love and Suffering*. Philadelphia: Westminster Press, 1971.

Gerstenberger, Erhard, and Schrage, Wolfang. *Suffering*. Translated by J. E. Steely. Nashville: Abingdon Press, 1980.

Hauerwas, S. "Reflections on Suffering, Death and Medicine." *Ethics in Science and Medicine* 6, no. 4 (1979): 229–37.

Hebblethwaite, Brian. *Evil, Suffering, and Religion*. New York: Hawthorn Books, 1976.

Hick, J. *Evil and the God of Love*. Revised. New York: Harper & Row, 1977.

Kahn, Jack Harold. *Job's Illness: Loss, Grief, and Integration, a Psychological*

Bibliography

Interpretation. New York: Pergamon Press, 1975.

Kazoh, Kitamori. *Theology of the Pain of God*. Richmond: John Knox Press, 1965.

Kierkegaard, Sören A. *The Gospel of Our Suffering: Christian Discourses*. 1847. Translated by A. J. Aldworth and W. S. Ferrie. Grand Rapids: Eerdmans, 1964.

Kuhlman, Franklin Robert. "The Ministry of Suffering in the Pauline Corpus, Hebrews, James, I Peter, and Revelation." Master's thesis, Northwestern University, 1962.

Lavelle, Louis. *Evil and Suffering*. New York: Macmillan Co., 1963.

McGill, A. *Suffering: A Test of Theological Method*. Philadelphia: Geneva Press, 1968.

Martin, James. *Suffering Man, Loving God*. Philadelphia: Westminster Press, 1969.

Moberly, Elizabeth R. *Suffering Innocent and Guilty*. London: S.P.C.K., 1978.

Paton, Alan, et al. *Creative Suffering: The Ripple of Hope*. New York: Pilgrim Press, 1970.

Proudfoot, Merrill. *Suffering: A Christian Understanding*. Philadelphia: Westminster Press, 1964.

Sellers, James Earl. *When Trouble Comes: A Christian View of Evil, Sin, and Suffering*. Nashville: Abingdon Press, 1960.

Soelle, Dorothee. *Suffering*. Philadelphia: Fortress Press, 1975.

Stuhmueller, Carroll. "Biblical Voices of Suffering and Prayer." Unpublished manuscript, 1979. Pp. 67ff. (Projected for publication in Proceedings of Stauros-Congress on Suffering.)

Taylor, Michael J., ed. *The Mystery of Suffering and Death*. Staten Island: Alba House, 1973.

Teilhard de Chardin, Pierre. *On Suffering*. New York: Harper & Row, 1974.

Unamuno, Miguel de. *The Agony of Christianity*. Translated by Pierre Loving. New York: Payson & Clarke, 1928.

Dying

Alger, William R. *Vesting of the Soul: A Critical History of the Doctrine of a Future Life*. 1880. 10th ed. Westport, Conn.: Greenwood Press, 1968.

Al-Najjar, Y. "Suicide and Islamic Law." *Mental Health and Society* 3, no. 3–4 (1976): 137–41.

Alvarez, A. *The Savage God: A Study of Suicide*. New York: Random House, 1972.

Aries, Philippe. *Western Attitudes Toward Death: From the Middle Ages to the Present*. Translated by Patricia M. Ranum. Baltimore: Johns Hopkins Press, 1974.

Augustine, Saint. "On the Immortality of the Soul." In *Basic Writings of St.*

Bibliography

Augustine, vol. 1. Edited by Whitney J. Oates, pp. 301–16. New York: Random House, 1948.

"Autopsies and Talmudic Teaching" (letter). *New England Journal of Medicine* 298, no. 14 (April 1978): 800.

Baquil, M. A. "Muslim Teaching Concerning Death." *Nursing Times* 75, no. 14 suppl. (April 1979): 43–44.

Barth, Karl. *The Resurrection of the Dead.* 1926. Translated by H. J. Stenning. London: Hodder & Stoughton, 1933.

Becker, Ernest. *The Denial of Death.* New York: Free Press, 1973.

Bixler, Julius S., et al. *In Search of God and Immortality.* Boston: Beacon Press, 1961.

Blauner, Robert. "Death and Social Structure." *Psychiatry* 29 (1966): 378–94.

Bluebond-Langner, Myra. "Meanings of Death of Children." In *New Meanings of Death.* Edited by Herman Feifel, pp. 48–66. New York: McGraw-Hill, 1977.

Brandon, S. G. F. *The Judgment of Death: The Idea of Life After Death in the Major Religions.* New York: Charles Scribner's Sons, 1967.

Bultmann, Rudolph, ed. *Life and Death.* London: A. & C. Black, 1965.

Byrne, P. A.; O'Reilly, S.; and Quay, P. M. "Brain Death—An Opposing Viewpoint." *Journal of the American Medical Association* 42, no. 18 (November 1979): 1985–90.

Cahill, Lisa Sowle. "A 'Natural Law' Reconsideration of Euthanasia." *Linacre Quarterly* 44 (February 1977): 47–63.

Cantero, Gomez F. "[The Struggle Against Death: Dysthanasia]." *Revista Española de Anestesiologia y Reanimacion* 19, no. 4 (October 1972): 495–504.

Choron, Jacques. *Suicide.* New York: Charles Scribner's Sons, 1972.

Cohn, H. "Suicide in Jewish Legal and Religious Tradition." *Mental Health and Society* 3, no. 3–4 (1976): 129–36.

Cronio, Daniel A. *The Moral Law in Regard to the Ordinary and Extraordinary Means of Conserving Life.* Rome: Pontificia Universitas Gregoriana, 1958.

Daube, David. "Limitations of Self-Sacrifice in Jewish Law and Tradition." *Theology* 72 (July 1969): 291–304.

Davidson, Glen W. "Histories and Rituals of Destiny: Implications for Thanatology." *Soundings* 54 (1971): 415–34.

Dijwi, Yusuf al-. "Hukm tashrih al-mayyit fi al-shari'ah al-Islamiyyah (Autopsy from the Islamic point of view)." *Majallat al-Azhar* (Journal of al-Azhar University) 6 (1935): 43–68.

"A Dispute over Suicide." Translated by John A. Wilson. *Ancient Near Eastern Texts.* Chicago: University of Chicago Press, 1959.

Enquist, Ray J., and Wildberger, Henry L. *Christian Faith and the Dying Patient.* New York: Lutheran Church in America, Board of Social Ministry, 1967.

Farraher, Joseph J. "Notes on Moral Theology: Suicide and Moral Principles."

Bibliography

Theological Studies 24 (1963): 69–79.

Feldman, David M. "Sefirah, Lag BaOmer, and Mourning Observances." *Proceedings of the Rabbinical Assembly,* 1962, pp. 201–24.

Freehof, Solomon B. "Death and Burial in the Jewish Tradition." In *Judaism and Ethics.* Edited by Daniel Jeremy Silver, pp. 201ff. New York: Ktav Publishing House, 1970.

Graziani, René. "Non-utopian Euthanasia: An Italian Report, c. 1554." *Renaissance Quarterly* 22 (1969): 167–85.

Halibard, G. G. "Euthanasia." *Jewish Law Annual* 1 (1978): 197.

Jakobovits, I. "The Dying and Their Treatment in Jewish Law: Preparation for Death and Euthanasia." *Hebrew Medical Journal* 2, no. 251 (1961).

James, William. *Human Immortality.* 1898. Folcroft, Pa.: Folcroft Library Editions, 1977.

Kübler-Ross, Elisabeth. *On Death and Dying.* New York: Macmillan Co., 1969.

Maguire, Daniel C. *Death by Choice.* Garden City, N.Y.: Doubleday & Co., 1974.

Pelikan, Jaroslav. *The Shape of Death.* Nashville: Abingdon Press, 1961.

Rahner, Karl. *On the Theology of Death.* Translated by Charles H. Henkey. In *Quaestiones disputatae* 3. New York: Herder & Herder, 1961. 2d ed. London: Burns & Oates, 1965.

Stendahl, Krister, ed. *Immortality and Resurrection: Four Essays.* Ingersoll Lectures, Harvard University, 1955–59. New York: Macmillan Co. 1965.

Thielicke, Helmut. *Death and Life.* Translated by E. H. Schroeder. Philadelphia: Fortress Press, 1970.

Veatch, Robert M. *Death, Dying, and the Biological Revolution: Our Last Quest for Responsibility.* New Haven: Yale University Press, 1976.

Addendum

Aware of the magnitude and importance of Project Ten, Lutheran General Hospital enlisted the support and counsel of internationally recognized authorities to shape the objectives and limits of the Project.

The Board of Advisors

Darrel W. Amundsen, Ph.D.
  Professor of Classics
  Western Washington University
  Bellingham, Washington

Robert Bellah, Ph.D.
  Professor of Sociology
  University of California
  Berkeley, California

Glen Davidson, Ph.D.
  Chairman, Department of Medical Humanities
  Southern Illinois University
  School of Medicine
  Springfield, Illinois

H. Tristram Engelhardt, Jr., Ph.D., M.D.
  Professor of Philosophy and Medicine
  Kennedy Institute, Georgetown University
  Washington, D.C.

Addendum

Daniel Foster, M.D.
 Professor of Internal Medicine
 University of Texas
 Southwestern Medical School
 Dallas, Texas

Karen Lebacqz, Ph.D.
 Professor of Religion and Society
 Pacific School of Religion
 Berkeley, California

F. Dean Lueking, Ph.D.
 Pastor, Grace Lutheran Church
 River Forest, Illinois

William C. Martin, Ph.D.
 Professor of Sociology
 Rice University
 Houston, Texas

Richard McCormick, S.J., S.T.D.
 Professor Christian Ethics
 Kennedy Institute, Georgetown University
 Washington, D.C.

Ronald L. Numbers, Ph.D.
 Professor of the History of Medicine
 University of Wisconsin
 Madison, Wisconsin

Fazlur Rahman, Ph.D.
 Professor of Near Eastern Languages
 University of Chicago
 Chicago, Illinois

Dietrich Ritschl, Ph.D.
 Professor of Systematic Theology
 University of Mainz
 Mainz, Germany

Addendum

Seymour Siegel, Ph.D.
Professor of Theology
Jewish Theological Seminary
New York, New York

Ernst Wynder, M.D.
President, The American Health Foundation
New York, New York

Responsibility for the management of Project Ten rests on the following Executive Staff persons:

Lawrence E. Holst, S.T.M., *Project Chairman*
Chairman, Division of Pastoral Care
Lutheran General Hospital
Park Ridge, Illinois

Kenneth L. Vaux, Th.D., *Project Director*
Professor of Ethics
Department of Internal Medicine
University of Illinois Medical Center
Chicago, Illinois

David T. Stein, Ph.D., *Project Administrator*
Director of Parish Relations and Lay Training
Lutheran General Hospital
Park Ridge, Illinois

Martin E. Marty, Ph.D., *Theological Consultant*
Professor of Modern Church History
University of Chicago, Divinity School
Chicago, Illinois

Martin L. Koehneke, LL.D., D.D., *Executive Consultant*
(Retired) Senior Vice-President
Aid Association for Lutherans
Appleton, Wisconsin

Addendum

Patrick R. Staunton, M.D., *Medical Consultant*
Chairman, Division of Psychiatry
Lutheran General Hospital
Park Ridge, Illinois

Mary-Carroll Sullivan, R.N., M.T.S., *Research Consultant*
University of Chicago
University of Illinois
Chicago, Illinois

Special appreciation is due Mary-Carroll Sullivan for the research support and bibliographic development of this book, and to Sara Vaux for her careful and comprehensive style editing of the manuscript.

Support Staff services for Project Ten have been ably provided by Jane Frey, Secretary to the Project Administrator, by Fay DiNino and Thelma Rudy, from the Pastoral Care Staff, and by Fern Crane and other volunteers at Lutheran General Hospital.

The final word acknowledges the generous and enthusiastic support given to Project Ten by George B. Caldwell, President of Lutheran General Hospital. His providing the milieu for the scholarly debate of medicine and religion is deeply appreciated by all who share the responsibility and accountability for the Project.